Atlas of Interventional EUS

Anthony Y.B. Teoh • Marc Giovaninni
Mouen A. Khashab • Takao Itoi
Editors

Atlas of Interventional EUS

Case-based Strategies

Springer

Editors
Anthony Y.B. Teoh
Department of Surgery
The Prince of Wales Hospital
The Chinese University of Hong Kong
Shatin, Hong Kong SAR, China

Mouen A. Khashab
Division of Gastroenterology and Hepatology
Johns Hopkins Hospital
Baltimore, MD, USA

Marc Giovaninni
Unit of Endoscopy
Institute Paoli-Calmettes
Marseille, France

Takao Itoi
Department of Gastroenterology and Hepatology
Tokyo Medical University
Tokyo, Japan

ISBN 978-981-16-9339-7 ISBN 978-981-16-9340-3 (eBook)
https://doi.org/10.1007/978-981-16-9340-3

This Springer imprint is published by the registered company Springer Nature Singapore Pte Ltd.
The registered company address is: 152 Beach Road, #21-01/04 Gateway East, Singapore 189721, Singapore

Preface

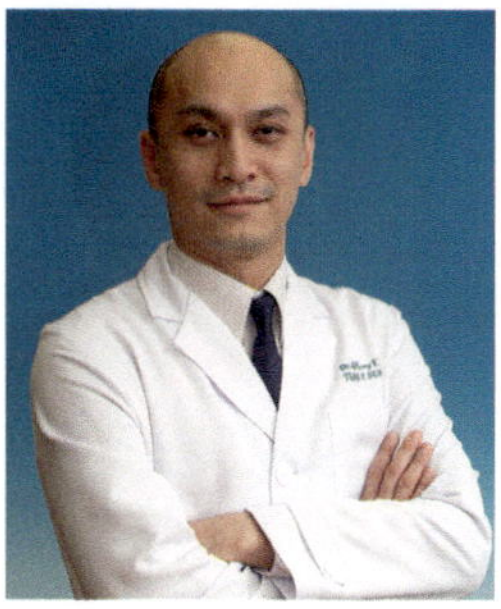

A handful of books on interventional EUS have been published in the field. Most of these only provide an overview on the technique, but none have taken a practical approach to discuss on how each procedure should be performed. As an interventionalist, I fully appreciate that each procedure performed on a patient would require different considerations and approaches. Hence, we decided to structure this book in the form of case-based strategies, to allow readers to understand what goes on in the mind of the endosonographer and to learn from their unique experiences.

I would like to thank all the co-editors and authors for their precious time, support, and patience in making this book happen. I also want to dedicate this book to my wife Yvonne, my two sons Shawn and Jake, for their limitless understanding, love, and support to allow me to pursue my passions in life.

Shatin, Hong Kong SAR, China Anthony Y.B. Teoh

Preface

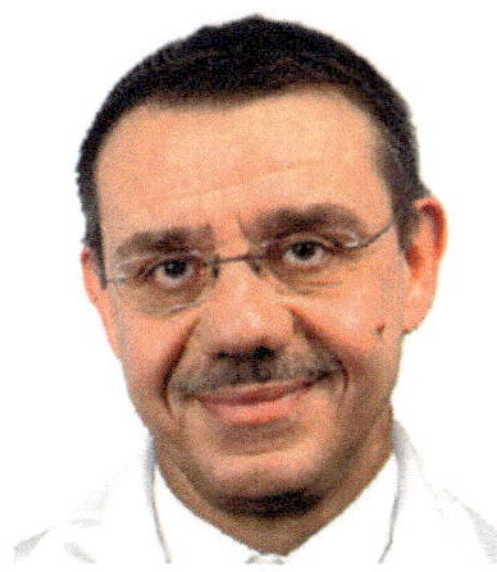

I would like to thank all the co-editors and authors for their precious time, support, and patience in making this book happen. I am sure this book would become an essential reading to all beginners and advanced endosonographers!

Marseilles, France — Marc Giovaninni

Preface

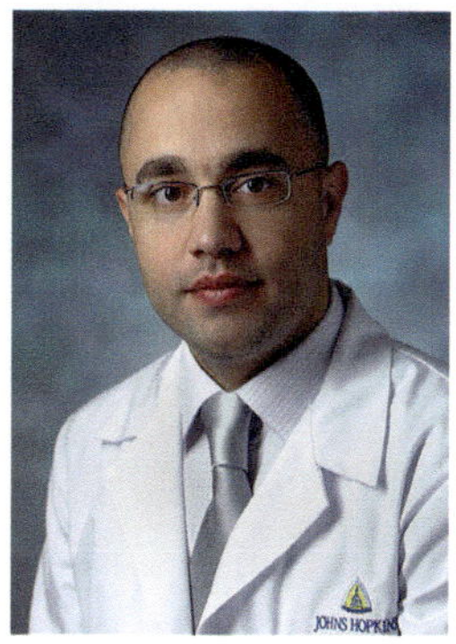

This book is dedicated to my family, trainees, nurses, colleagues, and mentors. I am grateful to both my personal family and my work family who allowed me to have the focus, dedication, and time to be a coeditor of this book.

Baltimore, MD, USA — Mouen A. Khashab

Preface

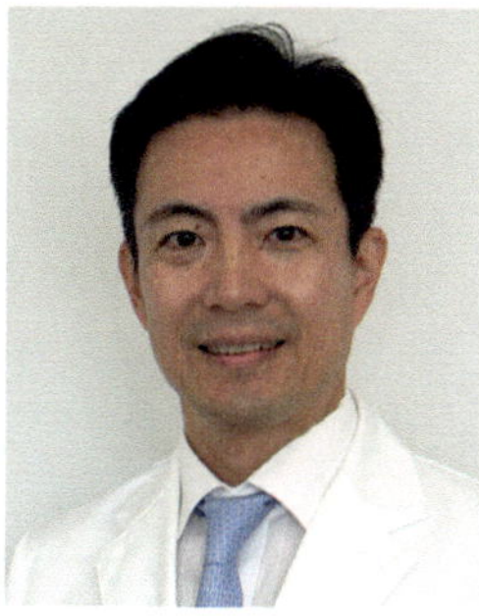

First of all, I would like to congratulate Professor Anthony Y.B. Teoh, on the completion and publication of this book and give him my warmest congratulations for his efforts.

This book is a practical textbook on the latest techniques of Interventional EUS, written by the world's leading experts in this field. This book must be a practical textbook for not only beginners but also senior endosonographers for Interventional EUS.

I hope you will learn a lot from this book. Practice makes perfect!

Tokyo, Japan　　　　　Takao Itoi

Contents

Part I

EUS-Guided Drainage of Pancreatic Fluid Collections

EUS-guided Drainage of a Pancreatic Pseudocyst with a Self Folding Lumen Apposing Stent

1

Yun Nah Lee and Jong Ho Moon

1.1 Background

A pancreatic pseudocyst (PPC) is a collection of fluid that develops as an adverse event (AE) of acute or chronic pancreatitis. PPCs are encapsulated collections of fluid with well-defined inflammatory walls and minimal or no necrosis. Large symptomatic PPCs must be drained, and endoscopic ultrasound (EUS)-guided drainage has become a standard treatment due to its inherent advantages. EUS allows the visualization of non-bulging collections and avoidance of intervening blood vessels and aids the determination of internal content type [1–4]. These factors enhance the success and safety of PPC drainage.

1.2 Case History

A 57-year-old man with a history of alcoholic acute pancreatitis was admitted for persistent abdominal pain and fever of 7 days' duration. He had been treated for acute pancreatitis with acute peripancreatic fluid collection 2 months previously. Physical examination demonstrated diffuse abdominal pain and exquisite back tenderness. CT showed a PPC measuring 8.2 × 7.6 cm on the pancreatic tail (Fig. 1.1a). The patient was offered EUS transmural drainage to treat the infected PPC.

1.3 Procedural Plan

Further characterization of PPCs by EUS is useful to guide the selection of stent type and number before drainage [5]. Distinguishing between types of PPC remains challenging and depends on high-quality imaging and an understanding of the natural history and physiology of the disease [6]. EUS is also used to measure the distance between the PPC and lumen wall (ideally < 10 mm) and to identify the intervening blood vessels, potentially reducing the risk of vessel puncture and bleeding [4, 7]. A 19G EUS needle was used to puncture the patient's pseudocyst wall under EUS guidance. Fluid can be aspirated from the cyst to confirm needle location and for microbial culture, particularly when an infection is clinically suspected. A guidewire (0.025 inch or 0.035 inch) can be placed and coiled multiple times in the cyst cavity under EUS and/or fluoroscopic guidance. Cystogastrostomy or cystoduodenostomy should be performed mechanically or with electrocautery. Graded tract dilation without cautery

Supplementary Information The online version contains supplementary material available at [https://doi.org/10.1007/978-981-16-9340-3_1].

Y. N. Lee · J. H. Moon (✉)
Department of Internal Medicine, Digestive Disease Center and Research Institute, SoonChunHyang University School of Medicine, Bucheon, Korea
e-mail: yunnah@schmc.ac.kr; jhmoon@schmc.ac.kr

A. Y.B. Teoh et al. (eds.), *Atlas of Interventional EUS*, https://doi.org/10.1007/978-981-16-9340-3_1

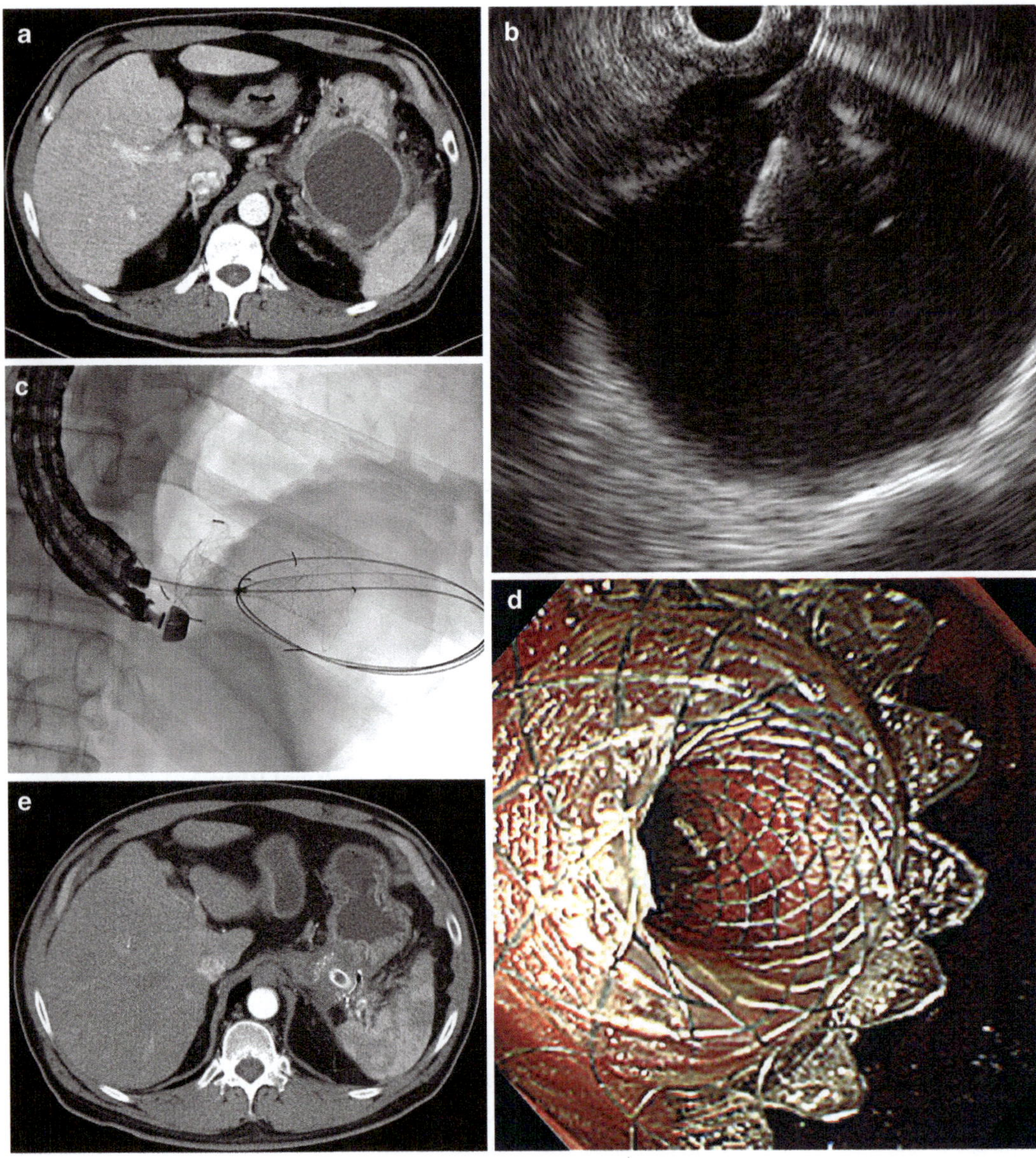

Fig. 1.1 EUS-guided transgastric drainage of pancreatic pseudocyst using a lumen-apposing metal stent. (**a**) Computed tomography (CT) showing the pseudocyst on the pancreatic tail. (**b**) EUS-guided transgastric puncture of the pseudocyst by using a 19-gauge needle. (**c**) Fluoroscopic imaging of the placement of a stent. (**d**) Endoscopic image of an inserted stent. (**e**) Follow-up CT showing complete resolution of the pseudocyst

requires the use of one or more endoscopic retrograde cholangiopancreatography (ERCP) cannulas (4.5–10F) to sequentially widen the tract until a balloon dilator can be inserted [8, 9]. The outer sheath of a fine-needle aspiration needle can also be used to dilate the tract. Tract dilation with electrocautery involves the use of a needle-knife sphincterotome (6F) or cystotome (10F). After the tract is dilated, further dilation to 4–8 mm using a biliary or luminal catheter balloon is required to permit placement of a plastic or metallic stent.

After proper tract dilation, the chosen stent is advanced into the PPC cavity along with the remaining guidewire and deployed under EUS and fluoroscopic guidance.

As the pseudocyst fluid is thin and watery, endoscopic drainage via the placement of one or more 7F or 10F double-pigtail plastic stents through a single transmural tract is usually effective [10]. However, plastic stents with small diameters may not allow adequate drainage, resulting in PPC superinfection, which typically occurs when plastic stents are obstructed. In addition, the placement of multiple plastic stents into a PPC can be technically challenging and time consuming, particularly when 10F stents are used [11, 12]. Fully covered, self-expanding metal stents (FCSEMSs) with larger lumen diameters (>10 mm) offer more rapid drainage and less likelihood of stent occlusion [13]. However, conventional biliary or esophageal FCSEMSs are often too long, they cannot be anchored in place, and they do not completely seal the transmural tract [4].

Lumen-apposing metal stents (LAMSs) are double-flanged FCSEMSs designed specifically for EUS drainage; they are short and have large diameters to promote lumen apposition and reduce the chance of leakage or stent migration [4, 14]. Two types of LAMS are currently popular: the AXIOS stent (Boston Scientific Corp., Natick, MA, USA) and the SPAXUS stent (Taewoong Medical, Gyeonggi-do, South Korea). The Hot AXIOS electrocautery-enhanced LAMS (Boston Scientific Corp.) allows single-step deployment and obviates the need for tract dilation, guidewire placement, and use of fluoroscopy. EUS drainage with LAMSs has yielded high clinical success rates for PPC management in prospective studies [15–17]. However, prospective data on the effectiveness of EUS-guided PPC drainage according to stent type and number are lacking.

1.4 Description of the Procedure

EUS transmural drainage of a PPC was performed with a LAMS (SPAXUS; Taewoong Medical) via the transgastric approach using a linear echoendoscope. Apparent bulging on the posterior wall of the stomach was observed on the endoscopic view. EUS revealed an 8.2 × 7.6 cm PPC with no solid internal component adjacent to the gastric wall. After the exclusion of interposing vessels by color Doppler, the PPC was punctured with a 19G needle (Fig. 1.1b). Subsequently, a 0.025 inch guidewire was inserted through the needle. Then, the needle was removed and the tract was dilated using a 6F cystotome with no dilating balloon. A LAMS (10 mm diameter, 2 cm length) was inserted and deployed under direct fluoroscopic and EUS guidance (Fig. 1.1c, d and Videos 1.1, 1.2).

1.5 Post-procedural Management

Most patients with uninfected PPCs do not require hospitalization after uncomplicated endoscopic drainage [18]. Oral intake can be resumed after this procedure, and oral antibiotics are typically prescribed [19, 20]. Some endoscopists continue antibiotic therapy until the collection has collapsed fully. However, we generally prescribe a 7–10-day course for patients with uninfected PPCs.

Although clear guidelines for follow-up after endoscopic PPC drainage are lacking, CT examination is often repeated 3–4 weeks later. If the PPC has resolved and there is no suspicion or evidence of pancreatic leakage, then the transmural drainage stent can be removed. If the PPC persists, then the transmural drainage stent should be assessed for patency and replaced if necessary; ERCP should be considered if not already performed. The persistent failure of a PPC to resolve should prompt rapid assessment to identify previously unrecognized cyst contents, such as necrotic tissue or blood, and the evaluation of pancreatic duct integrity [20]. In the case reported here, complete resolution of the PPC was confirmed by follow-up CT 3 weeks after drainage (Fig. 1.1e), and the LAMS was removed successfully by endoscopy (Video 1.3).

1.6 Potential Pitfalls

AEs related to endoscopic drainage occur in 5–20% of patients with PPCs [6, 21]. Potential AEs include bleeding, perforation, pseudocyst superinfection, and stent erosion, migration, and obstruction [6, 22]. If bleeding at the transmural entry site does not resolve or is of large volume, a dilating balloon can be used to temporarily tamponade the bleeding site. If needed, an FCSEMS can be deployed to stop the bleeding. LAMS use increases the risk of delayed bleeding [23–25]. Unlike double-pigtail plastic stents, which tend to migrate toward the gastrointestinal lumen when a PPC resolves, LAMSs remain anchored *in situ*. As a result, the edges of the stent can erode the vessels due to persistent contact with the PPC cavity, precipitating a bleeding episode or pseudoaneurysm. Such AEs occur when PPCs are ≤7 cm and LAMS removal is delayed beyond 4 weeks [26]. The consequences of pseudocyst superinfection can be severe and are almost always the result of inadequate drainage caused by stent dysfunction or jailing off of a compartment in the cavity. Perforations can occur in the retroperitoneal or peritoneal space, and the risk of such events is greatest for poorly adherent collections [6, 20].

References

1. Trikudanathan G, Attam R, Arain MA, et al. Endoscopic interventions for necrotizing pancreatitis. Am J Gastroenterol. 2014;109:969–81; quiz 982.
2. Bollen TL, Singh VK, Maurer R, et al. A comparative evaluation of radiologic and clinical scoring systems in the early prediction of severity in acute pancreatitis. Am J Gastroenterol. 2012;107:612–9.
3. Zerem E. Treatment of severe acute pancreatitis and its complications. World J Gastroenterol. 2014;20:13879–92.
4. Siddiqui UD, Levy MJ. EUS-guided transluminal interventions. Gastroenterology. 2018;154:1911–24.
5. Rana SS, Bhasin DK, Reddy YR, et al. Morphological features of fluid collections on endoscopic ultrasound in acute necrotizing pancreatitis: do they change over time? Ann Gastroenterol. 2014;27:258–61.
6. Holt BA, Varadarajulu S. The endoscopic management of pancreatic pseudocysts (with videos). Gastrointest Endosc. 2015;81:804–12.
7. Sriram PV, Kaffes AJ, Rao GV, et al. Endoscopic ultrasound-guided drainage of pancreatic pseudocysts complicated by portal hypertension or by intervening vessels. Endoscopy. 2005;37:231–5.
8. Monkemuller KE, Baron TH, Morgan DE. Transmural drainage of pancreatic fluid collections without electrocautery using the Seldinger technique. Gastrointest Endosc. 1998;48:195–200.
9. Varadarajulu S, Tamhane A, Blakely J. Graded dilation technique for EUS-guided drainage of peripancreatic fluid collections: an assessment of outcomes and complications and technical proficiency (with video). Gastrointest Endosc. 2008;68:656–66.
10. Varadarajulu S, Bang JY, Phadnis MA, et al. Endoscopic transmural drainage of peripancreatic fluid collections: outcomes and predictors of treatment success in 211 consecutive patients. J Gastrointest Surg. 2011;15:2080–8.
11. Sharaiha RZ, DeFilippis EM, Kedia P, et al. Metal versus plastic for pancreatic pseudocyst drainage: clinical outcomes and success. Gastrointest Endosc. 2015;82:822–7.
12. Binmoeller KF, Weilert F, Shah JN, et al. Endosonography-guided transmural drainage of pancreatic pseudocysts using an exchange-free access device: initial clinical experience. Surg Endosc. 2013;27:1835–9.
13. Talreja JP, Shami VM, Ku J, et al. Transenteric drainage of pancreatic-fluid collections with fully covered self-expanding metallic stents (with video). Gastrointest Endosc. 2008;68:1199–203.
14. Bang JY, Varadarajulu S. Lumen-apposing metal stents for endoscopic ultrasonography-guided interventions. Dig Endosc. 2019;31:619–26.
15. Walter D, Will U, Sanchez-Yague A, et al. A novel lumen-apposing metal stent for endoscopic ultrasound-guided drainage of pancreatic fluid collections: a prospective cohort study. Endoscopy. 2015;47:63–7.
16. Song TJ, Lee SS, Moon JH, et al. Efficacy of a novel lumen-apposing metal stent for the treatment of symptomatic pancreatic pseudocysts (with video). Gastrointest Endosc. 2019;90:507–13.
17. Moon JH, Choi HJ, Kim DC, et al. A newly designed fully covered metal stent for lumen apposition in EUS-guided drainage and access: a feasibility study (with videos). Gastrointest Endosc. 2014;79:990–5.
18. Baron TH, Harewood GC, Morgan DE, et al. Outcome differences after endoscopic drainage of pancreatic necrosis, acute pancreatic pseudocysts, and chronic pancreatic pseudocysts. Gastrointest Endosc. 2002;56:7–17.
19. Committee ASoP, Khashab MA, Chithadi KV, et al. Antibiotic prophylaxis for GI endoscopy. Gastrointest Endosc. 2015;81:81–9.
20. Elmunzer BJ. Endoscopic drainage of pancreatic fluid collections. Clin Gastroenterol Hepatol. 2018;16:1851–63, e3.
21. Varadarajulu S, Bang JY, Sutton BS, et al. Equal efficacy of endoscopic and surgical cystogastrostomy for pancreatic pseudocyst drainage in a randomized trial. Gastroenterology. 2013;145:583–90, e1.
22. Committee ASoP, Muthusamy VR, Chandrasekhara V, et al. The role of endoscopy in the diagnosis and treatment of inflammatory pancreatic fluid collections. Gastrointest Endosc. 2016;83:481–8.
23. DeSimone ML, Asombang AW, Berzin TM. Lumen apposing metal stents for pancreatic fluid collections:

Recognition and management of complications. World J Gastrointest Endosc. 2017;9:456–63.
24. Brimhall B, Han S, Tatman PD, et al. Increased incidence of pseudoaneurysm bleeding with lumen-apposing metal stents compared to double-pigtail plastic stents in patients with peripancreatic fluid collections. Clin Gastroenterol Hepatol. 2018;16:1521–8.
25. Bang JY, Navaneethan U, Hasan MK, et al. Non-superiority of lumen-apposing metal stents over plastic stents for drainage of walled-off necrosis in a randomised trial. Gut. 2019;68:1200–9.
26. Bang JY, Hawes RH, Varadarajulu S. Lumen-apposing metal stent placement for drainage of pancreatic fluid collections: predictors of adverse events. Gut. 2020;69(8):1379–81.

2 EUS-guided Drainage of a Pancreatic Pseudocyst with a Lumen Apposing Stent

Jennifer M. Kolb and Sachin Wani

2.1 Background

Pancreatic fluid collections (PFCs) are a common local complication of acute pancreatitis. The revised Atlanta classification categorizes PFCs according to the location (pancreatic or peripancreatic), the content (pure fluid versus necrosis), and the wall thickness [1]. A cutoff time of <4 weeks since the pancreatitis episode is used to delineate an acute collection. Most acute peripancreatic fluid collections that occur as a result of interstitial edematous pancreatitis will resolve. However, those that persist can develop into a well circumscribed, encapsulated collection called a pseudocyst. A pseudocyst is thought to occur as a result of a disrupted pancreatic duct leading to continued leakage of pancreatic juice into a collection. It is characterized by a well-defined, non-epithelialized wall and contains amylase rich pure fluid with minimal or no necrosis.

Pancreatic pseudocysts usually resolve on their own over time and can be followed with serial imaging to ensure eventual resolution. However, pseudocysts that persist for more than 4–6 weeks, continue to enlarge, are larger than 6 cm, lead to ongoing systemic illness, or cause clinical symptoms or complications warrant intervention [2, 3]. Symptomatic biliary or gastric outlet obstruction related to pseudocyst is an indication for drainage. Typical symptoms from gastric outlet obstruction include refractory abdominal pain, anorexia, or weight loss.

The traditional approaches for PFCs include percutaneous and surgical management. Percutaneous drainage still has a role in the acute setting when infection is suspected, though it is not commonly performed and carries a risk of pancreaticocutaneous fistula. Surgery had always been the mainstay of therapy, but the advent of endoscopic ultrasound (EUS)-guided drainage has revolutionized the management of patients with PFCs. A 2013 randomized controlled study demonstrated that endoscopic pseudocyst drainage provided similar treatment success and adverse events rates compared to surgery but with the additional benefit of shorter hospital length of stay, lower cost, and improved patient centered outcomes [4]. Marked advancements in endoscopic tools and improved techniques have led to endoscopic drainage becoming the predominant strategy for the majority of individuals with PFCs.

Endoscopic pseudocyst drainage is typically only performed after imaging shows a clearly defined, matured, and encapsulated wall which typically takes at least 1 month to develop.

Supplementary Information The online version contains supplementary material available at [https://doi.org/10.1007/978-981-16-9340-3_2].

J. M. Kolb · S. Wani (✉)
Division of Gastroenterology and Hepatology, University of Colorado Hospital Anschutz Medical Campus, Aurora, CO, USA
e-mail: jennifer.m.kolb@cuanschutz.edu

A. Y.B. Teoh et al. (eds.), *Atlas of Interventional EUS*, https://doi.org/10.1007/978-981-16-9340-3_2

Because of the location of most pseudocysts, endoscopic ultrasound (EUS) guided transmural drainage can typically be accomplished through either the stomach or the duodenum by creating a connection between the digestive tract and the collection (cystgastrostomy or cyst-duodenostomy). Small pseudocysts <5 cm can sometimes be managed via transpapillary drainage and stent placement [5]. There are multiple different approaches to transmural pseudocyst drainage each with its own advantages, risks, and unique features and endoscopist preference also plays a role [6]. In the traditional method, EUS guided needle puncture into the cyst is followed by wire guided dilation of the tract and placement of one or multiple double pigtail plastic stents. This approach has always been the cornerstone of endoscopic therapy given its high technical and procedural success rates. However, it can be labor intensive (requiring use of multiple wires for simultaneous access, difficult to deploy 10 French plastic stents through a small 3.7 mm channel) and plastic stents are prone to premature occlusion requiring frequent stent exchange or placement of additional stents. Fully covered self-expanding metal stents provide a larger diameter for drainage and can better maintain patency; however, they can cause bleeding and migrate [7, 8].

The more recent introduction of a dumbbell shaped fully covered lumen-apposing metal stent (LAMS) has dramatically changed the landscape for PFCs and in particular for necrotic collections by allowing for deployment followed by entrance into the cavity for debridement [9]. In the United States, we use the AXIOS stent (Boston Scientific) while various stents are available in other parts of the world including the Spaxus (Taewoong Medical), the Nagi (Taewoong Medical), the Aix (Luefen Medical), and the Hanaro (M.I. Tech) [10]. The AXIOS utilizes an innovative electrocautery platform that allows for efficient and seamless cyst puncture and stent deployment. The anchoring flanges are anti-migratory so a plastic stent may not be needed for anchoring; however, may be useful to prevent bleeding and solid material from entering the cavity [11]. Repeat imaging is usually performed within 2–4 weeks of LAMS placement and if resolution of the pseudocyst is confirmed, the stent can be removed.

2.2 Case History

A 40-year-old female with a history of alcohol related liver disease presented with acute pancreatitis complicated by portal vein and splenic vein thrombosis. This was her first episode of pancreatitis and she was managed with supportive care and discharged home on anticoagulation. Three months later she presents with worsening abdominal pain and inability to tolerate an oral diet. She denied fevers or chills. A computed tomography (CT) scan revealed a large pseudocyst measuring 12.7 × 10.8 cm with gastric compression (Fig. 2.1). The pseudocyst wall was mature and in close proximity to the stomach, thus endoscopic drainage was deemed appropriate.

2.3 Procedural Plan

Prior to any planned procedure the patient is evaluated for any ongoing medical problems and the medication list is reviewed. Our group follows the guidelines published by the American Society for Gastrointestinal Endoscopy related to peri-procedural management of antithrombotic agents which considers cystgastrostomy to be a high risk procedure for bleeding [12, 13]. The patient's subcutaneous therapeutic low molecular weight heparin was held for 24 hours prior to the procedure. In our endoscopy lab, transmural drainage of PFCs is performed under general endotracheal anesthesia to limit the risk of aspiration. A prophylactic dose of antibiotics is also given [14]. As is our usual practice, we went through a detailed consent process with the patient and discussed procedural risk as well as alternative treatments.

The first step is to review the patient's cross-sectional imaging to ensure wall maturity for puncture. We utilize EUS to determine the best access site which is dependent on the location of the cyst. In this case, the large pseudocyst was seen best from the body of the stomach, so we chose a

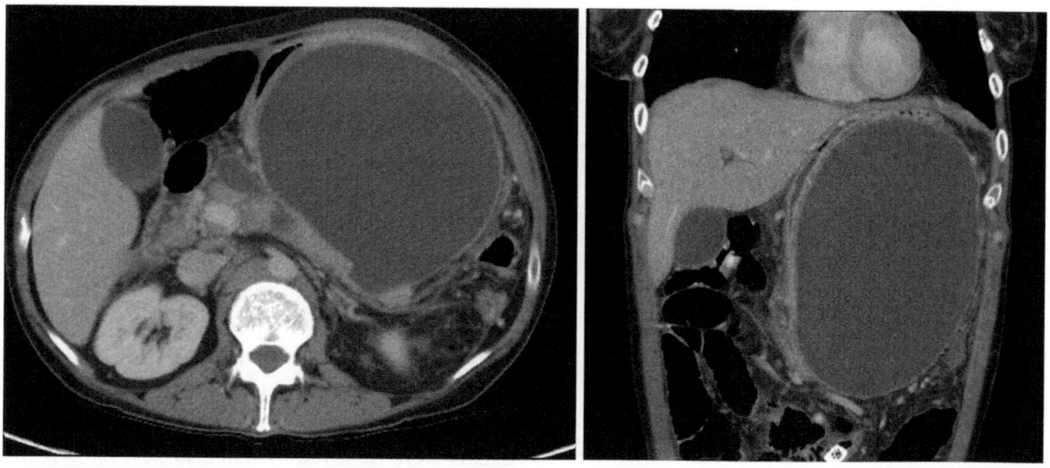

Fig. 2.1 Computed tomography shows a large loculated fluid filled collection in the gastrosplenic space causing significant mass effect with anterior displacement of the stomach and posterior displacement of the pancreas tail and contiguous with the focal defect in the pancreas tail

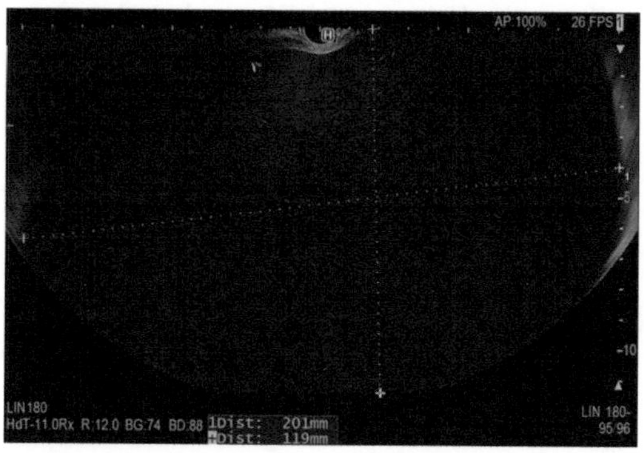

Fig. 2.2 EUS demonstrates a 20.1 × 11.9 cm pseudocyst

transgastric approach. As described above, there are several possible approaches for transmural drainage. We acknowledge that there are no randomized controlled trials comparing the traditional approach of EUS-guided drainage using double pigtail stents to LAMS. There is some comparative data to guide this decision but most of these studies focus on pancreatic necrosis. Over the past few years at our tertiary care high volume center our practice has evolved to using LAMS for drainage of most pancreatic or peripancreatic fluid collections. The advantages of LAMs include ease of deployment and shorter procedural time. It is our routine practice to place one or two 7 French plastic stents through the LAMS.

2.4 Description of the Procedure

During endoscopy, extrinsic compression was noted in the gastric body. EUS demonstrated an anechoic lesion in the pancreatic body with a thick outer wall that measured 20.1 cm by 11.9 cm in maximal cross-sectional diameter (Fig. 2.2). There was a single compartment without septae and <10% internal debris. An appropriate position in the stomach was identified for creation of cystgastrostomy. The distance between the transducer and the wall of the collection was confirmed <10 mm which is critical to ensure the cyst wall remains closely apposed to the gastrointestinal tract. We interrogated this area with color Doppler imaging, and an avascular plane was confirmed.

EUS-guided cystgastrostomy was performed using an electrocautery enhanced LAMS (AXIOS 15 mm by 10 mm, Boston Scientific) (Video 2.1). The device was advanced into the cyst and the stent was placed with the flanges in close approximation to the walls of the cyst and the stomach. A large amount of brown fluid immediately drained through the cystgastrostomy and nearly 2000 mL was aspirated through the endoscope (Fig. 2.3). A long Jag guidewire was inserted through the AXIOS stent into the pseudocyst

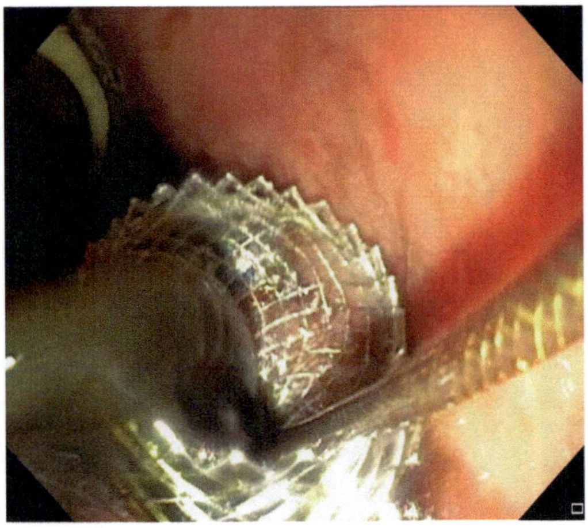

Fig. 2.3 Dark fluid draining from pseudocyst

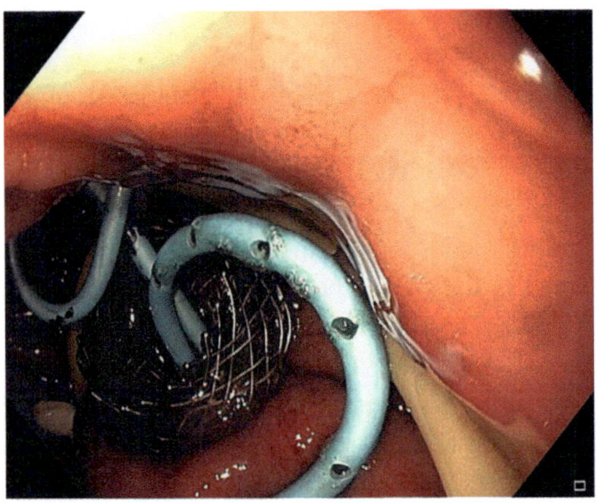

Fig. 2.4 Cystgastrostomy created using AXIOS and two plastic stents

under fluoroscopic guidance and two 5 cm by 7 Fr double pigtail stents were placed (Fig. 2.4).

2.5 Post-procedural Management

Post-procedure a clear liquid diet is recommended and advanced as soon as tolerated. She was continued on antibiotics to complete a 5-day course of ciprofloxacin. These patients are scheduled for repeat cross-sectional imaging 2–4 weeks post procedure to assess for pseudocyst resolution and tentatively planned for a repeat upper endoscopy at that time. The decision to perform ERCP is individualized based on pseudocyst resolution versus recurrence post drainage which should prompt assessment of the pancreas to evaluate for the presence of pancreatic duct stricture or disconnected duct syndrome. This patient had a CT scan one month later which demonstrated complete collapse of the pseudocyst (Fig. 2.5). She underwent endoscopy which confirmed that the cavity had completely collapsed, and all three stents were removed (Video 2.1).

2.6 Potential Pitfalls

The most common adverse events related to endoscopic drainage of PFCs include bleeding, stent occlusion, stent migration, buried stent syndrome, and infection. The adverse event rate for LAMS in PFCs is around 6–7% in most series and is higher for walled-off necrosis compared to pseudocyst and in cases where the tract is dilated [15–17]. Because the LAMS is designed to stay in place, many of the adverse events occur as a result of PFC resolution. When the PFC shrinks, the LAMS then comes in direct contact with the wall cavity and can erode into the vasculature and cause bleeding. Bleeding associated with LAMS is typically in the 4–5% range but even lower with a protocol of early stent removal [16–18]. It can be catastrophic if a pseudoaneurysm is present. Buried stent syndrome similarly occurs as the PFC resolves and the mucosa heals over it. LAMS removal beyond 4 weeks has been associated with adverse events and PFC ≤7 cm is a predictor of delayed bleeding since a smaller cavity drains faster and brings the stent into contact with the wall [16]. It is our practice to remove these stents as soon as possible, ideally in 3–4 weeks.

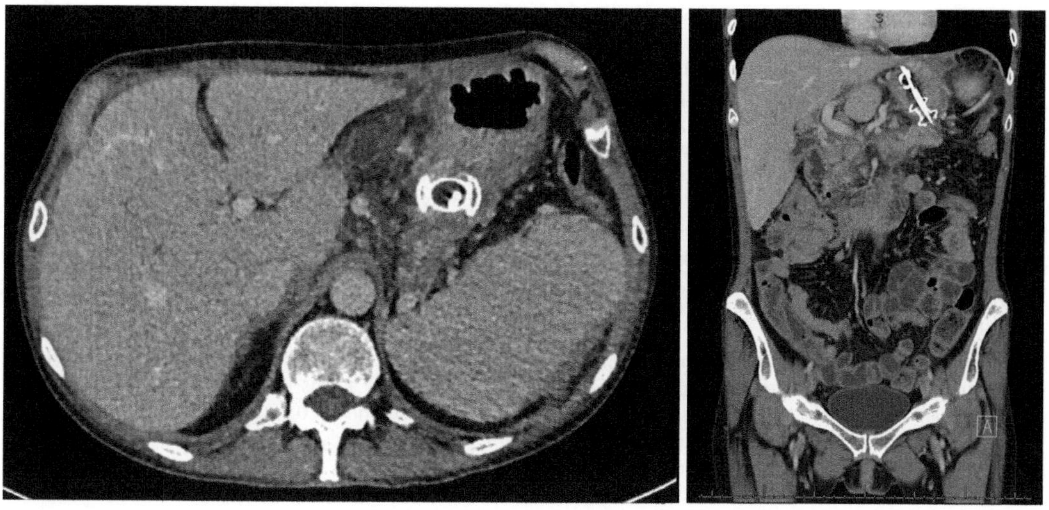

Fig. 2.5 Computed tomography 1 month later shows cystgastrostomy with complete collapse of previously seen pseudocyst

Disclosures SW is a consultant for Medtronic, Boston Scientific, and Interpace.

Funding JK is supported in part by a training grant (T32-DK007038)

SW is supported by the University of Colorado Department of Medicine Outstanding Early Scholars Program.

References

1. Banks PA, Bollen TL, Dervenis C, Gooszen HG, Johnson CD, Sarr MG, et al. Classification of acute pancreatitis--2012: revision of the Atlanta classification and definitions by international consensus. Gut. 2013;62(1):102–11.
2. Committee ASoP, Muthusamy VR, Chandrasekhara V, Acosta RD, Bruining DH, Chathadi KV, et al. The role of endoscopy in the diagnosis and treatment of inflammatory pancreatic fluid collections. Gastrointest Endosc. 2016;83(3):481–8.
3. Teoh AYB, Dhir V, Kida M, Yasuda I, Jin ZD, Seo DW, et al. Consensus guidelines on the optimal management in interventional EUS procedures: results from the Asian EUS group RAND/UCLA expert panel. Gut. 2018;67(7):1209–28.
4. Varadarajulu S, Bang JY, Sutton BS, Trevino JM, Christein JD, Wilcox CM. Equal efficacy of endoscopic and surgical cystogastrostomy for pancreatic pseudocyst drainage in a randomized trial. Gastroenterology. 2013;145(3):583–90, e1.
5. Elmunzer BJ. Endoscopic drainage of pancreatic fluid collections. Clin Gastroenterol Hepatol. 2018;16(12):1851–63 e3.
6. Teoh AY, Ho LK, Dhir VK, Jin ZD, Kida M, Seo DW, et al. A multi-institutional survey on the practice of endoscopic ultrasound (EUS) guided pseudocyst drainage in the Asian EUS group. Endosc Int Open. 2015;3(2):E130–3.
7. Penn DE, Draganov PV, Wagh MS, Forsmark CE, Gupte AR, Chauhan SS. Prospective evaluation of the use of fully covered self-expanding metal stents for EUS-guided transmural drainage of pancreatic pseudocysts. Gastrointest Endosc. 2012;76(3):679–84.
8. Dhir V, Teoh AY, Bapat M, Bhandari S, Joshi N, Maydeo A. EUS-guided pseudocyst drainage: prospective evaluation of early removal of fully covered self-expandable metal stents with pancreatic ductal stenting in selected patients. Gastrointest Endosc. 2015;82(4):650–7; quiz 718 e1–5.
9. Shah RJ, Shah JN, Waxman I, Kowalski TE, Sanchez-Yague A, Nieto J, et al. Safety and efficacy of endoscopic ultrasound-guided drainage of pancreatic fluid collections with lumen-apposing covered self-expanding metal stents. Clin Gastroenterol Hepatol. 2015;13(4):747–52.
10. Anderloni A, Troncone E, Fugazza A, Cappello A, Blanco GDV, Monteleone G, et al. Lumen-apposing metal stents for malignant biliary obstruction: Is this the ultimate horizon of our experience? World J Gastroenterol. 2019;25(29):3857–69.
11. Aburajab M, Smith Z, Khan A, Dua K. Safety and efficacy of lumen-apposing metal stents with and without simultaneous double-pigtail plastic stents for draining pancreatic pseudocyst. Gastrointest Endosc. 2018;87(5):1248–55.
12. Committee ASoP, Acosta RD, Abraham NS, Chandrasekhara V, Chathadi KV, Early DS, et al. The management of antithrombotic agents for patients

undergoing GI endoscopy. Gastrointest Endosc. 2016;83(1):3–16.

13. Chan FKL, Goh KL, Reddy N, Fujimoto K, Ho KY, Hokimoto S, et al. Management of patients on antithrombotic agents undergoing emergency and elective endoscopy: joint Asian Pacific Association of Gastroenterology (APAGE) and Asian Pacific Society for Digestive Endoscopy (APSDE) practice guidelines. Gut. 2018;67(3):405–17.
14. Committee ASoP, Khashab MA, Chithadi KV, Acosta RD, Bruining DH, Chandrasekhara V, et al. Antibiotic prophylaxis for GI endoscopy. Gastrointest Endosc. 2015;81(1):81–9.
15. Fugazza A, Sethi A, Trindade AJ, Troncone E, Devlin J, Khashab MA, et al. International multicenter comprehensive analysis of adverse events associated with lumen-apposing metal stent placement for pancreatic fluid collection drainage. Gastrointest Endosc. 2020;91(3):574–83.
16. Bang JY, Hawes RH, Varadarajulu S. Lumen-apposing metal stent placement for drainage of pancreatic fluid collections: predictors of adverse events. Gut. 2020;69(8):1379–81.
17. Teoh AYB, Bapaye A, Lakhtakia S, Ratanachu T, Reknimitr R, Chan SM, et al. Prospective multicenter international study on the outcomes of a newly developed self-approximating lumen-apposing metallic stent for drainage of pancreatic fluid collections and endoscopic necrosectomy. Dig Endosc. 2020;32(3):391–8.
18. Ahmad W, Fehmi SA, Savides TJ, Anand G, Chang MA, Kwong WT. Protocol of early lumen apposing metal stent removal for pseudocysts and walled off necrosis avoids bleeding complications. Scand J Gastroenterol. 2020;55(2):242–7.

3 EUS-guided Drainage of Walled-off Pancreatic Necrosis

Andrew Nett and Kenneth F. Binmoeller

3.1 Background

A step-up approach regarding invasiveness of procedural intervention is standard in the management of necrotizing pancreatitis. EUS-guided drainage of WOPN is a critical treatment modality within this approach and is becoming the first-line therapy. Compared to open or minimally invasive surgical necrosectomy, an endoscopic-assisted minimally invasive step-up approach results in fewer adverse events, major complications, and death in patients with necrotizing pancreatitis [1–3]. While endoscopic and percutaneous drainage of WOPN may both be appropriate first-line therapies individually or pursued complementary, endoscopic step-up therapy also appears to carry advantage over percutaneous step-up therapy. In cases of infected pancreatic necrosis, an endoscopic approach (EUS-guided drainage followed by direct endoscopic necrosectomy, if necessary) results in fewer pancreatic fistulae and a shorter hospital stay compared to a percutaneous step-up approach (percutaneous drainage followed by VARD if necessary) [4].

Indications for EUS-guided drainage of WOPN include suspected infection, complicating symptomatic mass effects including biliary or gastric outlet obstruction or significant vascular compression, or refractory symptoms such as pain, anorexia, early satiety, or weight loss. After endosonographic examination, if the collection is amenable to endoscopic therapy, transmural puncture of the collection is performed under EUS guidance. When the electrocautery-enhanced delivery system is used, current is run through diathermic wires at the tip of the catheter as it penetrates the WOPN cavity. Catheter advancement is immediately followed by deployment of the lumen-apposing metal stent (LAMS). While LAMS is increasingly the stent of choice for WOPN, fully covered self-expanding tubular metal stents or plastic stents may be used as well. For these stents, a 19 gauge FNA needle or a cystotome may be used to puncture the WOPN cavity, followed by guidewire advancement into the cavity, over-the-wire tract dilation, and then over-the-wire stent deployment (i.e., Seldinger technique).

Post-procedure, several variables in management must be determined, including timing of initial or subsequent endoscopic necrosectomy sessions, duration of antibiotics, and timing of cystenterostomy stent exchange or removal. If clinical improvement does not occur, the cysten-

Supplementary Information The online version contains supplementary material available at [https://doi.org/10.1007/978-981-16-9340-3_3].

A. Nett · K. F. Binmoeller (✉)
Paul May and Frank Stein Interventional Endoscopy Center (IES), California Pacific Medical Center, San Francisco, CA, USA
e-mail: NettAS@sutterhealth.org; BinmoeK@sutterhealth.org

A. Y.B. Teoh et al. (eds.), *Atlas of Interventional EUS*, https://doi.org/10.1007/978-981-16-9340-3_3

terostomy stent should be assessed for lumen occlusion. Additional drainage may be necessary as well. Adjunct percutaneous drain placement is one option, but multi-gated therapy with additional EUS-guided stent placement into the WOPN, and/or endoscopic nasocystic catheter drain placement for continuous irrigation of the collection may also be considered.

3.2 Case History (Figures 3.1, 3.2, 3.3, 3.4, and 3.5, Video 3.1)

A 55-year-old female with a history of schizoaffective disorder, methamphetamine abuse, and alcohol dependence developed necrotizing pancreatitis complicated by portal vein and superior mesenteric vein thrombosis. She had severe persistent abdominal pain 4 weeks after her initial presentation. A CT scan at that time showed a rim-enhancing fluid collection present in the central abdomen in close contiguity with the pancreatic body and tail. The collection measured 13.3 × 7.8 × 8.7 cm and contained a small focus of gas (Fig. 3.1). EUS-guided cystgastrostomy and direct endoscopic necrosectomy were offered.

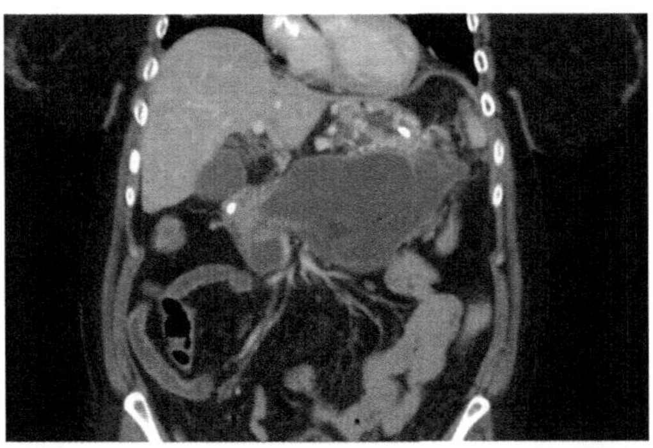

Fig. 3.1 CT showing a 13.3 × 7.8 × 8.7 cm WOPN containing a small focus of gas (arrow)

3.3 Procedural Plan

Endosonographic examination of WOPN first ensures the appropriateness for transmural intervention, determining: (1) the distance of the collection from the gastric or enteral wall; (2) adherence of the bowel and cyst walls; (3) the degree of solid necroses within the fluid collection cavity; and (4) the presence of any significant vessels (interposed between the GI tract and the WOPN, or coursing through the WOPN itself). If the collection is > 1 cm from the GI tract wall and/or there is poor adherence of the walls, endoscopic intervention may result in perforation and leak of cavity contents. Poor adherence would be an indication for use of a LAMS to retain wall apposition, ideally delivered with the one-step, one-device electrocautery-enhanced system. With the exception of progressive deterioration from uncontrolled sepsis, drainage of WOPN cavities predominantly comprised of solid necrosis should be delayed to allow for further content liquefaction. Premature drainage in this situation is likely to result in frequent and recurrent cystenterostomy occlusion with resultant superinfection risking patient decompensation.

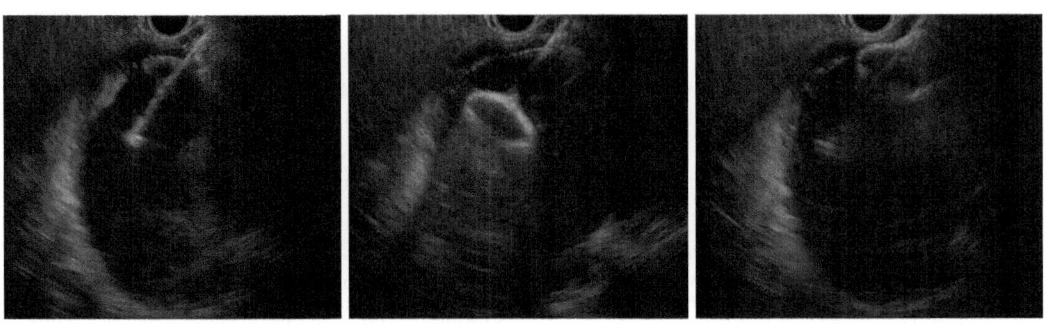

Fig. 3.2 Puncture of the WOPN with the electrocautery-enhanced delivery system. The distal flange (arrow) of a 15 × 10 mm LAMS was deployed and retracted back until it was hubbed against the WOPN wall

EUS-guided drainage of WOPN may be performed with a transgastric or transenteric approach. In general, drainage across the gastric wall is easier due to a straighter, more stable echoendoscope positioning. Greater integrity of the thicker gastric wall may also protect against stent maldeployment and complications such as perforation and bleeding. Transenteric drainage may be necessary to achieve a safe therapeutic window, for example, to avoid interposed blood vessels between the stomach and the WOPN, or due to a more inferior or caudal WOPN location, a requirement for multi-gated therapy, or the presence of surgically altered anatomy.

For drainage of WOPN, the larger lumen diameter and short length of a LAMS has conceptual advantages over pigtail stents and a tubular SEMS. Retrospective comparisons of metal stents versus plastic stents have suggested higher rates of long-term WOPN resolution with metal stents [5, 6]. A large international retrospective multicenter comparison of LAMS and plastic stents for WOPN management found that use of LAMs results in improved clinical success, shorter procedure time, lower need for surgery, and lower rates of WOPN recurrence [7]. However, a single-center randomized controlled-trial comparing EUS-guided drainage of WOPN using LAMS versus plastic stents suggested equivalent rates of treatment success, clinical adverse events, hospital re-admission, length of stay, overall treatment cost, and total number of procedures performed [8]. Comparable rates of clinical success and adverse events were also noted by a systematic review and meta-analysis examining use of LAMS versus plastic stents for WOPN drainage. Most recently, a 2020 retrospective analysis of patients undergoing direct endoscopic necrosectomy showed LAMS achieved faster resolution, lower recurrence, and decreased need for surgery, but higher rates of adverse events, compared to double pigtail stents [9].

Retrospective comparison of LAMS versus tubular fully covered self-expanding metal stents (FCSEMS) has suggested that LAMS may achieve complete WOPN resolution in fewer procedures, though with potentially more early adverse events [5]. One advantage of a LAMS over tubular SEMS is that the lumen can be

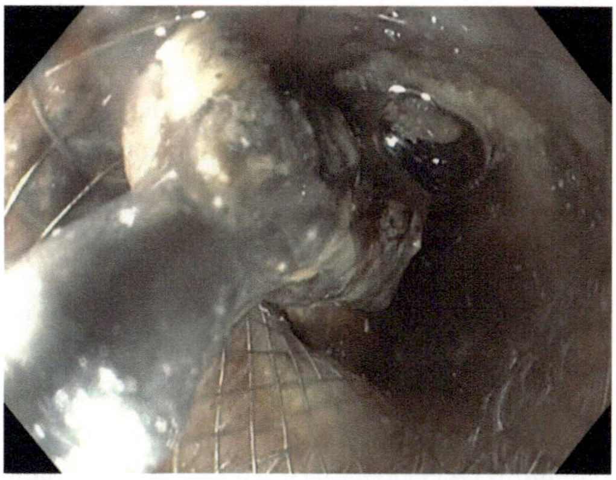

Fig. 3.4 Direct endoscopic necrosectomy using a rat-toothed forceps

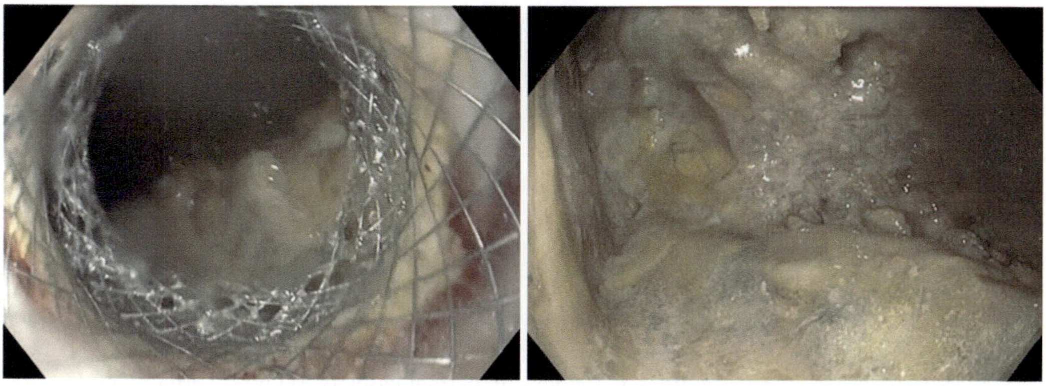

Fig. 3.3 Trans-LAMS intubation of the WOPN cavity for direct exploration and removal of loose necroses

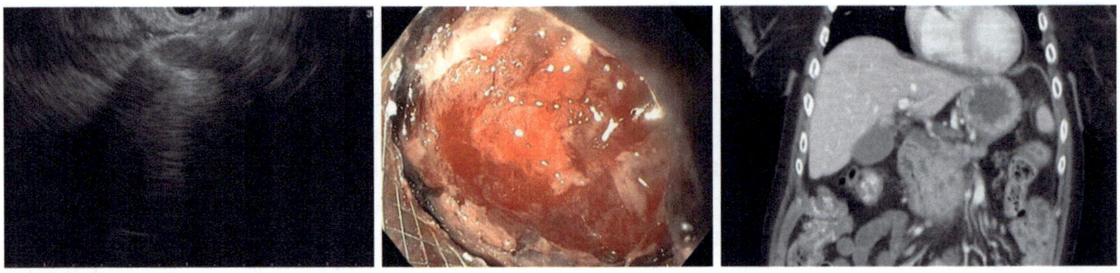

Fig. 3.5 WOPN cavity resolution noted on EUS and CT

dilated and immediately traversed to enable same-session direct endoscopic exploration of the necrotic cavity and necrosectomy using a variety of tools. The biflanged conformation of LAMS reduces risk of stent dislodgement during these index session transluminal manipulations. The stent's bilateral flanges approximate structures in order to protect against perforation or leak, particularly when the WOPN collection is not completely adherent to the gastrointestinal wall. In contrast to tubular SEMS, the LAMS is short in length with limited extension into the WOPN cavity or GI tract lumen, potentially mitigating the risk of injury to contralateral wall tissue. The shorter stent lumen length also creates less physical predisposition to stent clogging by WOPN cavity contents or food debris [10, 11].

Deployment of plastic stents or LAMS may be performed over a guidewire initially introduced into the WOPN cavity through a 19 gauge needle under EUS guidance. The needle is then exchanged out over the wire. The cystenterostomy tract is then dilated, and the stent(s) are introduced over the guidewire. Use of the electrocautery-enhanced delivery system simplifies LAMS introduction, however, eliminating the steps of 19-gauge needle puncture, guidewire insertion, and tract dilation. Instead, the electrocautery-enhanced delivery system enables single-step, single-device WOPN cavity puncture and LAMS delivery catheter introduction followed by immediate deployment of the LAMS, avoiding multi-step exchanges with the intent of making WOPN drainage technically easier, faster, and safer [10, 11].

LAMS most typically have a 10 mm saddle length. If a WOPN cavity is more distant from the GI tract wall, a longer saddle LAMS (15 mm lumen diameter × 15 mm saddle length) is also available for initial drainage. The standard 10 mm length LAMS comes with 10, 15, or 20 mm lumen diameters. Use of at least a 15 mm lumen diameter enables dilation of the stent lumen following deployment and same-session endoscopic necrosectomy with a therapeutic gastroscope. Though the 15 mm diameter is frequently sufficient, there is theoretical benefit to use of the 20 mm LAMS for treatment of WOPN if the cavity depth permits (given that the 20 mm deployment catheter must be introduced deeper into the WOPN cavity to ensure intra-cavity deployment of the distal stent flange). A retrospective case-matched study has shown equivalent rates of clinical success and similar safety with use of the 20 mm and 15 mm diameter LAMS. Fewer sessions of direct endoscopic necrosectomy were necessary with 20 mm LAMS use, despite the average WOPN cavity size being larger [12]. Use of a 20 mm diameter LAMS should therefore be considered if the WOPN is predominantly occupied by solid necroses in an effort to reduce the risk of stent dysfunction from clogging of the lumen and resultant WOPN superinfection. The benefit of adding one or more double pigtail plastic stents deployed across the LAMS lumen for the purpose of preventing stent dysfunction due to clogging remains to be proven. Double pigtail stents placed through a LAMS may be beneficial for drainage of more loculated areas within a large WOPN collection, which can reduce the need for concomitant percutaneous drainage [13].

Multiple cystenterostomies may be beneficial in certain cases of WOPN. Termed "multi-gate" therapy, deployment of multiple transmural plastic stents for creation of multiple internal fistulae for WOPN drainage in conjunction with nasocystic catheter drainage may enhance rates of collection resolution [14]. The benefits of multi-gate therapy have not been specifically established with the use of multiple LAMS, but may be considered in cases of larger WOPN with multiple septated compartments [15].

3.4 Description of the Procedure

Under endosonographic examination, a transgastric window was identified in which the WOPN collection was <1 cm from the gastric wall. The collection measured ~ 9 cm in maximum diameter, endosonographically. Doppler effect confirmed the absence of mural and interposed vessels between the GI tract wall and WOPN collection. Solid necroses occupied ~ 20% of the cavity volume. EUS-guided WOPN drainage was then performed. Using a therapeutic linear echoendoscope, the WOPN cavity was punctured under endosonographic visualization using the electrocautery-enhanced delivery system. The distal flange of a 15 × 10 mm LAMS was then deployed under continued endosonographic visualization (Fig. 3.2). The distal flange was then retracted back until it was hubbed against the WOPN wall, and further gentle retraction apposed the cavity toward the gastric wall. The proximal flange was then deployed completely within the echoendoscope channel before being pushed out of the channel by advancing the delivery catheter while pulling back the echoendoscope. Contents of the WOPN immediately entered the stomach and were suctioned. A sample was sent for routine fluid characterization (CEA, amylase, cytology). Using a through-the-scope dilating balloon, the LAMS lumen was dilated fully to 15 mm.

3.5 Post-procedural Management

After EUS-guided cystgastrostomy, in the case presented, the echoendoscope was exchanged for the therapeutic gastroscope, which was used to intubate and directly explore the WOPN cavity (Fig. 3.3). Removal of loose necroses was performed by vigorous lavage of the WOPN cavity followed by instillation of dilute hydrogen peroxide. Prior published comparison of direct endoscopic necrosectomy versus cavity irrigation has shown improved therapeutic outcomes if necrosectomy is performed, albeit specifically in the context of plastic stent use (16—Gardner et al). Following EUS-guided LAMS cystenterostomy, however, it is not fully established if necrosectomy should be performed at the index session, at regularly scheduled intervals, or on an as-needed basis when patients develop signs of LAMS occlusion or fail to progressively improve clinically [16, 17]. While index session debridement can risk stent dislodgement, it may reduce total necrosectomy sessions and improve overall clinical success (Yan et al). In the case presented, suction of loose necroses was performed during the initial procedure. Subsequent scheduled necrosectomy was performed at 3 weeks and at 6 weeks using a rat-toothed forceps (Fig. 3.4) and a polypectomy snare. At 9 weeks, endoscopy and endosonography confirmed WOPN cavity resolution and the LAMS was removed. CT confirmed resolution of the WOPN cavity after removal of the LAMS (Fig. 3.5).

Diet initiation is guided by the patient's clinical status with oral intake initiated and advanced as tolerated. Frequently, pain and nausea improvement following decompression of the WOPN and relief of mass effect will permit oral nutrition. In cases of ileus or persistent severe symptomatology from the WOPN, enteral feeding may be necessary. The presence of the cystenterostomy stent itself, however, does not dictate need for any dietary restriction or modification.

Given the high risk of stent occlusion from necrotic debris between serial necrosectomies, an argument can be made to continue antibiotics until complete WOPN cavity resolution and stent removal have occurred. There are no data in the literature to guide antimicrobial therapy duration. Sampling of WOPN for culturing can be performed at the time of endoscopic intervention to shape antimicrobial agent choice, though it is unreliable given the method of sampling from within the contaminated GI lumen.

In our patients, we also hold acid suppression medications until cavity resolution so that gastric acid can potentially aid in digestion and dissolution of necrotic contents within the collection. Gastric acid may also buffer and neutralize bicarbonate-rich fluid seeping into the cavity from a persistent pancreatic fistula. Proton pump inhibitor (PPI) discontinuation during LAMS-mediated endoscopic drainage and debridement of WOPN has been reported to be associated with fewer endoscopic necrosectomy sessions required to achieve cavity resolution [18]. Though no differences in overall adverse event rates have been reported, the same study did show increased episodes of stent occlusion in association with PPI cessation. There also has been speculation that entry of stomach acid into a WOPN may increase the risk of bleeding.

Prolonged indwelling stents carry risk of tissue erosion, bleeding, and stent ingrowth and burial. In the trial published by Bang et al comparing LAMS and plastic stents for WOPN drainage, high initial rates of delayed complications due to persistent indwelling LAMS were observed. Stent-related bleeding, stent burial, and stent-induced biliary obstruction occurred in 50% of patients, but all such events occurred longer than 3 weeks after stent placement [8, 19]. As such, the trial protocol was modified to include earlier imaging assessment at 3 weeks post LAMS placement, with stent removal if WOPN resolution had occurred. Other studies have not observed delayed adverse events rates nearly as high [20, 21], but higher rates of bleeding noted with LAMS compared to plastic cystenterostomy stents do raise alarm that the distal stent flange can erode into vasculature and precipitate life-threatening bleeding [22]. Prospective evaluation of an early LAMS removal protocol suggests efficacy of this strategy in preventing delayed bleeding [8, 21]. It is our practice to repeat endosonography or cross-sectional MRI imaging to assess for fluid collection resolution within 3 weeks of LAMS cystenterostomy placement if the patient is not already undergoing serial necrosectomy. If longer stenting duration is required, the LAMS is exchanged for double pigtail stents for maintenance of the cystenterostomy tract. Of note, use of long-term indwelling double pigtails stents for symptomatic peripancreatic fluid collections is also not entirely free of complication, carrying risk of delayed intestinal perforation caused by the extraluminal stent ends [23].

3.6 Potential Pitfalls

During EUS-guided cystenterostomy for WOPN, potential complications include stent maldeployment and related perforation. If the distal end is maldeployed external to the GI tract lumen, but not within the WOPN cavity, the proximal end should be deployed within the GI tract lumen to enable removal with a rat-toothed forceps. The perforation can then be closed using clips or sutures. If the distal end is initially deployed successfully within the WOPN cavity, but inadvertently becomes dislodged out of the WOPN before full LAMS deployment, a guidewire may be introduced through the delivery catheter for salvage of access through the same cystenterostomy tract. The proximal stent end is then deployed and the LAMS is removed over the guidewire. A new LAMS can then be delivered over the guidewire through the same cystenterostomy tract, sealing any perforation. If the proximal end of the stent inadvertently deploys or migrates outside of the GI tract wall, advancement of a guidewire through the delivery catheter into the WOPN can be followed by over-the wire deployment of a tubular SEMS through the maldeployed stent to bridge the GI lumen and WOPN cavities. Alternatively, once a guidewire has been passed through the delivery catheter into the WOPN cavity the catheter can be exchanged for a through-the-scope dilating balloon to dilate the cystenterostomy tract to enable access to the migrated proximal end of the stent for subsequent repositioning of the stent across the bowel and WOPN cavities.

Immediate bleeding can occur during EUS-guided cystenterostomy, most frequently after dilation of the stent lumen. If a LAMS or tubular SEMS was used, bleeding is typically self-limited by the tamponade effect at the site of insertion. If plastic stents were deployed, immediate exchange for a covered metal stent for tamponade hemostasis may be necessary.

Rapid decompression and resultant collapse of the WOPN after drainage may bring a vessel along the contralateral cavity wall into close proximity of the distal end of a tubular SEMS or LAMS, which may result in vascular erosion and delayed bleeding. If the WOPN cavity is fully adherent to the gastric or duodenal wall with low concern for risk of leak, immediate LAMS removal and plastic stent placement should be considered. If the collection is poorly adherent, deployment of double pigtail stents through the metal stent helps to maintain separation between the contralateral wall vessel and the stent end as the cavity collapses further. The metal stent should thereafter be removed and exchanged for plastic stents alone as soon as possible.

Delayed complications include bleeding, as well as stent erosion, migration, occlusion, or burial. Delayed bleeding can be massive and may require emergent radiographic angiography and embolization. Stent complications can be managed endoscopically with stent clearance, exchange, or removal as appropriate.

References

1. Gurusamy KS, et al. Interventions for necrotising pancreatitis. Cochrane Database Syst Rev. 2016;4:pCD011383.
2. Bakker OJ, et al. Endoscopic transgastric vs surgical necrosectomy for infected necrotizing pancreatitis: a randomized trial. JAMA. 2012;307(10):1053–61.
3. Bang, J.Y., et al., An endoscopic transluminal approach, compared with minimally invasive surgery, reduces complications and costs for patients with necrotizing pancreatitis. Gastroenterology. 2019;156(4):1027–40. e3.
4. van Brunschot S, et al. Endoscopic or surgical step-up approach for infected necrotising pancreatitis: a multicentre randomised trial. Lancet. 2018;391(10115):51–8.
5. Siddiqui AA, et al. Fully covered self-expanding metal stents versus lumen-apposing fully covered self-expanding metal stent versus plastic stents for endoscopic drainage of pancreatic walled-off necrosis: clinical outcomes and success. Gastrointest Endosc. 2017;85(4):758–65.
6. Abu Dayyeh BK, et al. Large-caliber metal stents versus plastic stents for the management of pancreatic walled-off necrosis. Gastrointest Endosc. 2018;87(1):141–9.
7. Chen YI, et al. Lumen apposing metal stents are superior to plastic stents in pancreatic walled-off necrosis: a large international multicenter study. Endosc Int Open. 2019;7(3):E347–54.
8. Bang JY, et al. Non-superiority of lumen-apposing metal stents over plastic stents for drainage of walled-off necrosis in a randomised trial. Gut. 2019;68(7):1200–9.
9. Ge PS, et al. Comparative study evaluating lumen apposing metal stents versus double pigtail plastic stents for treatment of walled-off necrosis. Pancreas. 2020;49(2):236–41.
10. Sharaiha RZ, et al. Endoscopic therapy with lumen-apposing metal stents is safe and effective for patients with pancreatic walled-off necrosis. Clin Gastroenterol Hepatol. 2016;14(12):1797–803.
11. Nett A, Binmoeller KF. Pancreatic fluid collections and leaks. In: Chandrasekhara V, et al., editors. Clinical Gastrointestinal Endoscopy. Philadelphia, PA: Elsevier; 2018.
12. Parsa N, et al. Endoscopic ultrasound-guided drainage of pancreatic walled-off necrosis using 20-mm versus 15-mm lumen-apposing metal stents: an international, multicenter, case-matched study. Endoscopy. 2020;52(3):211–9.
13. Jagielski M, Smoczyński M, Adrych K. Single transluminal gateway transcystic multiple drainage for extensive walled-off pancreatic necrosis—a single-centre experience. Prz Gastroenterol. 2018;13(3):242–8.
14. Varadarajulu S, et al. Multiple transluminal gateway technique for EUS-guided drainage of symptomatic walled-off pancreatic necrosis. Gastrointest Endosc. 2011;74(1):74–80.
15. Bang JY, Varadarajulu S. Management of walled-off necrosis using the multiple transluminal gateway technique with the Hot AXIOS System. Dig Endosc. 2016;28(1):103.
16. Gardner TB, et al. A comparison of direct endoscopic necrosectomy with transmural endoscopic drainage for the treatment of walled-off pancreatic necrosis. Gastrointest Endosc. 2009;69(6):1085–94.
17. Baron TH, et al. American gastroenterological association clinical practice update: management of pancreatic necrosis. Gastroenterology. 2020;158(1):67–75. e1.
18. Powers PC, et al. Discontinuation of proton pump inhibitor use reduces the number of endoscopic procedures required for resolution of walled-off pancreatic necrosis. Endosc Ultrasound. 2019;8(3):194–8.
19. Bang JY, et al. Lumen-apposing metal stents (LAMS) for pancreatic fluid collection (PFC) drainage: may not be business as usual. Gut. 2017;66(12):2054–6.
20. Yang D, et al. Safety and rate of delayed adverse events with lumen-apposing metal stents (LAMS) for pancreatic fluid collections: a multicenter study. Endosc Int Open. 2018;6(10):E1267–75.

21. Ahmad W, et al. Protocol of early lumen apposing metal stent removal for pseudocysts and walled off necrosis avoids bleeding complications. Scand J Gastroenterol. 2020;55(2):242–7.
22. Lang GD, et al. EUS-guided drainage of peripancreatic fluid collections with lumen-apposing metal stents and plastic double-pigtail stents: comparison of efficacy and adverse event rates. Gastrointest Endosc. 2018;87(1):150–7.
23. Yamauchi H, et al. Complications of long-term indwelling transmural double pigtail stent placement for symptomatic peripancreatic fluid collections. Dig Dis Sci. 2019;64(7):1976–84.

Endoscopic Access and Drainage of Walled-off Pancreatic Necrosis

4

Elena Gibson and Douglas G. Adler

4.1 Background

The revised Atlanta classification defines WOPN as a necrotic pancreatic fluid collection (PFC) with a well-defined wall that occurs ≥ 4 weeks after an episode of acute pancreatitis [1]. Indications for drainage of WOPN include infection, obstruction, nutritional failure, and ongoing pain [2]. In recent years, EUS-guided drainage has become a preferred treatment for the endoscopic access and drainage of WOPN with a reported clinical success rate of 88–90% [2]. Compared to surgical and percutaneous approaches, EUS-guided drainage provides comparable success rates with fewer complications and lower costs, and can be performed on an outpatient basis [3–5]. EUS-guided drainage of WOPN is performed with the creation of a cystgastrostomy or cystduodenostomy with subsequent transmural stent placement to establish transluminal drainage followed by repeat necrosectomy procedures as needed to ensure resolution of the PFC [2].

Supplementary Information The online version contains supplementary material available at [https://doi.org/10.1007/978-981-16-9340-3_4].

E. Gibson · D. G. Adler (✉)
Gastroenterology and Hepatology, Center for Advanced Therapeutic Endoscopy (CATE), Porter Adventist Hospital, Denver, CO, USA
e-mail: douglas.adler@centura.org

4.2 Case History

Two months after developing acute pancreatitis of unclear etiology, a 78-year-old male presented to our clinic for evaluation of PFCs, ongoing abdominal pain and distention, and weight loss. Computed tomography was notable for a rim-enhancing PFC measuring 28 × 16 cm, consistent with WOPN (Fig. 4.1). Indications for drainage included the patient's symptoms, as well as the age and size of the PFC. Surgical, percutaneous, and endoscopic approaches were discussed with the patient, and the patient elected to pursue endoscopic drainage.

4.3 Procedural Plan

EUS-guided drainage and debridement of WOPN is currently most commonly performed via the creation of a cystgastrostomy or a cystduodenostomy using lumen-apposing, self-expandable metal stents (LAMS), although a few centers still use double pigtail stents (DPS) for drainage [6]. PFC location is confirmed on cross sectional imaging and endosonographically. The PFC can be accessed with a fine-needle aspiration device followed by guidewire insertion and sequential tract dilation. Either LAMS or one or more DPS are advanced across the tract for drainage. Use of the newer electrocautery-enhanced LAMS (HOT AXIOS) (Boston Scientific, Natick MA) with an electrocautery wire in the delivery system allows

A. Y.B. Teoh et al. (eds.), *Atlas of Interventional EUS*, https://doi.org/10.1007/978-981-16-9340-3_4

for direct access without needle aspiration, guidewire insertion, or dilation (Boston Scientific, Natick MA).

The advantages of LAMS include a larger stent diameter for drainage and the ability of the endoscope to advance through the LAMS to facilitate direct necrosectomy. Although no differences in efficacy or adverse outcomes have been identified between LAMS and DPS for EUS-guided WOPN drainage, LAMS are associated with fewer mean procedures to resolution and are currently the most widely used tool in this setting [7]. Following initial stent placement and debridement, multiple repeat necrosectomy procedures are usually necessary to obtain resolution of WOPN [8]. No current guidelines exist, but necrosectomy procedures are often performed at intervals of 1–3 weeks using a variety of devices such as rat-toothed forceps, snares, and stone-retrieval baskets to remove necrotic debris from a PFC through a LAMS [2, 9]. Other techniques such as diluted hydrogen peroxide washes, 3% diluted at 1:5 or 1:10, and saline irrigation are also used to facilitate debridement [9, 10]. Necrosectomy procedures are repeated until resolution of the PFC is confirmed on cross sectional imaging and/or via direct endoscopic and fluoroscopic visualization.

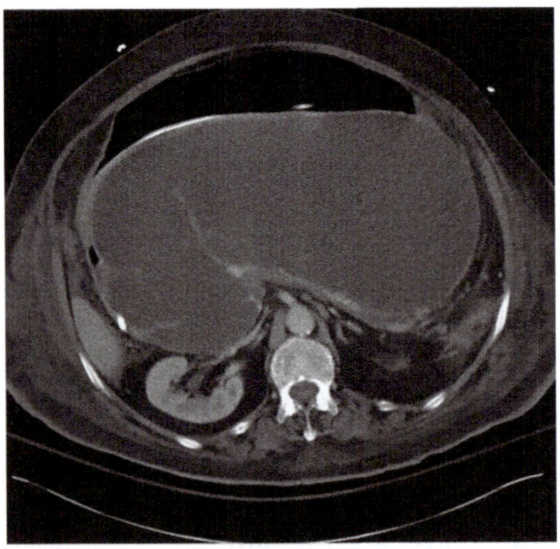

Fig. 4.1 CT scan showing very large PFC/WON

4.4 Description of the Procedure

The stomach was markedly compressed by the PFC. EUS identified a 28 × 16 cm fluid-filled cavity with copious solid debris in the expected location of the head, genu, and body of the pancreas, concordant with prior imaging (Fig. 4.2). Doppler ultrasound identified an area between the stomach and the PFC that was devoid of interposed vessels, and a cystgastrostomy was created using an electrocautery-enhanced 20 mm AXIOS LAMS and delivery system (Boston Scientific, Natick, MA) (Fig. 4.3). The LAMS were deployed across the cystgastrostomy tract without difficulty under endoscopic and EUS guidance (Fig. 4.4). Copious fluid and debris drained

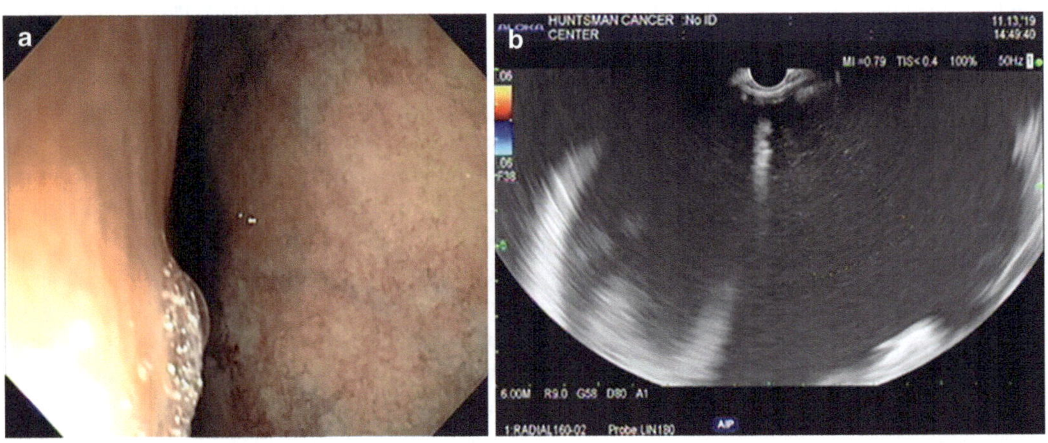

Fig. 4.2 (**a**) Gastric compression from PFC/WON; (**b**) EUS image of large PFC/WON prior to cystgastrostomy

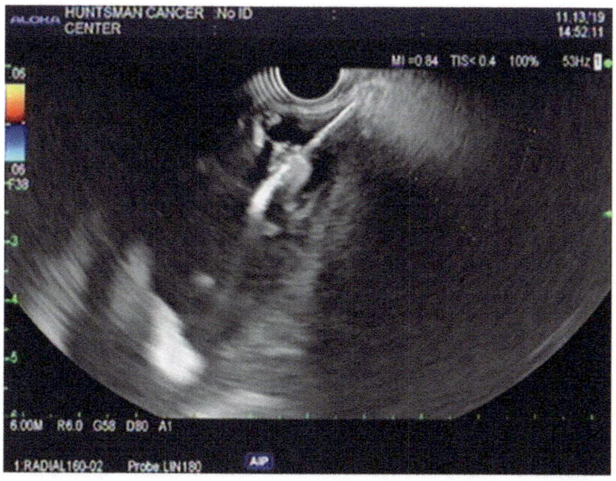

Fig. 4.3 Cystgastrostomy created via Hot AXIOS Catheter

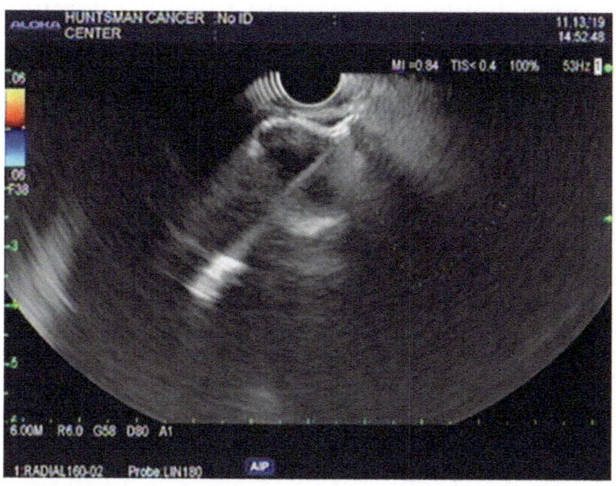

Fig. 4.4 EUS view of deployment of distal flange of lumen-apposing metal stent

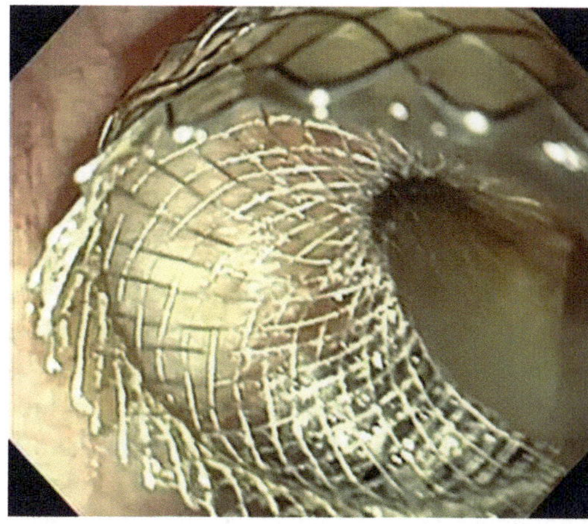

Fig. 4.5 Endoscopic view of lumen-apposing metal stent following deployment of proximal flange. (Note PFC fluid draining rapidly)

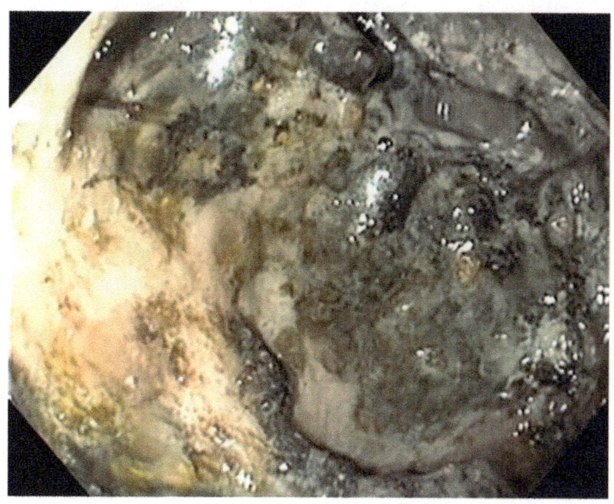

Fig. 4.6 Endoscopic appearance of PFC/WON cavity on subsequent procedure with dense necrotic tissue seen throughout

spontaneously into the stomach, and proper positioning of the stent was confirmed on endoscopic and EUS evaluation (Fig. 4.5).

One week later, a repeat endoscopy with necrosectomy was performed using rat-tooth forceps, a biliary stone basket, and diluted hydrogen peroxide lavage to remove purulent fluid and solid, adherent necrotic debris from the cyst (Fig. 4.6). To maximize drainage, a 0.035" guidewire was advanced through the stent under fluoroscopic visualization, and two 7 Fr × 7 cm DPS were placed with each DPS having one pigtail in the PFC and one pigtail in the gastric lumen (Fig. 4.7).

One month later, as the patient needed a rehabilitation stay, a repeat endoscopy revealed mucosal congestion and stenosis in the first and second portion of the duodenum from PFC compression. The two DPS were removed for necrosectomy. Contrast injected into the PFC under fluoroscopic and endoscopic visualization revealed a deep tract extending into the right, inferolateral abdomen. Guidewire advancement into the tract expulsed purulent fluid, and necrosectomy was performed with a trapezoid basket and hydrogen peroxide lavage to good effect. One 7 Fr x10 cm DPS was inserted into the tract with drainage into the gastric body.

Three weeks later, repeat endoscopy identified a small amount of solid debris in the PFC, which was cleared with diluted hydrogen peroxide and manual debridement. The DPS were removed.

CT scan obtained 2 weeks later showed resolution of the PVC cavity. A subsequent repeat endoscopy showed essential resolution of the WOPN and the patient underwent removal of the previously placed LAMS using rat-tooth forceps (Fig. 4.8). Before removing the LAMS, endoscopic visualization of a closed PFC with well-healed mucosa was confirmed, and no evidence of a residual cavity and no residual necrotic debris was identified with fluoroscopy.

The patient was seen for follow-up 4 months later after additional rehabilitation treatment. He was home, able to perform all of his activities of daily living, and eating well. He did require pancreatic enzyme replacement therapy to treat exocrine pancreatic insufficiency.

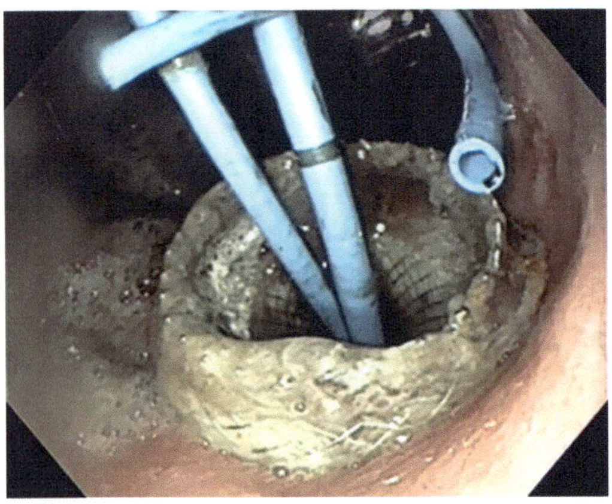

Fig. 4.7 Two double pigtail plastic stents placed through the lumen-apposing metal stent

4.5 Post-procedural Management

Initial LAMS placement and repeat necrosectomy procedures can be performed on an outpatient or inpatient basis with similar efficacy and long-term outcomes. However, any clinically concerning symptom (acute systemic illness, fever, inability to tolerate oral intake) or procedural complication should prompt further consideration for hospital admission [5]. Although there is limited research regarding the duration of antibiotic use for EUS-guided drainage of WOPN, broad spectrum antibiotics, such as fluoroquinolones, are typically administered during the procedure and prescribed for a short period of time following each procedure to prevent secondary infection given manipulation of the contents of the WOPN [11, 12]. In patients with no ongoing signs or symptoms of gastrointestinal obstruction, a clear liquid diet is recommended for the first twenty four hours with subsequent advancement as tolerated [2]. If oral intake is not tolerated or obstruction is present, enteral nutrition should be initiated, most commonly with a feeding tube with the tip beyond the ligament of Treitz.

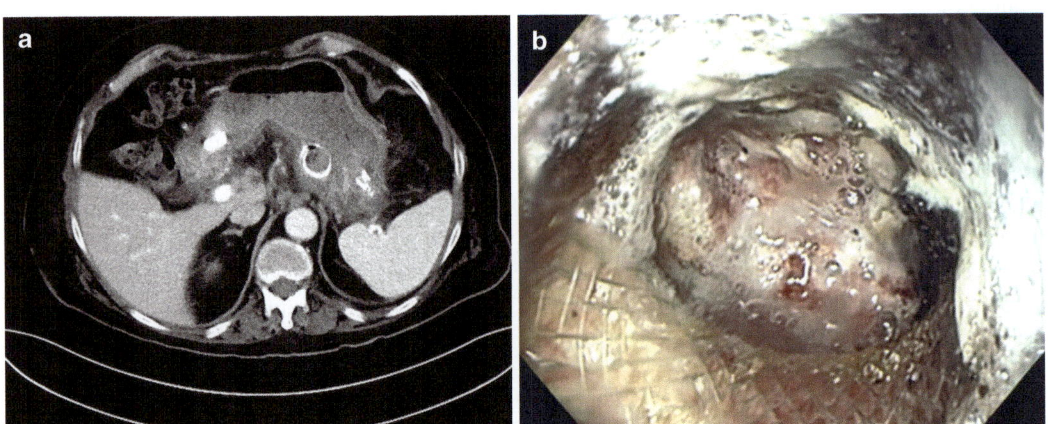

Fig. 4.8 (**a**) CT scan showing resolution of the PFC/WON; (**b**) Endoscopy showing resolution of the PFC/WON. The lumen-apposing stent was then removed

Reported clinical success rates following EUS-guided drainage of WOPN are high (88–95%), and the median duration of stent implantation ranges from 1 to 2 months with an average of 2 to 3 procedures completed prior to resolution, recognizing that some patients will have much longer durations of treatment if the WOPN is extensive or subtotal [5, 7, 13, 14]. To evaluate for improvement, the PFC size and characteristics should be assessed during each repeat procedure, and a contrast-enhanced CT is typically repeated every 4 to 8 weeks following initial stent placement [5, 10]

4.6 Potential Pitfalls

Potential adverse events associated with EUS-guided drainage of WOPN include infection, bleeding, perforation of the PFC or bowel lumen, sepsis, stent obstruction, and/or stent migration [7, 13]. Pre-procedural imaging and EUS should be used to ensure a safe distance between the luminal wall and WOPN to reduce the risk of perforation and ensure proper stent placement. LAMS have been associated with improved stent deployment and reduced bleeding, possibly due to the tamponade-like forces applied by a larger diameter self-expanding metal stent [15]. Furthermore, DPS can be placed within LAMS to help prevent stent migration and occlusion. DPS can also reduce the risk of bleeding and help break up solid necrotic material in WOPN.

Bleeding and perforation are two of the most clinically concerning complications associated with drainage of WOPN, although both only occur rarely. Bleeding can occur at the time of stent placement, during repeat necrosectomy procedures, or at the time of stent removal [7]. To reduce the risk of bleeding with initial stent placement, Doppler ultrasound is used to identify and avoid interposing vasculature. When bleeding events do occur, the vast majority are managed endoscopically using epinephrine injections, endo-clips, or stent/balloon tamponade [7, 15]. However, severe bleeding may require coil embolization or, in extremely rare cases, surgical intervention [13, 16]. Perforation should be suspected in patients with severe post-procedural pain or any sign of peritonitis. Peritonitis requires immediate surgical evaluation and possible intervention, and perforation without evidence of peritonitis is often treated effectively with conservative management [13].

References

1. Banks PA, Bollen TL, Dervenis C, Gooszen HG, Johnson CD, Sarr MG, Tsiotos GG, Vege SS. Classification of acute pancreatitis--2012: revision of the Atlanta classification and definitions by international consensus. Gut. 2013;62(1):102–11. https://doi.org/10.1136/gutjnl-2012-302779.
2. Baron TH, DiMaio CJ, Wang AY, Morgan KA (2020) American Gastroenterological Association Clinical Practice Update: management of pancreatic necrosis. Gastroenterology. 158 (1):67–75. e61. https://doi.org/10.1053/j.gastro.2019.07.064
3. van Brunschot S, van Grinsven J, van Santvoort HC, Bakker OJ, Besselink MG, Boermeester MA, Bollen TL, Bosscha K, Bouwense SA, Bruno MJ, Cappendijk VC, Consten EC, Dejong CH, van Eijck CH, Erkelens WG, van Goor H, van Grevenstein WMU, Haveman JW, Hofker SH, Jansen JM, Lameris JS, van Lienden KP, Meijssen MA, Mulder CJ, Nieuwenhuijs VB, Poley JW, Quispel R, de Ridder RJ, Romkens TE, Scheepers JJ, Schepers NJ, Schwartz MP, Seerden T, Spanier BWM, Straathof JWA, Strijker M, Timmer R, Venneman NG, Vleggaar FP, Voermans RP, Witteman BJ, Gooszen HG, Dijkgraaf MG, Fockens P. Endoscopic or surgical step-up approach for infected necrotising pancreatitis: a multicentre randomised trial. Lancet. 2018;391(10115):51–8. https://doi.org/10.1016/s0140-6736(17)32404-2.
4. Bakker OJ, van Santvoort HC, van Brunschot S, Geskus RB, Besselink MG, Bollen TL, van Eijck CH, Fockens P, Hazebroek EJ, Nijmeijer RM, Poley JW, van Ramshorst B, Vleggaar FP, Boermeester MA, Gooszen HG, Weusten BL, Timmer R. Endoscopic transgastric vs surgical necrosectomy for infected necrotizing pancreatitis: a randomized trial. JAMA. 2012;307(10):1053–61. https://doi.org/10.1001/jama.2012.276.
5. Adler DG, Shah J, Nieto J, Binmoeller K, Bhat Y, Taylor LJ, Siddiqui AA. Placement of lumen-apposing metal stents to drain pseudocysts and walled-off pancreatic necrosis can be safely performed on an outpatient basis: A multicenter study. Endosc Ultrasound. 2019;8(1):36–42. https://doi.org/10.4103/eus.eus_30_17.
6. Guo J, Saftoiu A, Vilmann P, Fusaroli P, Giovannini M, Mishra G, Rana SS, Ho S, Poley JW, Ang TL, Kalaitzakis E, Siddiqui AA, De La Mora-Levy JG, Lakhtakia S, Bhutani MS, Sharma M, Mukai S, Garg

PK, Lee LS, Vila JJ, Artifon E, Adler DG, Sun S. A multi-institutional consensus on how to perform endoscopic ultrasound-guided peri-pancreatic fluid collection drainage and endoscopic necrosectomy. Endosc Ultrasound. 2017;6(5):285–91. https://doi.org/10.4103/eus.eus_85_17.
7. Mohan BP, Jayaraj M, Asokkumar R, Shakhatreh M, Pahal P, Ponnada S, Navaneethan U, Adler DG. Lumen apposing metal stents in drainage of pancreatic walled-off necrosis, are they any better than plastic stents? A systematic review and meta-analysis of studies published since the revised Atlanta classification of pancreatic fluid collections. Endosc Ultrasound. 2019;8(2):82–90. https://doi.org/10.4103/eus.eus_7_19.
8. Yan L, Dargan A, Nieto J, Shariaha RZ, Binmoeller KF, Adler DG, DeSimone M, Berzin T, Swahney M, Draganov PV, Yang DJ, Diehl DL, Wang L, Ghulab A, Butt N, Siddiqui AA. Direct endoscopic necrosectomy at the time of transmural stent placement results in earlier resolution of complex walled-off pancreatic necrosis: Results from a large multicenter United States trial. Endosc Ultrasound. 2019;8(3):172–9. https://doi.org/10.4103/eus.eus_108_17.
9. Shahid H. Endoscopic management of pancreatic fluid collections. Transl Gastroenterol Hepatol. 2019;4:15. https://doi.org/10.21037/tgh.2019.01.09.
10. Siddiqui AA, Easler J, Strongin A, Slivka A, Kowalski TE, Muddana V, Chennat J, Baron TH, Loren DE, Papachristou GI. Hydrogen peroxide-assisted endoscopic necrosectomy for walled-off pancreatic necrosis: a dual center pilot experience. Dig Dis Sci. 2014;59(3):687–90. https://doi.org/10.1007/s10620-013-2945-x.
11. Sahar N, Kozarek RA, Kanji ZS, Chihara S, Gan SI, Gluck M, Larsen M, Ross AS, Irani S. Duration of antibiotic treatment after endoscopic ultrasound-guided drainage of walled-off pancreatic necrosis not affecting outcomes. J Gastroenterol Hepatol. 2018;33(8):1548–52. https://doi.org/10.1111/jgh.14111.
12. Khashab MA, Chithadi KV, Acosta RD, Bruining DH, Chandrasekhara V, Eloubeidi MA, Fanelli RD, Faulx AL, Fonkalsrud L, Lightdale JR, Muthusamy VR, Pasha SF, Saltzman JR, Shaukat A, Wang A, Cash BD. Antibiotic prophylaxis for GI endoscopy. Gastrointest Endosc. 2015;81(1):81–9. https://doi.org/10.1016/j.gie.2014.08.008.
13. Rana SS, Shah J, Kang M, Gupta R. Complications of endoscopic ultrasound-guided transmural drainage of pancreatic fluid collections and their management. Ann Gastroenterol. 2019;32(5):441–50. https://doi.org/10.20524/aog.2019.0404.
14. Siddiqui AA, Adler DG, Nieto J, Shah JN, Binmoeller KF, Kane S, Yan L, Laique SN, Kowalski T, Loren DE, Taylor LJ, Munigala S, Bhat YM. EUS-guided drainage of peripancreatic fluid collections and necrosis by using a novel lumen-apposing stent: a large retrospective, multicenter U.S. experience (with videos). Gastrointest Endosc. 2016;83(4):699–707. https://doi.org/10.1016/j.gie.2015.10.020.
15. Abu Dayyeh BK, Mukewar S, Majumder S, Zaghlol R, Vargas Valls EJ, Bazerbachi F, Levy MJ, Baron TH, Gostout CJ, Petersen BT, Martin J, Gleeson FC, Pearson RK, Chari ST, Vege SS, Topazian MD. Large-caliber metal stents versus plastic stents for the management of pancreatic walled-off necrosis. Gastrointest Endosc. 2018;87(1):141–9. https://doi.org/10.1016/j.gie.2017.04.032.
16. van Brunschot S, Fockens P, Bakker OJ, Besselink MG, Voermans RP, Poley JW, Gooszen HG, Bruno M, van Santvoort HC. Endoscopic transluminal necrosectomy in necrotising pancreatitis: a systematic review. Surg Endosc. 2014;28(5):1425–38. https://doi.org/10.1007/s00464-013-3382-9.

5 EUS-guided Drainage of Postoperative Fluid Collections

Auke Bogte and Frank P. Vleggaar

5.1 Background

EUS-guided postoperative drainage (EUS-POD) of postoperative fluid collections (POFCs) is increasingly popular as an alternative to percutaneous drainage in the management of patients with fluid collections after surgery. The technique involves placement of plastic double-pigtail stents or lumen-apposing metal stents (LAMS) and can be performed via a transgastric, transduodenal, or transrectal approach. Usually, EUS-POD is performed when a wall surrounding the collection has formed to optimize the safety of the procedure. Earlier data suggest that EUS-POD may be comparable to percutaneous drainage with regard to safety and effectivity [1]. In addition, recent data imply that early EUS-guided drainage of postoperative fluid collections (without the formation of a surrounding wall) is also safe and effective [2]. Many different types of postoperative fluid collections could be candidates for EUS-POD, such as collections after hepatopancreatobiliary, bariatric, or colorectal surgery [3–5].

5.2 Case History

A 56-year-old woman underwent an extended left hemihepatectomy because of a large intrahepatic cholangiocarcinoma. Although initial recovery was uneventful, she developed abdominal pain and fever. Computed tomography showed a subphrenic postoperative fluid collection containing air bubbles of 8 × 6 cm adjacent to the liver remnant, its features compatible with an infected biloma (Fig. 5.1). Percutaneous drainage was deemed impossible due to the location. Instead, EUS-guided drainage (EUS-POD) was proposed as an alternative.

5.3 Procedural Plan

EUS-POD can be performed via transgastric, transduodenal, or transrectal access. The POFCs can be located anywhere in the abdominal cavity, dictating an individualized approach. We chose to drain the biloma via the transgastric route, as there appeared to be a window for transmural drainage in the wall of the stomach. Technical considerations for drainage involve the size, shape, accessibility, and proximity (preferably less than 1 cm) to the gastrointestinal tract. All these can best be determined with CT and during

Supplementary Information The online version contains supplementary material available at [https://doi.org/10.1007/978-981-16-9340-3_5].

A. Bogte (✉) · F. P. Vleggaar
Department of Gastroenterology and Hepatology, University Medical Center Utrecht, Utrecht, The Netherlands
e-mail: a.bogte@umcutrecht.nl; f.vleggaar@umcutrecht.nl

A. Y.B. Teoh et al. (eds.), *Atlas of Interventional EUS*, https://doi.org/10.1007/978-981-16-9340-3_5

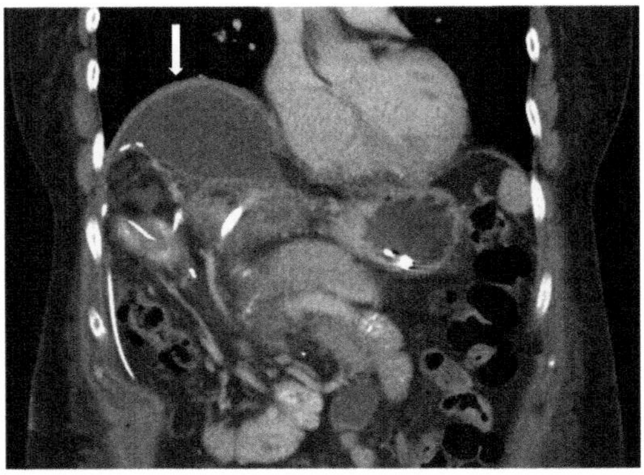

Fig. 5.1 Computed tomography demonstrating a postoperative fluid collection (biloma)

the EUS-procedure. In addition, the position of the echoendoscope needs to be preferably straight for LAMS placement. Ideally, the final position of the LAMS should not block the pylorus.

We prefer to drain postoperative fluid collections using lumen-apposing metal stents (LAMS). The advantage of the cautery enhanced system with HotAXIOS (Boston Scientific, Marlborough, MA, USA) is that it allows direct puncture of the POFC and reduces the procedural time and need for exchange of devices. Furthermore, the risk of stent dislodgement is reduced with LAMS. Alternatively, a 19-gauge fine needle can be used to get access to the POFC, through which a guidewire can be put in place, and after tract dilation, placement of plastic double-pigtail stents.

5.4 Description of the Procedure

The EUS-POD was performed under sedation with propofol via the transgastric approach using a linear echoendoscope. The fluid collection was identified and measured at 3 × 6 cm (Video 5.1, Fig. 5.2). There were no intervening blood vessels. The biloma was directly punctured with the cautery enhanced delivery system (Boston Scientific, Marlborough, MA, USA) with a 10 × 10 mm LAMS. The distal flange was deployed under EUS guidance. The stent was then pulled back to appose the two walls. Thereafter, the proximal flange was opened in the echoendoscope instrumentation channel ("blind" part of the procedure) and pushed outwards under endoscopic guidance to deploy in the gastric lumen. Figure 5.3 depicts the position of the echoendoscope with X-ray. It is paramount that the tip of the echoendoscope is in a straight position to insure proper deployment of the LAMS. However, the endoscope itself does not necessarily have to be. Figure 5.4 shows the position of the LAMS with respect to the pylorus. Caution is warranted, as a deployed LAMS may occlude the pylorus if placed too near to it.

We do not routinely dilate the stent after placement as it should be completely deployed within 24 hours. A double-pigtail plastic stent can be inserted after dilation to prevent obstruction of the lumen of the stent, particularly when the LAMS is placed transgastrically and there is a risk of food obstruction. LAMS removal is usually performed after 3–6 weeks, after a CT scan shows complete resolution of the POFC.

5.5 Post-procedural Management

Antibiotics were discontinued a day after drainage. The patient suffered from severe postoperative gastroparesis, which lasted for three weeks until complete resolution of the biloma. After that she recovered well. Figure 5.5a shows the content of the biloma 3 days after stent deployment. Figure 5.5b shows the collapsed biloma, with surgical clips of the previously performed extended hemihepatectomy protruding in the opposing wall upon LAMS removal 3 weeks later.

5.6 Potential Pitfalls

The potential adverse events after EUS-POD using LAMS include maldeployment of the stent, migration, buried stent syndrome, perforation, bleeding, stent occlusion, and occlusion of the pylorus. A recent multicenter retrospective review for pancreatic fluid collection drainage showed excellent technical and clinical success rates, but the named complications are not negli-

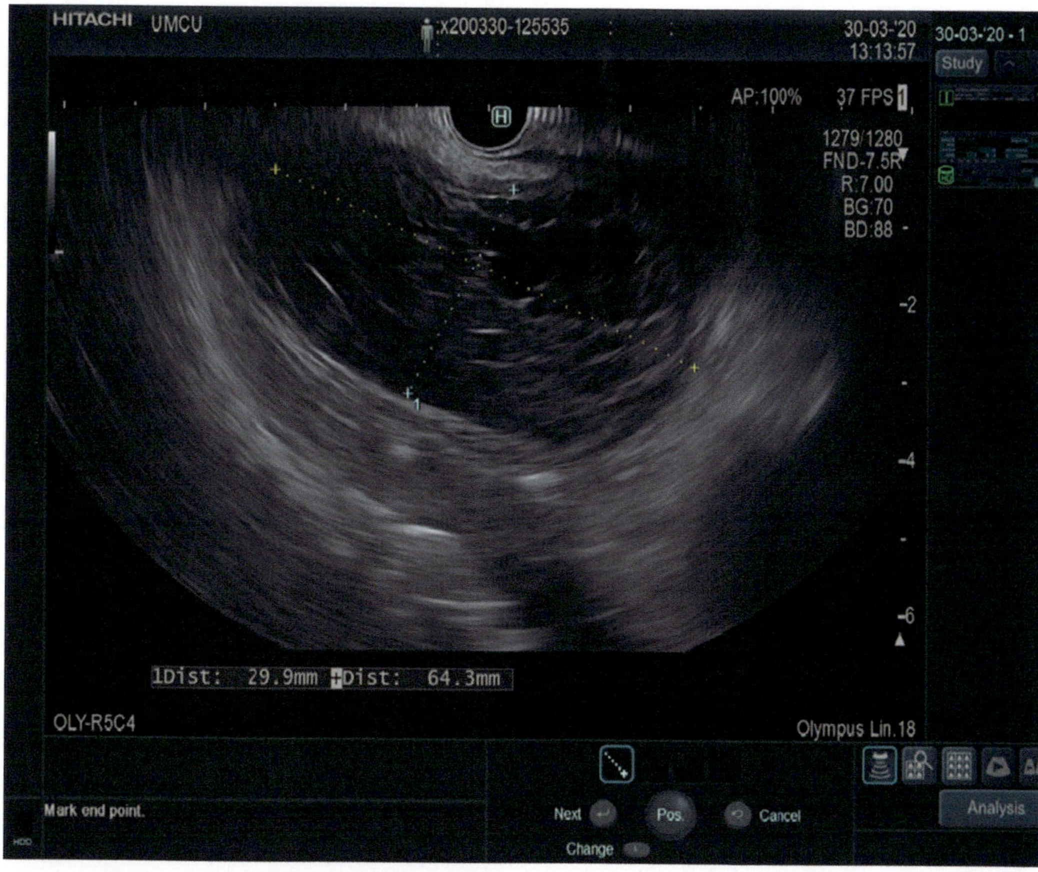

Fig. 5.2 EUS-image of the corresponding fluid collection

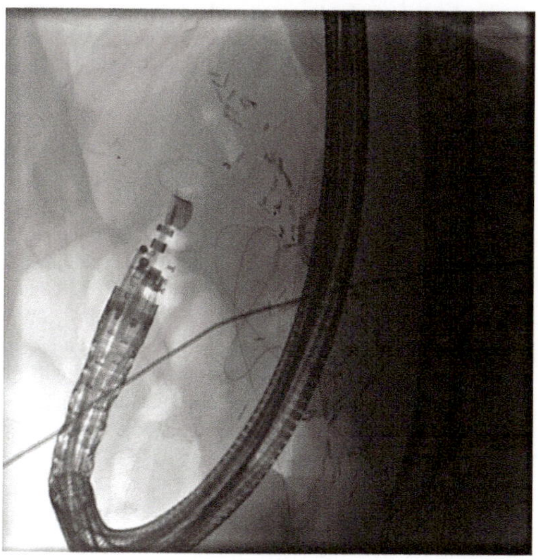

Fig. 5.3 X-ray showing the position of the scope during stent deployment

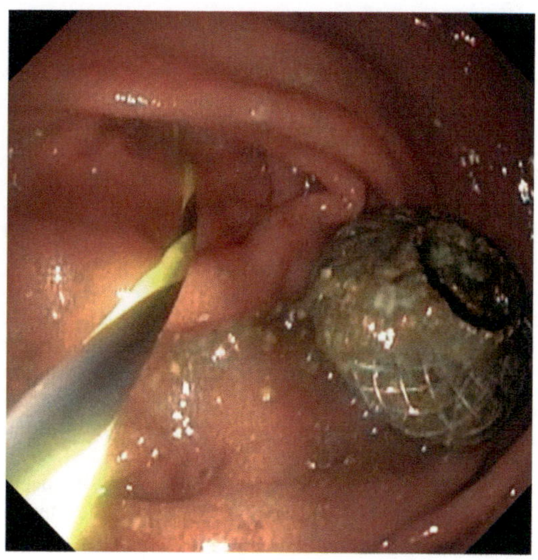

Fig. 5.4 Position of the LAMS in respect to the pylorus

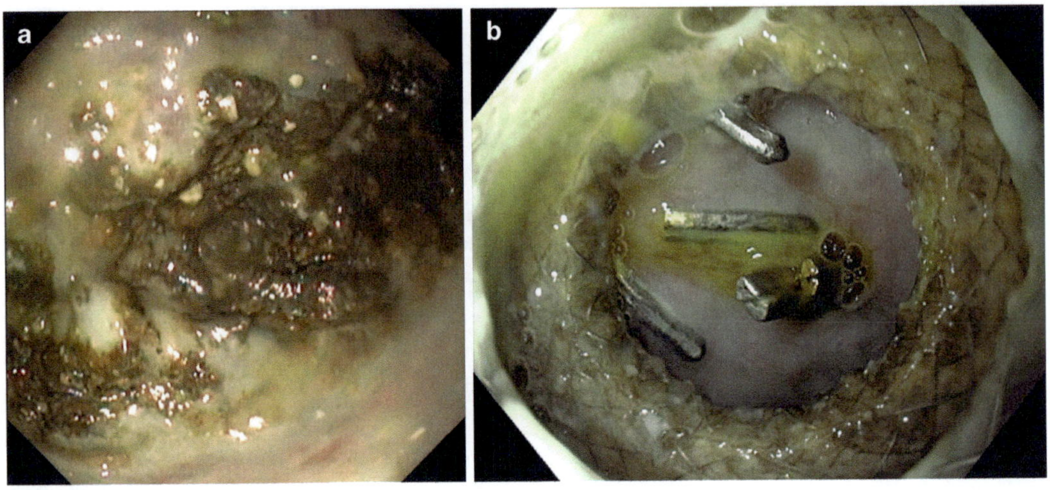

Fig. 5.5 (**a**) Endoscopic view of the inside of the biloma 3 days later; (**b**) Endoscopic view of the collapsed biloma upon LAMS removal, showing surgical clips of the previous extended hemihepatectomy through the opposing wall

gible [6]. When looking at adverse events in postoperative fluid collections instead, a recent international multicenter study on safety and efficacy of LAMS in POFCs showed markedly lower adverse events (12.9%) [7]. Experienced endoscopists will be able to treat these adverse events accordingly.

References

1. Tellez-Avila F, Carmona-Aguilera GJ, Valdovinos-Andraca F, et al. Postoperative abdominal collections drainage: percutaneous versus guided by endoscopic ultrasound. Dig Endosc. 2015;27:762–6.
2. Storm AC, Levy MJ, Kaura K, Abu Dayyeh BK, Cleary SP, Kendrick ML, Truty MJ, Vargas EJ, Topazian M, Chandrasekhara V. Acute and early EUS-guided transmural drainage of symptomatic postoperative fluid collections. Gastrointest Endosc. 2019; https://doi.org/10.1016/j.gie.2019.11.045.
3. Machlab S, Pascua-Solé M, Hernández L, Lira A, Vives J, Pedregal P, Luna A, Junquera F. Endoscopic Ultrasound (EUS)-guided drainage of a postsleeve gastrectomy subphrenic collection using a lumen apposition stent. Obes Surg. 2020 Mar 18. https://doi.org/10.1007/s11695-020-04553-w.
4. Donatelli G, Fuks D, Cereatti F, Pourcher G, Perniceni T, Dumont JL, Tuszynski T, Vergeau BM, Meduri B, Gayet B. Endoscopic transmural management of abdominal fluid collection following gastrointestinal, bariatric, and hepato-bilio-pancreatic surgery. Surg Endosc. 2018;32(5):2281–7.
5. Cassis P, Shah-Khan SM, Nasr J. EUS-guided drainage of a 20-cm biloma by use of a lumen-apposing metal stent. VideoGIE. 2019;5(1):20–1.
6. Fugazza A, Sethi A, Trindade AJ, Troncone E, Devlin J, Khashab MA, Vleggaar FP, Bogte A, Tarantino I, Deprez PH, Fabbri C, Aparicio JR, Fockens P, Voermans RP, Uwe W, Vanbiervliet G, Charachon A, Packey CD, Benias PC, El-Sherif Y, Paiji C, Ligresti D, Binda C, Martínez B, Correale L, Adler DG, Repici A, Anderloni A. International multicenter comprehensive analysis of adverse events associated with lumen-apposing metal stent placement for pancreatic fluid collection drainage. Gastrointest Endosc. 2020;91(3):574–83.
7. Yang J, Kaplan JH, Sethi A, Dawod E, Sharaiha RZ, Chiang A, Kowalski T, Nieto J, Law R, Hammad H, Wani S, Wagh MS, Yang D, Draganov PV, Messallam A, Cai Q, Kushnir V, Cosgrove N, Ahmed AM, Anderloni A, Adler DG, Kumta NA, Nagula S, Vleggaar FP, Irani S, Robles-Medranda C, El Chafic AH, Pawa R, Brewer O, Sanaei O, Dbouk M, Singh VK, Kumbhari V, Khashab MA. Safety and efficacy of the use of lumen-apposing metal stents in the management of postoperative fluid collections: a large, international, multicenter study. Endoscopy. 2019;51(8):715–21.

Transgastric Necrosectomy

6

Andrea Anderloni, Alessandro Fugazza, Matteo Colombo, and Alessandro Repici

6.1 Background

Walled-off necrosis (WON) is defined as one of the possible local complications occurring after a necrotizing pancreatitis and it is characterized by the presence of necrotic material contained within a wall of reactive tissue [1]. There is a general consensus that WON has to be drained when it becomes infected or when it causes symptoms due to increased volume, such as abdominal pain, nausea, and vomiting. In the past years, the most commonly used approach for symptomatic necrotic collections was major intervention as surgical debridement, while nowadays a minimally invasive approach such as endoscopic and/or percutaneous is favored [2].

Supplementary Information The online version contains supplementary material available at [https://doi.org/10.1007/978-981-16-9340-3_6].

A. Anderloni (✉) · A. Fugazza · M. Colombo
Division of Gastroenterology and Digestive Endoscopy, Humanitas Research Hospital - IRCCS, Rozzano (MI), Italy
e-mail: andrea.anderloni@humanitas.it; alessandro.fugazza@humanitas.it; matteo.colombo@humanitas.it

A. Repici
Division of Gastroenterology and Digestive Endoscopy, Humanitas Research Hospital - IRCCS, Rozzano (MI), Italy

Department of Biomedical Sciences, Humanitas University, Pieve Emanuele (MI), Italy
e-mail: alessandro.repici@hunimed.eu

Endoscopic transmural drainage for pancreatic necrosis was first described in 1996 [3]. Since then, endosonography (EUS)-guided drainage of WON has become the procedure of choice, being characterized by a high success rate with low adverse event and mortality rates [4]. More recently, with the introduction in clinical practice of a novel "saddle-shaped" lumen-apposing, fully covered, self-expandable metal stent (LAMS), the endoscopic management of WON has become simpler and faster, maintaining high technical and long-term success rates [5]. Due to their specific antimigratory design, this type of stents could ensure a more stable access to the cavity in order to facilitate a possible session of direct endoscopic necrosectomy (DEN). Moreover, the large caliber of the stent, that in the greater version can reach 20 mm, is of paramount importance as it allows for the withdrawal of larger necrotic debris, avoiding the risk of stent occlusion due to necrotic tissue impaction.

6.2 Case History

A 46-year-old man had experienced severe acute biliary pancreatitis, requiring admission to the Intensive Care Unit (ICU) where he was treated conservatively with fluid resuscitation and broad-spectrum antibiotics. 6-weeks after being discharged, due to the onset of abdominal pain and early satiety, he underwent an abdomen computed tomography (CT) which showed an

A. Y.B. Teoh et al. (eds.), *Atlas of Interventional EUS*, https://doi.org/10.1007/978-981-16-9340-3_6

increase in size of the WON (110 × 60 mm) with signs of infection and compression of the superior mesenteric and spleen vein (Fig. 6.1).

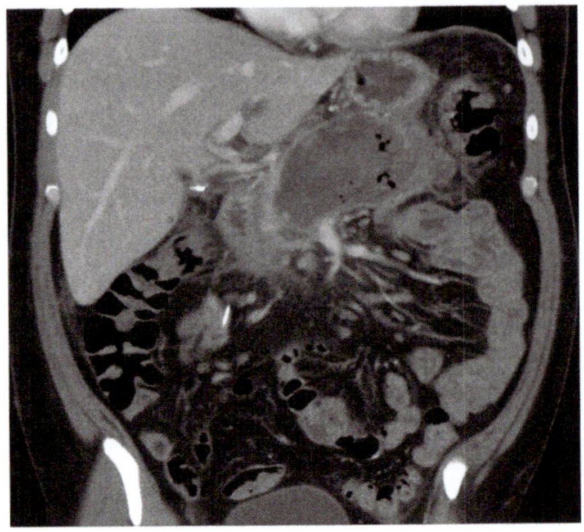

Fig. 6.1 Computed tomography demonstrating the peri-pancreatic collection

6.3 Procedural Plan

After a multidisciplinary team discussion, in conjunction with surgeons and radiologist, it was decided to perform an endoscopic ultrasound-guided drainage of the fluid collection. Considering the location of the latter, a transgastric approach was chosen. To provide a better access to the cavity after deployment of the stent, a pneumatic dilation of the LAMS was planned; subsequently, a concomitant direct endoscopic necrosectomy (DEN) session was scheduled, as it allows for early mobilization and debridement of solid debris within the WON. Published data confirm that this approach reduces the number of DEN required for successful resolution of WON and the risk of AE [6, 7].

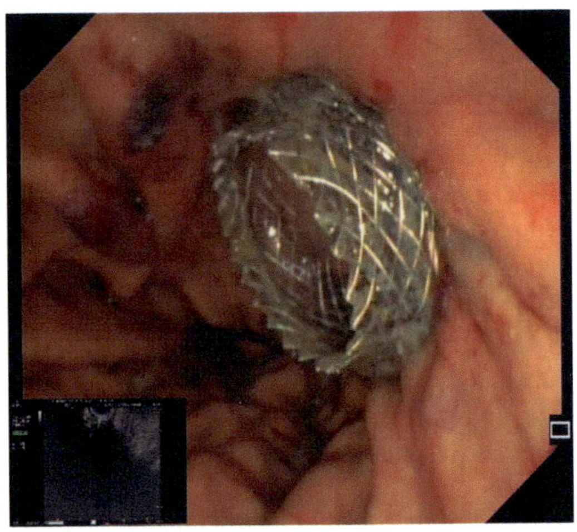

Fig. 6.2 Endoscopic view from the stomach of the lumen-apposing metal stent

6.4 Description of the Procedure

The procedure was performed with the patient in spontaneous breath under deep sedation, in an endoscopic room with all fluoroscopic equipment assembled before the procedure. An EUS examination should always be performed in order to localize vessels and other structures which may be located on the intended path. WON drainage was performed with a cautery enhanced LAMS 15 × 10 mm (EC-LAMS; Hot-AXIOS, Boston Scientific, Corp Natick MA, USA), using a linear echoendoscope (Fig. 6.2). The outflow of clear liquid and necrotic debris through the stent confirmed its correct positioning. Subsequently, the newly created fistulous tract between the collection and the gastric cavity was dilated pneumatically using a balloon, up to 15 mm. After obtaining a wider access, the inner part of the collection was reached with an operative gastroscope under CO2 insufflation showing large amount of necrotic material (Fig. 6.3). DEN was carried out using different accessories: firstly a Dormia basket, then a tripod and finally a snare with partial removal of the necrotic material (Fig. 6.4—Video 6.1). Post-procedural course was uneventful. A CT-scan 3 weeks later showed reduction of the WON size with minimal amount of necrosis. A second procedure was then scheduled with DEN, LAMS removal and placement of 2 plastic double pig-tail stent. After 1 month, a subsequent CT-scan showed complete resolution of the collection with plastic stent still in place that were removed few days later with a snare. No recurrence of the WON occurred during follow-up.

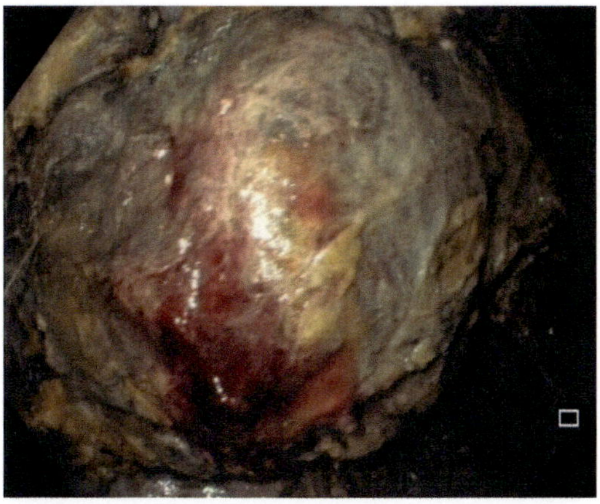

Fig. 6.3 Endoscopic "through-the-stent" view of the necrotic material inside the collection

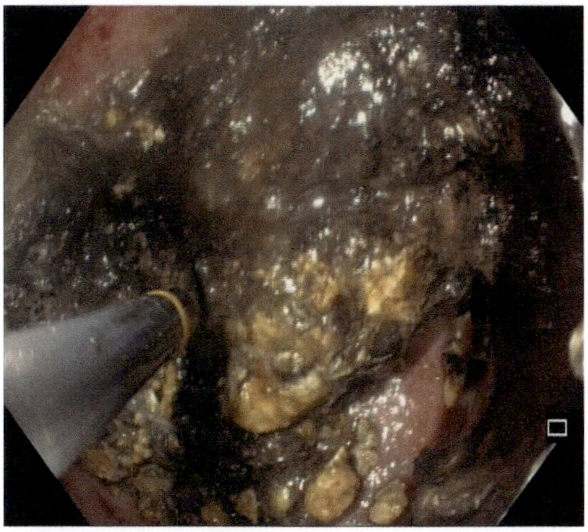

Fig. 6.4 Endoscopic "through-the-stent" view of a endoscopic necrosectomy using a Dormia

6.5 Post-procedural Management

Oral in-take can be resumed when the patients tolerate it. Antibiotics should be administered intravenously until necessary. According to Bang et al. [8], we usually schedule an abdomen CT-scan at 3–4 weeks in all patients treated with LAMS, followed by stent removal if the collection has resolved. This approach is particularly useful in avoiding stent-related AEs (e.g., bleeding and buried LAMS syndrome) when the cavity starts to shrink. In case of incomplete drainage of the WON, a second session of DEN can be performed. After stent removal, double pig-tail plastic stents (7 Fr or 10 Fr) may be left in place to allow complete resolution of the collection.

6.6 Potential Pitfalls

Potential AEs related to endoscopic treatment of WON are usually stent occlusion, stent dislodgment, stent migration, bleeding, and infection. Interestingly in 2019, Wang et al reported no significant difference in terms of stent-related AEs between different stent types, except for LAMS which had the lowest risk of stent migration [9]. Stent occlusion and migration may be manageable with endoscopy and usually do not require surgery. In case of bleeding could be managed by endoscopy [10] whereas if a massive bleeding from a large pseudoaneurysm is encountered, angiographic embolization is needed. Sometimes during a session of DEN the stent can be grasped and dislodged by one of the accessories used for removing necrotic debris. To manage this procedure-related AE recently a new technique has been proposed, which allows to reuse the stent previously placed avoiding the need of using a new LAMS [11]. The risk of infection and stent occlusion could be reduced using pneumatic dilation after LAMS deployment as described in a recent multicenter study [7]. However, randomized controlled studies are needed in order to confirm this data.

References

1. Banks PA, Bollen TL, Dervenis C, et al. Classification of acute pancreatitis–2012: revision of the Atlanta classification and definitions by international consensus. Gut. 2013;62:102–11.
2. Baron TH, DiMaio CJ, Wang AY, Morgan KA. American Gastroenterological Association Clinical Practice Update: management of pancreatic necrosis. Gastroenterology. 2020;158(1):67–75.e1.
3. Baron TH, Thaggard WG, Morgan DE, et al. Endoscopic therapy for organized pancreatic necrosis. Gastroenterology. 1996;111:755–64.
4. Varadarajulu S, Bang JY, Phadnis MA, et al. Endoscopic transmural drainage of peripancreatic

fluid collections: outcomes and predictors of treatment success in 211 consecutive patients. J Gastrointest Surg. 2011;15:2080–8.
5. Siddiqui AA, Adler DG, Nieto J, et al. EUS-guided drainage of peripancreatic fluid collections and necrosis by using a novel lumen-apposing stent: a large retrospective, multicenter U.S. experience (with videos). Gastrointest Endosc. 2016;83(4): 699–707.
6. Yan L, Dargan A, Nieto J, et al. Direct endoscopic necrosectomy at the time of transmural stent placement results in earlier resolution of complex walled-off pancreatic necrosis: Results from a large multicenter United States trial. Endosc Ultrasound. 2019;8(3):172–9.
7. Fugazza A, Sethi A, Trindade AJ, et al. International multicenter comprehensive analysis of adverse events associated with lumen-apposing metal stent placement for pancreatic fluid collection drainage. Gastrointest Endosc. 2020;91(3):574–83.
8. Bang JY, Hasan M, Navaneethan U, et al. Lumen-apposing metal stents (LAMS) for pancreatic fluid collection (PFC) drainage: may not be business as usual. Gut. 2017;66(12):2054–6.
9. Wang Z, Zhao S, Meng Q, et al. Comparison of three different stents for endoscopic ultrasound-guided drainage of pancreatic fluid collection: a large retrospective study. J Gastroenterol Hepatol. 2019;34:791–8.
10. Auriemma F, Anderloni A, Carrara S, et al. Cyanoacrylate hemostasis for massive bleeding after drainage of pancreatic fluid collection by lumen-apposing metal stent. Am J Gastroenterol. 2018;113(11):1582. https://doi.org/10.1038/s41395-018-0266-6.
11. Fugazza A, Colombo M, Gabbiadini R, et al. Repositioning rather than replacing: the management of a dislodged lumen-apposing metal stent (LAMS) in a Walled Off Necrosis. Am J Gastroenterol. 2020;115(6):811.

Part II

EUS-Guided Biliary Drainage

7 EUS-guided Rendezvous ERCP

Hiroyuki Isayama and Shigeto Ishii

7.1 Background

ERCP related procedures are still standard techniques to treat pancreato-biliary diseases. However, biliary access was sometimes difficult, and there are many tips to overcome these situations [1, 2]. Recently, the technique of EUS-guided rendezvous (EUS-RV) technique assisted biliary access was indicated to the failed biliary cannulation cases with accessible papilla. There are 3 approach routes: trans-gastric (TG), trans-duodenal with short scope position (TDS), and trans-duodenal with long scope position (TDL) [3]. There are some pros and cons of each procedure, therefore we should select the available route to obtain acceptable success rate [4]. TDS is the first-choice approach route because of short distance between the puncture point and the papilla, and manipulation of guide-wire (GW) is easier than the other route. Other reason was the discrepancy in the direction between the puncture and GW insertion was smaller than the other route. This discrepancy made GW manipulation difficult. Scope stability was little bit more difficult in TDS route.

Basically, after puncturing the bile duct, guidewire was inserted into the bile duct and advanced toward to the duodenum through the stricture and papilla. GW manipulation was the most difficult step with naked GW. Insertion of catheter or thin boogie dilator was helpful to pass the stricture/papilla. Iwashita T, et al. reported this method as "EUS-guided Hybrid RV (EUS-HRV)" [5]. Original method of biliary cannulation after insertion of GW into the duodenum was as follows; (1) withdrawing echoendoscope remaining GW, (2) grasping the GW with forceps/snare, (3) pulling back the GW into accessory channel and out from the proximal site, and (4) catheter insertion along the GW and cannulation. Three types of cannulation techniques using GW protruding from the papilla; along the GW, besides the GW, and "Hitch and ride" technique. Success rate of besides the GW was low. The technique of "Hitch and ride" was a new concept of cannulation using GW [6]. The catheter with slit on the tip hitch the GW, and insert the catheter ride on the GW

Supplementary Information The online version contains supplementary material available at [https://doi.org/10.1007/978-981-16-9340-3_7].

H. Isayama (✉) · S. Ishii
Department of Gastroenterology, Graduate School of Medicine, Juntendo University, Tokyo, Japan
e-mail: h-isayama@juntendo.ac.jp; sishii@juntendo.ac.jp

7.2 Case History

An old female, 93 y.o., had admitted to a hospital due to cholangitis caused by common bile duct stone (CBDS) (Fig. 7.1). Endoscopic biliary cannulation was failed because of intra-diverticulum

A. Y.B. Teoh et al. (eds.), *Atlas of Interventional EUS*, https://doi.org/10.1007/978-981-16-9340-3_7

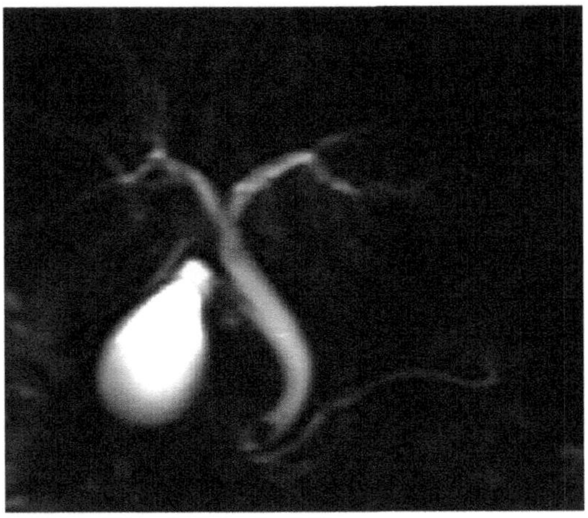

Fig. 7.1 MRCP image revealed stone as a defect at the distal common bile duct

papilla. After improvement of cholangitis with antibiotics, she was referred to our hospital for the removal of CBDS.

7.3 Procedural Plan

EUS-guided rendezvous technique for biliary cannulation for the patient. Standard endoscopic biliary cannulation and precutting technique were sometimes very difficult in the cases with intra-diverticulum papilla. In this case, it was difficult to face to the papilla, recognize the direction of the axis and manipulate the scope and catheter.

The Difficulty of EUS-RV lies in Guidewire (GW) manipulation to pass the stricture and papilla. Torque ability of VisiGlide 2 (0.025 inch, Olympus Medical Devices) which we selected for this procedure was good and useful in this procedure. After GW insertion into the duodenum, a modified ERCP catheter was used for the "Hitch and ride" cannulation technique. We made the slit for attaching the GW with a surgical scalpel.

7.4 Description of the Procedure (Video 7.1)

We checked the possibility of puncturing through the 1st and 2nd portion of the duodenum and decided on a TDS procedure. Puncture of distal part of CBD was done with 19 Gauge EUS-FNA needle (EZ Shot-3; Olympus Medical Corporation, Tokyo, Japan) (Fig. 7.2a, b, and c). After injection of contrast for performance of a cholangiogram. A GW was inserted into the CBD and it passed to the papilla easily. The GW was then advanced towards to the anal side of duodenum as far as possible (Fig. 7.2d). The echoendoscope was then carefully withdrawn, and the duodenoscope (EG 580T, Fujifilm Corp) was inserted under fluoroscopic guidance to avoid the disolodging the GW during scope insertion (Fig. 7.3a). The duodenoscope was then advanced to the papilla and a GW was noted to be protruding from the orifice of the papilla which was located in the diverticulum completely (Fig. 7.3b). We inserted the special catheter with slit on the tip for the "Hitch and ride" technique (Fig. 7.3c) and successfully cannulated the bile duct (Fig. 7.3d). Cannulation with the "Hitch and ride technique" could be made easier by adjusting the catheter direction with scope manipulation.

After biliary cannulation, an additional GW was inserted into CBD from the catheter, and the previous GW was removed. A Small sphincterotomy following balloon dilation (ESBD) was performed and CBDS was removed with retrieval balloon catheter.

7.5 Post-procedural Management

No adverse event was observed in the patient. A follow-up plain CT was routinely taken for all patients that received interventional EUS on the

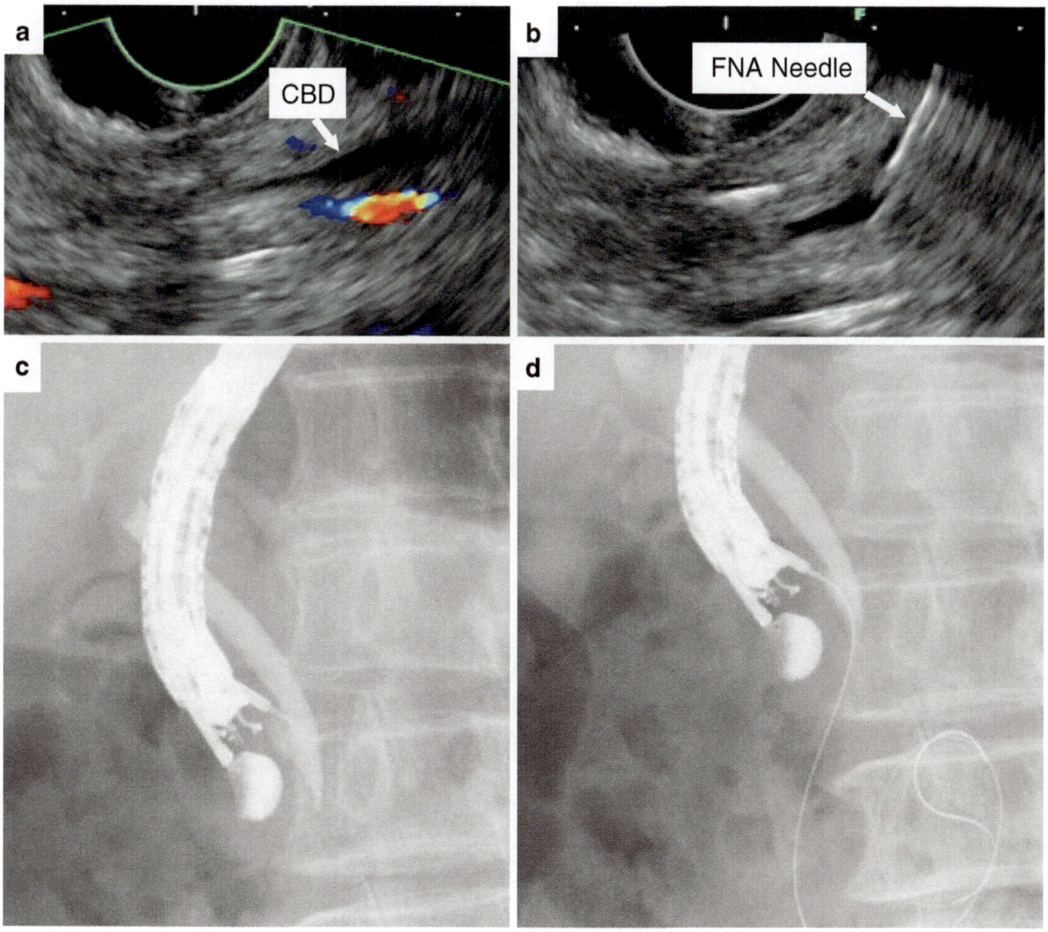

Fig. 7.2 EUS-guided rendezvous procedure: (**a**) EUS image of distal common bile duct (CBD); (**b**) EUS guided puncturing the CBD; (**c**) Cholangiogram by EUS-guided puncture; (**d**) GW insertion into the duodenum pass the papilla

next morning to detect the adverse event in our center. But, if the patients showed severe symptoms (high fever, severe pain with insufficient effect of NSAID, and any symptoms which required immediately procedure), we may arrange contrast-enhanced CT.

7.6 Potential Pitfalls

The Most difficult step of this procedure was passing the GW through the stricture or papilla. If this step was unsuccessful with standard GW, then there are 2 options. First, you can change to a hydrophilic GW to allow easier manupilation through the papilla [7]. Second, a catheter or dilator can be along the GW to make manipulation easier and allow exchange of the GW [5]. Regarding retrieval of the GW, usually it is grasped with a forceps or snare. However, sometimes the GW is dislodged inside the duodenoscope channel and one method is to lock it using the elevator and pull it out of the mouth together with the endoscope. Afterwards, the duodenoscope could be reinserted on GW and use it to facilitate cannulation.

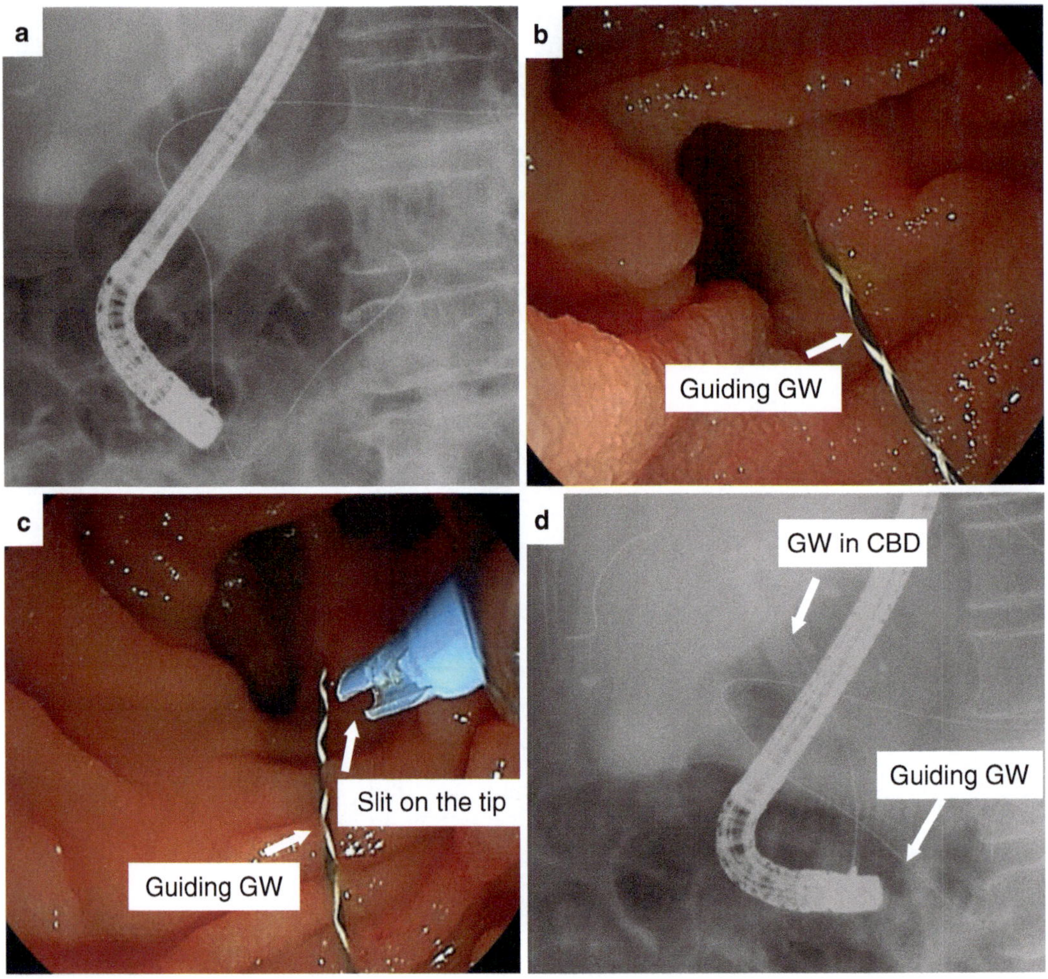

Fig. 7.3 Biliary cannulation of "Hitch and ride" technique. (**a**) X-ray image of duodenoscope and guiding GW; (**b**) Endoscopic image of GW coming out from the papilla which is located in the diverticulum; (**c**) Endoscopic image of ERCP catheter with slit on the tip; (**d**) Successful biliary cannulation

References

1. Liao WC, Angsuwatcharakon P, Isayama H, Dhir V, Devereaux B, Khor CJ, Ponnudurai R, Lakhtakia S, Lee DK, Ratanachu-Ek T, Yasuda I, Dy FT, Ho SH, Makmun D, Liang HL, Draganov PV, Rerknimitr R, Wang HP. International consensus recommendations for difficult biliary access. Gastrointest Endosc. 2016 Oct 5;85(2):295–304.
2. Dhir V, Isayama H, Itoi T, Almadi M, Siripun A, Teoh AYB, Ho KY. Endoscopic ultrasonography-guided biliary and pancreatic duct interventions. Dig Endosc. 2017 May;29(4):472–85.
3. Isayama H, Nakai Y, Kawakubo K, Kawakami H, Itoi T, Yamamoto N, Kogure H, Koike K. The endoscopic ultrasonography-guided rendezvous technique for biliary cannulation: a technical review. J Hepatobiliary Pancreat Sci. 2013 Apr;20(4):413–20.
4. Kawakubo K, Isayama H, Sasahira N, Nakai Y, Kogure H, Hamada T, Miyabayashi K, Mizuno S, Sasaki T, Ito Y, Yamamoto N, Hirano K, Tada M, Koike K. Clinical utility of an endoscopic ultrasound-guided rendezvous technique via various approach routes. Surg Endosc. 2013 Sep;27(9):3437–43.
5. Iwashita T, Uemura S, Yoshida K, Mita N, Tezuka R, Yasuda I, Shimizu M. EUS-guided hybrid rendezvous technique as salvage for standard rendezvous with intra-hepatic bile duct approach. PLoS One. 2018;13(8):e0202445.
6. Nakai Y, Isayama H, Matsubara S, Kogure H, Mizuno S, Hamada T, Takahara N, Nakamura T, Sato T, Takeda

T, Hakuta R, Ishigaki K, Saito K, Tada M, Koike K. A novel "hitch-and-ride" deep biliary cannulation method during rendezvous endoscopic ultrasound-guided ERCP technique. Endoscopy. 2017 Oct;49(10):983–8.

7. Dhir V, Bhandari S, Bapat M, Maydeo A. Comparison of EUS-guided rendezvous and precut papillotomy techniques for biliary access (with videos). Gastrointest Endosc. 2012;75:354–9.

EUS-guided Choledochoduodenostomy

8

Kazuo Hara, Nozomi Okuno, Shin Haba, and Takamichi Kuwahara

8.1 Background

EUS-guided choledochoduodenostomy (EUS-CDS) is gaining popularity as a rescue in patients with failed ERCP and the procedure is also considered as an option for primary biliary drainage [1–3]. The procedure has been shown to be associated with higher success rate, lower adverse events, shorter hospital stays, and fewer reinterventions [3]. An important advantage of EUS-CDS is no risk of pancreatitis and a permanent fistula may be created in some patients [2, 4]. Apart from malignant conditions, EUS-CDS can also be performed in selected benign diseases.

8.2 Case History

A 56-year-old female with a pancreatic head cancer was admitted for obstructive jaundice.

Computed tomography showed a dilated extrahepatic bile duct. The tumor has invaded into the duodenum and surrounding tissue. EUS-CDS was performed as primary drainage as ERCP was anticipated to be difficult. Extensive ascites could be a contraindication for EUS-guided biliary drainage but this was absent in this patient.

8.3 Procedural Plan

A cautery-enhanced one step system with the lumen apposing stent could be used EUS-CDS. The device can prevent bile leakage and make the procedure easier. However, the short length of the stent may result in easier stent dysfunction due to retrograde cholangitis or food debris. So, we selected a laser-cut fully covered metal stent. Laser-cut metal stents are easy to be deployed because there is no shortening. Additionally, the mesh of laser-cut metal stent was very sharp, so this can prevent stent migration. After deployment, the distal end of the stent should be pushed down to the D2 to prevent the retrograde flow of gastrointestinal contents into the stent. Plastic stents are generally not recommended for EUS-CDS as the risk of adverse events are higher in particular for bile peritonitis [5].

8.4 Description of the Procedure

EUS-CDS was performed using a linear echoendoscope. The extrahepatic bile duct was first identified and an area without intervening blood vessels was located. The extrahepatic bile duct

Supplementary Information The online version contains supplementary material available at [https://doi.org/10.1007/978-981-16-9340-3_8].

K. Hara (✉) · N. Okuno · S. Haba · T. Kuwahara
Department of Gastroenterology, AICHI Cancer Center, Nagoya City, Japan
e-mail: khara@aichi-cc.jp; nokuno@aichi-cc.jp; s.haba@aichi-cc.jp; kuwa_tak@aichi-cc.jp

A. Y.B. Teoh et al. (eds.), *Atlas of Interventional EUS*, https://doi.org/10.1007/978-981-16-9340-3_8

was directly punctured with 19G needle as shown in Fig 8.1. After complete aspiration of the bile. A cholangiogram was performed to confirm the location of the hepatic hilum. A 0.025 inch guidewire was inserted into the intrahepatic bile duct deeply. A 6 Fr cautery dilator was used to create the fistula as shown in Fig. 8.2. Finally, a metal stent was inserted under EUS and X-ray guidance as shown in Fig. 8.3. After opening the distal portion, the metal stent was then pulled back to appose the two organs as shown in Fig. 8.4. Nearly 80~90% of the proximal portion was opened in the instrument channel and pushed out to the anal side in the duodenum as shown in Fig. 8.5 [5].

8.5 Post-procedural Management

In the day after EUS-CDS, we should check the patient's condition bloods and X-ray. If possible, a CT scan is recommended. Diets can usually be resumed the next day. The patient could be discharged if liver functions improve without sepsis.

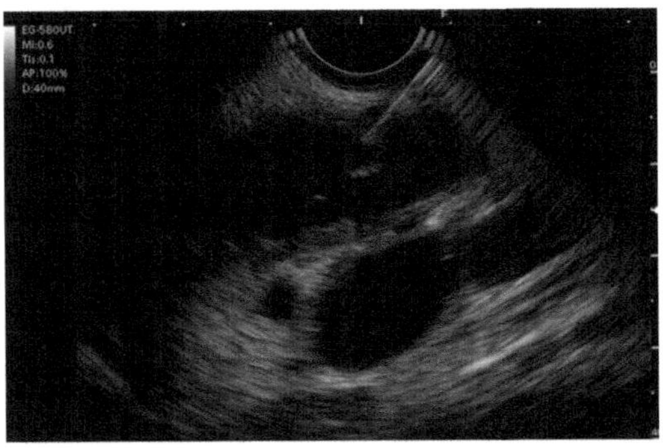

Fig. 8.1 Puncture the dilated CBD under EUS guidance

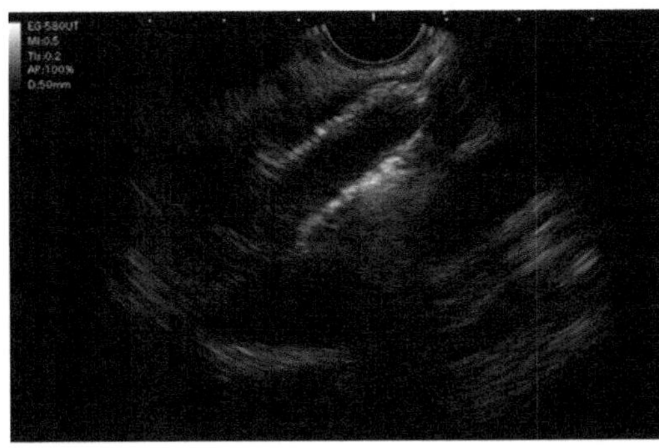

Fig. 8.3 Laser-cut metal stent deployed under EUS guidance

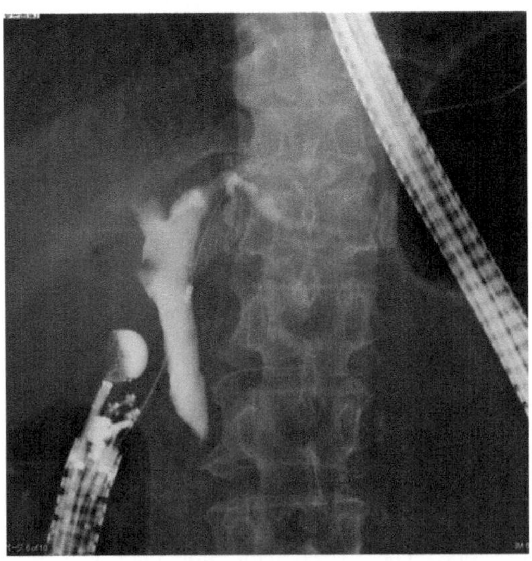

Fig. 8.2 Cautery dilation using co-axial dilator

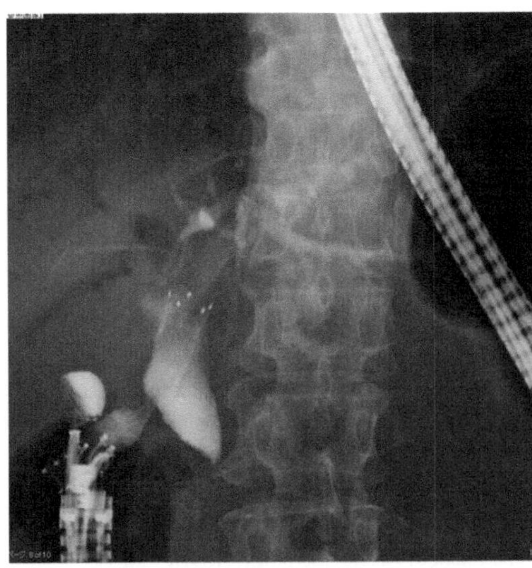

Fig. 8.4 Proximal of the metal stent deployed in the channel of the echoendoscope and pushed out of the endoscope

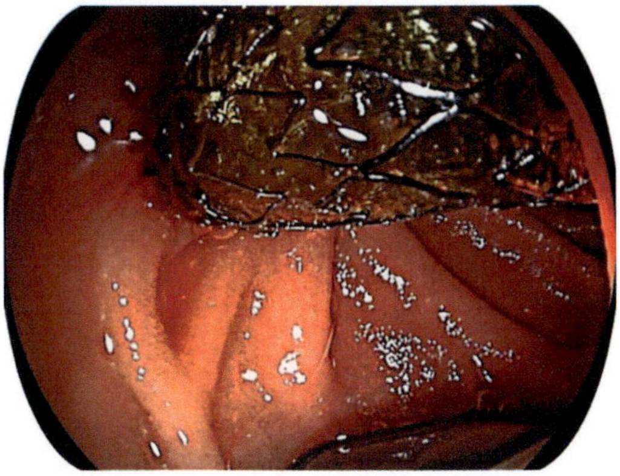

Fig. 8.5 The stent direction to the anal side in the duodenum

8.6 Potential Pitfalls

The potential adverse events after EUS-CDS include misdeployment of the stent, perforation, and bleeding. Double penetration of the duodenum is the unique complication in EUS-CDS [6]. The use of Forward-viewing EUS could avoid double penetration of the duodenum in EUS-CDS [5]. If adverse events occur, then an experienced interventional endosonographer should be consulted for management of the condition. Percutaneous biliary drainage may be required in some cases. In some patients, surgery may be required.

References

1. Hara K, Yamao K, Hijioka S, et al. Prospective clinical study of endoscopic ultrasound-guided choledochoduodenostomy with direct metallic stent placement using a forward-viewing echoendoscope. Endoscopy. 2013;45:392–6.
2. Hara K, Okuno N, Yamao K. De novo EUS-guided biliary drainage. Endosc Ultrasound. 2019;8:S14–6.
3. Paik WH, Lee TH, Park DH, et al. EUS-guided biliary drainage versus ERCP for the primary palliation of malignant biliary obstruction: a multicenter randomized clinical trial. Am J Gastroenterol. 2018;113:987–97.
4. Iwai T, Kida M, Yamauchi H, et al. Long-lasting patent fistula after EUS-guided choledochoduodenostomy in a patient with refractory benign biliary stricture. VideoGIE. 2018;3:193–5.
5. Matsumoto S, Hara K, Mizuno N, et al. Risk factor analysis for adverse events and stent dysfunction of Endoscopic ultrasound-guided choledochoduodenostomy. Dig Endosc. 2019;32(6):957–66.
6. Hara K, Yamao K, Mizuno N, et al. Endoscopic ultrasonography-guided biliary drainage: Who, when, which, and how? World J Gastroenterol. 2016;3:1297–303.

9 EUS-guided Choledochoduodenostomy with Lumen Apposing Stent

En-Ling Leung Ki and Bertrand Napoleon

9.1 Background

Endoscopic ultrasound guided-biliary drainage (EUS-BD) has been developed as an alternative for failed ERCP in malignant biliary obstruction (MBO) [1–3]. The most frequently used techniques are EUS-guided choledochoduodenostomy (EUS-CDS) and EUS-guided hepaticogastrostomy (EUS-HGS), which achieve extra-papillary drainage by trans-mural stenting [3]. Compared to percutaneous biliary drainage (PTBD), EUS-BD is as effective with less adverse events (AE), and lower re-intervention rates [4].

The advent of novel EUS-specific stent designs such as electrocautery enhanced lumen apposing metal stents (ECE-LAMS) has been revolutionary and has largely simplified the technique for EUS-CDS in distal MBO.

The Hot AXIOS™ is the only ECE-LAMS to be custom-designed and evaluated in EUS-CDS (Fig. 9.1). Recent data show excellent efficiency and safety profile [5–10]. The result of randomized studies comparing EUS-CDS with ECE-LAMS versus ERCP for distal MBO is still pending. Nevertheless, we strongly suggest considering the former when it is available, in particular for surgical candidates as it does not hinder surgery and also reduces the risk of post-ERCP pancreatitis which delays surgery [10–12].

Supplementary Information The online version contains supplementary material available at [https://doi.org/10.1007/978-981-16-9340-3_9].

E.-L. L. Ki
Department of Hepato-Gastroenterology, Private Hospital Jean-Mermoz, Ramsay Generale de Santé, Lyon, France

Department of Hepato-Gastroenterology, La Tour Hospital, Geneva, Switzerland

B. Napoleon (✉)
Department of Hepato-Gastroenterology, Private Hospital Jean-Mermoz, Ramsay Generale de Santé, Lyon, France

9.2 Case History

An 85 year-old poly-morbid man with a previous history of cholecystectomy was admitted for jaundice. Abdominal computed tomography (CT) showed a 4 cm pancreatic head tumor with portal vein infiltration and common bile duct (CBD) obstruction. Intra and extra-hepatic bile ducts were significantly dilated (Fig. 9.2). ERCP was not possible because of tumor induced duodenal stenosis. Subsequently, EUS-CDS was performed with Hot AXIOS™ in the same session.

9.3 Procedural Plan

The Hot AXIOS™ consists of a flexible, fully silicone covered, self-expanding nitinol stent that is pre-loaded within the ECE delivery system. A cautery enhanced system allows direct puncture of the dilated CBD. We systematically use the cautery system to enter the CBD. Conventional puncture with a 19G needle with insertion of a

A. Y.B. Teoh et al. (eds.), *Atlas of Interventional EUS*, https://doi.org/10.1007/978-981-16-9340-3_9

Fig. 9.1 Hot AXIOS™ fully deployed (*left*) and with electrocautery enhanced delivery system (*right*). Image provided by courtesy of Boston Scientific ©2019 Boston Scientific Corporation or its affiliates. All rights reserved

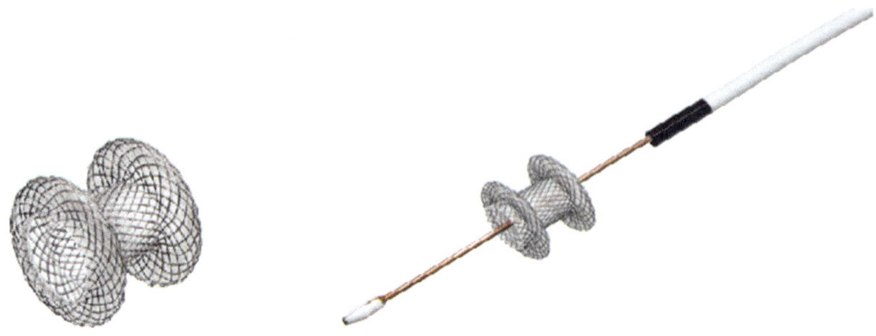

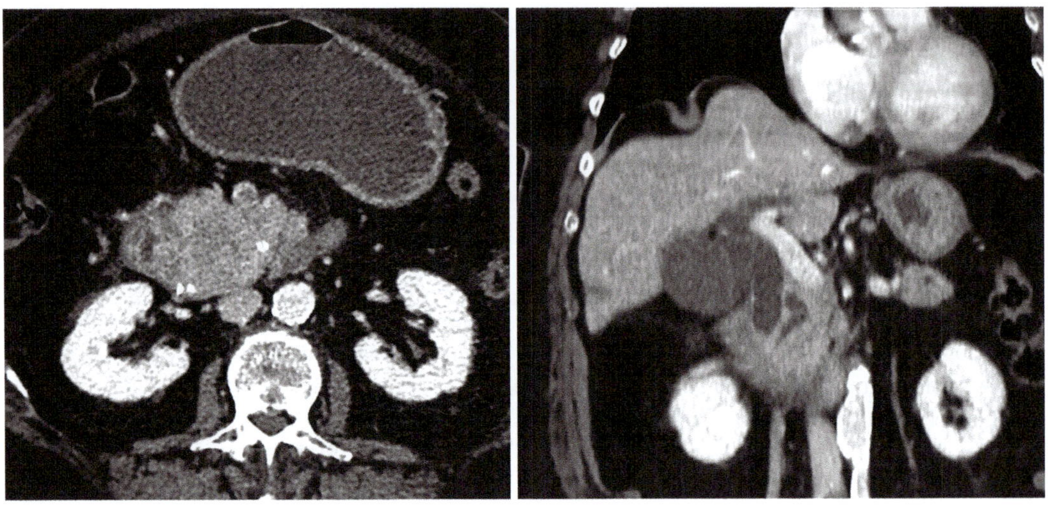

Fig. 9.2 Computed tomography demonstrating dilated biliary ducts with pancreatic tumor

guidewire is not recommended [9, 10]. The choice of the puncture site is particularly important: interposing vessels and the cystic duct must be avoided (Figs. 9.3 and 9.4). Ideally the tract of the puncture is performed close to a 90° angle and with at least 20 mm insertion of the system inside the CBD (Fig. 9.5) to reduce the risk of opening the distal flange outside the CBD. For beginners, we recommend performing EUS-CDS with a dilated CBD of at least 15 mm. If the duct diameter is <15 mm, we pre-insert a stiff 0.025″ guidewire in the channel of the Hot AXIOS™ and push it into the CBD after direct fistulotomy. The catheter can then be introduced over the wire. Fluoroscopy is required in this case. The choice of stent size can be adapted to the diameter of the CBD, nevertheless we recommend a 6 mm diameter stent particularly for CBD diameters <15 mm. We recommend proximal flange deployment in the working canal of the endoscope. We prefer to push the stent under EUS than endoscopic control to avoid the risk of misdeployment when pulling back the endoscope to get the endoscopic vision. In case of symptomatic duodenal stenosis a duodenal stent can be inserted during the same session.

9.4 Description of the Procedure (Video 9.1)

EUS-CDS was performed under general anesthesia with endotracheal intubation. A therapeutic linear echoendoscope with a long-route technique was used to facilitate stabilization in the duodenal bulb and to ensure that the transducer is well positioned close to the CBD. A suitable window for puncture was chosen in order to avoid interposing vessels including the gastroduodenal artery. The puncture was per-

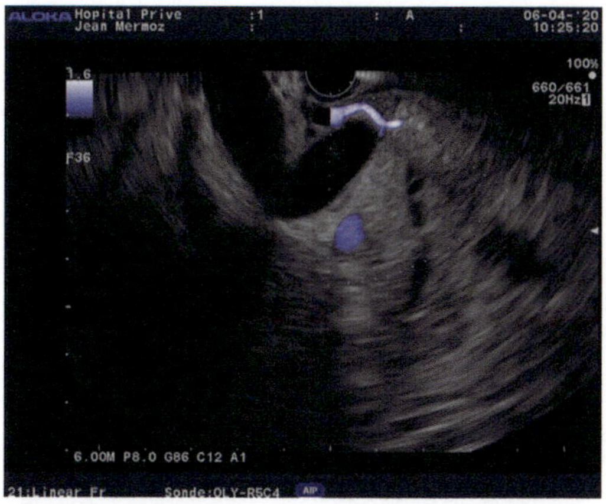

Fig. 9.3 Interposing vessels (gastroduodenal artery and aberrant arterial branch)

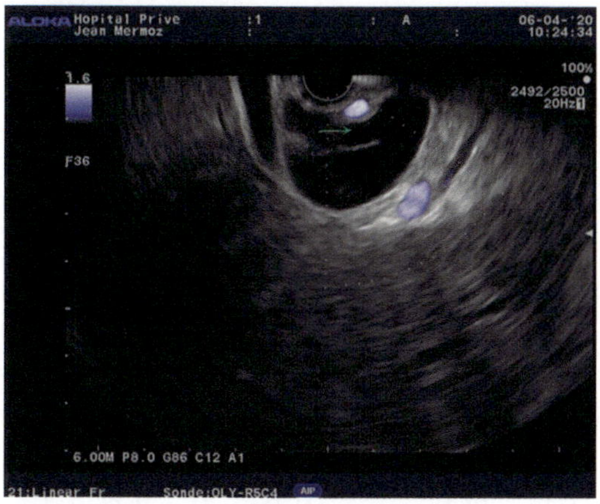

Fig. 9.4 Interposing cystic duct (*green arrow*)

formed with the ECE delivery system. Once introduced the catheter was prudently pushed slightly against the opposing wall of the CBD to obtain 20 mm insertion inside the CBD lumen. The distal flange was open under EUS guidance. The catheter was then pulled back to the proximal wall of the CBD until a slight deformation of the flange was obtained. The proximal flange was deployed in the working canal of the endoscope and pushed out of the endoscope in the duodenal bulb under EUS control. Finally, the catheter was removed. After stent deployment we aspirated in the duodenal bulb to ensure appropriate bile drainage through the proximal flange under endoscopic control. As the duodenal stenosis was not symptomatic we did not insert a duodenal stent.

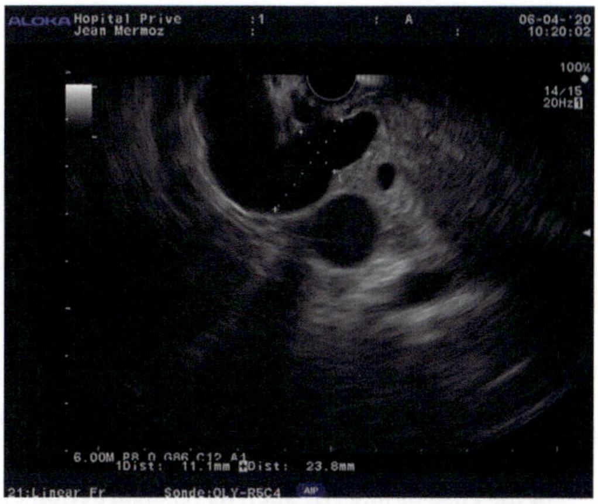

Fig. 9.5 The CBD is only slightly dilated (diameter 11.1 mm) but the ideal tract to insert the catheter and deploy the distal flange is twice as long (23.8 mm)

9.5 Post-Procedural Management

EUS-CDS can be performed as an inpatient or outpatient procedure. Patients may stay longer depending on medical conditions, and procedure-related or early AE. Diet can be resumed 6 h after the procedure. Antibiotic prophylaxis is administered.

If the patient presents pain or fever, liver function tests, blood count, and abdominal CT scan are requested.

9.6 Potential Pitfalls

Procedural and early AE include misdeployment of the stent, perforation, and bleeding. Late complications include stent migration, re-obstruction, and sump syndrome [5–10].

One possible pitfall is to puncture the dilated cystic duct instead of the CBD so care should be taken to follow the CBD to the hilum to ensure correct targeting. In the case of misdeployment of a flange in the duodenal wall or peritoneum, a guidewire can be inserted, and a fully covered self-expandable metal stent (FC-SEMS) can be inserted as a bridge. When the position is not secured with a guidewire a new procedure must be done to insert a FC-SEMS (EUS-CDS in another site, EUS-HGS, new attempt of ERCP).

If the drainage is efficient with a stent covering the initial hole in the CBD, the Hot AXIOS™ can be removed and the hole in the duodenal bulb can be close with a clip. Technical failure has been shown to be mostly related to poor manipulation of the device by operators who did not adhere strictly to all recommended steps of the procedure [9, 10] rather than to a lack of expertise.

In the case of bleeding, stent deployment with subsequent vascular compression can be sufficient for hemostasis, hence the procedure should not be prematurely abandoned.

In the case of late AE such as re-obstruction or migration, an endoscopy can be performed to gage if another stent can be placed in a patent fistulous tract. Otherwise alternative routes of drainage such as EUS-HGS, ERCP, or PTBD may be considered. The immediate placement of an axial oriented plastic stent within the ECE-LAMS and new designs of LAMS may reduce re-obstruction rates [5, 12].

In summary, ECE-LAMS in EUS-CDS reduces complications as well as procedure time. The widespread commercialization of ECE-LAMS will enable further studies to be performed on their efficacy and safety.

References

1. Giovannini M, Moutardier V, Pesenti C, et al. Endoscopic ultrasound-guided bilioduodenal anastomosis: a new technique for biliary drainage. Endoscopy. 2001;33:898–900–930.
2. Teoh AYB, Dhir V, Kida M, et al. Consensus guidelines on the optimal management in interventional EUS procedures: results for the Asian EUS group RAND/UCLA expert panel. Gut. 2018;67:1209–28.
3. Minaga K, Kitano M. Recent advances in endoscopic ultrasound-guided biliary drainage. Dig Endosc. 2018;30:38–47.
4. Sharaiha RZ, Khan MA, Kamal F, et al. Efficacy and safety of EUS-guided biliary drainage when ERCP fails: a systematic review and meta-analysis. Gastrointest Endosc. 2017;85:904–14.
5. El Chafic AH, Shah JN, Hamerski C, et al. EUS-guided choledochoduodenostomy for distal malignant biliary obstruction using electrocautery-enhanced lumen-apposing metal stents: first US, multicentre experience. Dig Dis Sci. 2019; (epub ahead of print)
6. Anderloni A, Fugazza A, Troncone E, et al. Single-stage EUS-guided choledochoduodenostomy using a lumen-apposing metal stent for malignant distal biliary obstruction. Gastrointest Endosc. 2019;89:69–76.
7. Tsuchiya T, Teoh AYB, Yamo K, et al. Long-term outcomes of EUS-guided choledochoduodenostomy using a lumen-apposing metal stent for malignant distal biliary obstruction: a prospective multicenter study. Gastrointest Endosc. 2018;87:1138–46.
8. Kunda R, Perez-Miranda M, Will U, et al. EUS-guided choledochoduodenostomy for malignant distal biliary obstruction using a lumen-apposing fully covered metal stent after failed ERCP. Surg Endosc. 2016;30:5002–8.
9. Jacques J, Privat J, Pinard F, et al. Endoscopic ultrasound-guided choledochoduodenostomy with electrocautery-enhanced lumen-apposing stents: a retrospective analysis. Endoscopy. 2019;51:540–7.
10. Jacques J, Fumex F, Privat J, et al. EUS-guided choledocho-duodenostomy using hot-AXIOS: a French multi-centric evaluation of its efficacy after training. Gastrointest Endosc. 2020; (in press)
11. Bang JY, Navaneethan U, Hasan M, et al. Stent placement by EUS or ERCP for primary biliary decompression in pancreatic cancer: a randomized trial. Gastrointest Endosc. 2018;88:9–17.
12. Paik WH, Lee TH, Park DH, et al. EUS-guided biliary drainage versus ERCP for the primary palliation of malignant biliary obstruction: a multicenter randomized clinical trial. Am J Gastroenterol. 2018;113:987–97.

10 Endoscopic Ultrasound-Guided Hepaticogastrostomy

Takeshi Ogura and Kazuhide Higuchi

10.1 Background

Endoscopic ultrasound-guided (EUS) hepaticogastrostomy (HGS) is indicated for patients with advanced malignant tumors as an alternative to failed ERCP or an inaccessible ampulla of Vater due to surgically altered anatomy [1]. The indications for EUS-HGS have recently expanded to include benign biliary stricture [2]. Various techniques such as transluminal cholangioscopy can proceed after an access route is created between the intrahepatic bile duct and the stomach. However, EUS-HGS is associated with critical adverse events such as stent migration into the abdominal cavity [3]. Therefore, it is extremely important to ensure successful EUS-HGS.

10.2 Case History

An 82-year-old man was admitted with obstructive jaundice. Contrast-enhanced computed tomography (CT) imaging revealed a tumor of the pancreatic head with liver metastasis and the result of EUS-guided FNA was adenocarcinoma. Therefore, unresectable pancreatic cancer was diagnosed. Although a duodenoscope was advanced into the second part of the duodenum, biliary cannulation failed due to duodenal invasion. Therefore, EUS-guided biliary drainage (BD) was attempted after duodenal metal stent deployment.

10.3 Procedure Planning

The main approach routes for EUS-BD are transduodenal or transgastric. A recent randomized controlled trial [4] found no significant difference in the rates of technical and clinical success and adverse events between these routes. However, if patients are complicated with a duodenal obstruction, the transgastric approach might be preferable to prevent adverse events such as reflux cholangitis [5]. Because duodenal obstruction in the present patient will soon become a complication, we selected EUS-HGS for biliary drainage.

We applied EUS-HGS using a balloon catheter to dilate the fistula. During EUS-HGS, the bile duct and stomach wall must be dilated to insert stent delivery systems. Electrocautery dilation might confer risk of adverse events such as bleeding due to burning [6]. A novel fine-gauge electrocautery dilator has recently become available in Japan [7]. Although an additional prospective comparison study is needed, this device might be

Supplementary Information The online version contains supplementary material available at [https://doi.org/10.1007/978-981-16-9340-3_10].

T. Ogura (✉) · K. Higuchi
2nd Department of Internal Medicine, Osaka Medical College, Osaka, Japan
e-mail: kazuhide.higuchi@ompu.ac.jp

A. Y.B. Teoh et al. (eds.), *Atlas of Interventional EUS*, https://doi.org/10.1007/978-981-16-9340-3_10

useful for dilation because the burning effect is reduced. Although balloon dilation is safe, bile leakage after balloon dilation is a disadvantage. A sufficient amount of hepatic parenchyma might be important to avoid this adverse event [8], but if hepatic parenchyma is insufficient, electrocautery dilation might be suitable.

Stent selection and technical tips for stent deployment are important for EUS-HGS. A dedicated plastic stent has recently become available in Japan [9]. Although this stent has clinical impact, its disadvantages include the following. Stent patency might be shorter than that of partially covered self-expandable metal stents (PCSEMS). Secondly, a stent that malfunctions before a fistula is created might lead to difficulties with stent exchange. Therefore, some operators use PCSEMS. During EUS-HGS using SEMS, stents can migrate due to stent shortening. Intra-scope channel release [10, 11] and a long metal stent (10 or 12 cm) have been recommended to prevent stent migration [12, 13].

10.4 Description of Procedure (Video 10.1)

An echoendoscope was advanced into the stomach, and the left hepatic lobe was identified. The intrahepatic bile duct was punctured at B3 or at the confluence of B2 and B3 using a 19 G needle (Fig. 10.1). Contrast medium was injected into the bile duct through the needle, and a cholangiographic image was obtained. A 0.025-inch guidewire was then inserted into the intrahepatic bile duct (Fig. 10.2) which, along with the stomach wall, was dilated using a 4-mm balloon catheter (Fig. 10.3). A PCSEMS delivery system was inserted into the intrahepatic bile duct, and the stent was carefully released from the intrahepatic bile duct up to 3–4 cm inside the echoendoscope. The echoendoscope was gently pulled up, and the stent delivery system was gently pushed. Finally, the stent was completely released under endoscopic visualization (Figs. 10.4 and 10.5).

10.5 Postprocedural Management

If infected bile juice leaks from the fistula before stent deployment using EUS-HGS, antibiotics are administered for up to two days. If inflammatory indicators are elevated, suggesting bile peritonitis, continuous antibiotics are administered. We assess stent migration or shortening using CT on the day after the procedure. If the stent is appropriately positioned, and infection is not evident, oral intake is started. If the stent is inappropriately positioned, re-intervention is attempted.

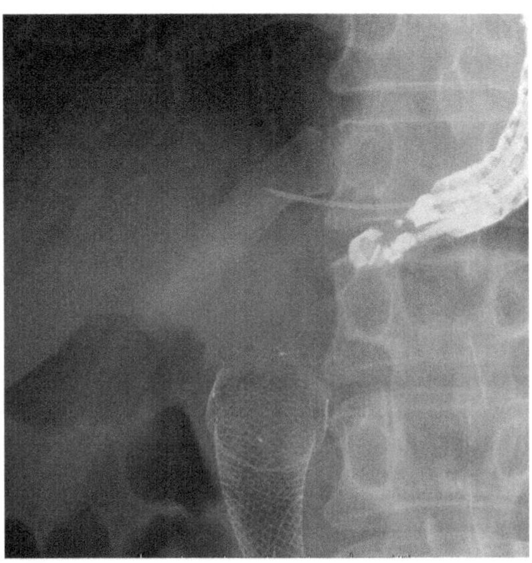

Fig. 10.1 The intrahepatic bile duct is punctured using 19G needle

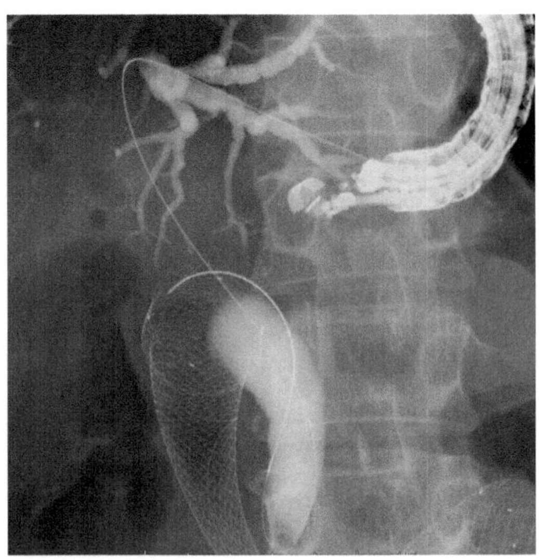

Fig. 10.2 The guidewire is inserted into the bile duct

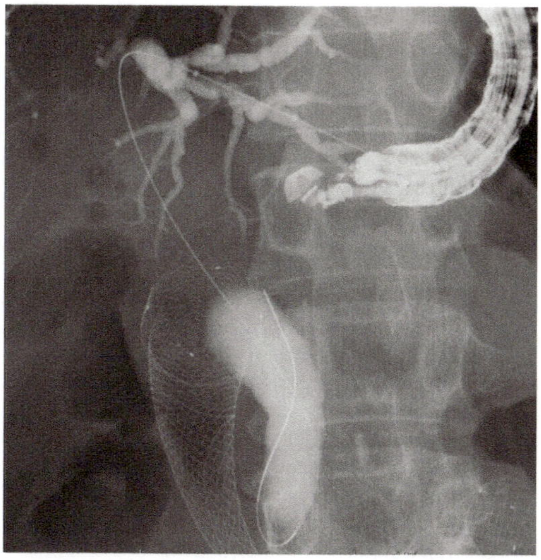

Fig. 10.3 The intrahepatic bile duct is dilated using a balloon catheter

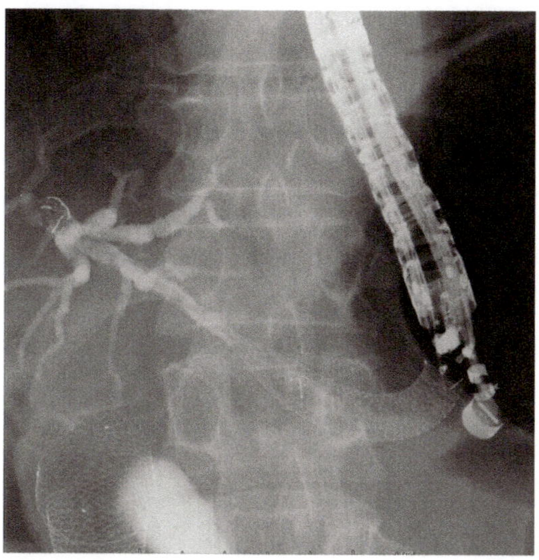

Fig. 10.4 Stent deployment is successfully performed (Fluoroscopic image)

After one month, we re-examine the stent position using CT and evaluate the resolution of obstructive jaundice from laboratory findings.

10.6 Potential Pitfalls

Potential adverse events after EUS-HGS include bile peritonitis, bleeding, bile leakage, and stent migration. Bile peritonitis can be usually treated conservatively. Bleeding can also be conservatively treated if a covered SEMS is deployed due to its tamponade effect. However, an endoscopic approach or endovascular intervention is sometimes needed if bleeding cannot be conservatively treated. Bile leakage can be also conservatively treated if a SEMS is deployed. However, if infection arises, additional intervention such as EUS-guided transluminal drainage should be considered.

On the other hand, conservative treatment is challenging when stents migrate. If a guidewire remains in the bile duct after stent deployment during EUS-HGS, an additional stent can be deployed. Therefore, the guidewire should be removed after the endoscopist ensures that the proximal end of the stent is indeed located in the stomach. However, if a stent migrates after the guidewire is removed or on the day after the procedure, percutaneous or surgical treatment should be considered. Therefore, the relationship between the endoscopist and radiologist or surgeon is extremely important.

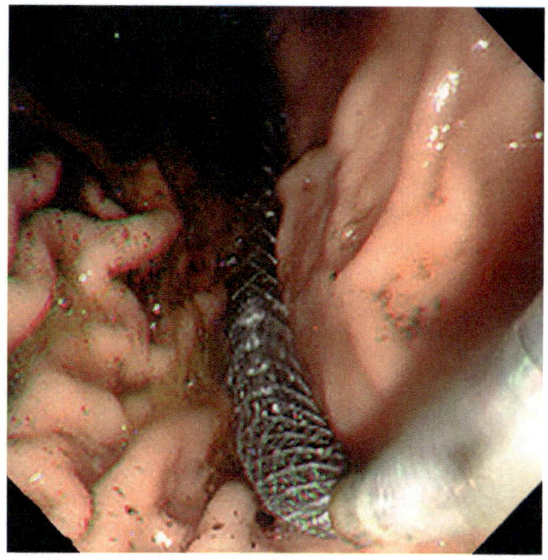

Fig. 10.5 Stent deployment is successfully performed (Endoscopic image)

References

1. Teoh AYB, Dhir V, Kuda M, Yasuda I, Jin ZD, Seo DW, et al. Consensus guidelines in the optimal management in interventional EUS procedures: results from the Asian EUS group RAND/UCLA expert panel. Gut. 2018;67:1209–28.

2. Ogura T, Takenaka M, Shiomi H, Goto D, Tamura T, Hisa T, et al. Long-term outcomes of EUS-guided transluminal stent deployment for benign biliary disease: multicenter clinical experience (with videos). Endosc Ultrasound. 2019;8:398–403.
3. Martins FP, Rossini LG, Ferrari AP. Migration of a covered metallic stent following endoscopic ultrasound-guided hepaticogastrostomy: fatal complication. Endoscopy. 2010;42:126–7.
4. Minaga K, Ogura T, Shiomi H, Imai H, Hoki N, Takenaka M, et al. Comparison of the efficacy and safety of endoscopic ultrasound-guided choledochoduodenostomy and hepaticogastrostomy for malignant biliary obstruction: multicenter, randomized, clinical trial. Dig Endosc. 2019;31:575–82.
5. Ogura T, Chiba Y, Masuda D, Kitano M, Sano T, Saori O, et al. Comparison of the clinical impact of endoscopic ultrasound-guided choledochoduodenostomy and hepaticogastrostomy for bile duct obstruction with duodenal obstruction. Endoscopy. 2016;48:156–63.
6. Honjo M, Itoi T, Tsuchiya T, Tanaka R, Tonozuka R, Mukai S, et al. Safety and efficacy of ultra-tapered mechanical dilator for EUS-guided hepaticogastrostomy and pancreatic duct drainage compared with electrocautery dilator (with video). Endosc Ultrasound. 2018;7:376–82.
7. Ogura T, Nakai Y, Iwashita T, Higuchi K. Novel fine gauge electrocautery dilator for endoscopic ultrasound-guided biliary drainage: experimental and clinical evaluation study (with video). Endosc Int Open. 2019;7:E1652–7.
8. Yamamoto Y, Ogura T, Nishioka N, Yamada T, Yamada M, Ueno S, et al. Risk factors for adverse events associated with bile leak during endoscopic ultrasound-guided hepaticogastrostomy. Endosc Ultrasound [Epub ahead of print].
9. Umeda J, Itoi T, Tsuchiya T, Sofuni A, Itokawa F, Ishii K, et al. A newly designed plastic stent for EUS-guided hepaticogastrostomy: a prospective preliminary feasibility study (with videos). Gastrointest Endosc. 2015;82:390–6.
10. Paik WH, Park DH, Choi JH, Choi JH, Lee SS, Seo DW, et al. Simplified fistula dilation technique and modified stent deployment maneuver for EUS-guided hepaticogastrostomy. World J Gastroenterol. 2014;7:5051–9.
11. Miyano A, Ogura T, Yamamoto K, Okuda A, Nishioka N, Higuchi K. Clinical impact of the intra-scope channel stent release technique in preventing stent migration during EUS-guided hepaticogastrostomy. J Gastrointest Surg. 2018;22:1312–8.
12. Ogura T, Yamamoto K, Sano T, Onda S, Imoto A, Masuda D, et al. Stent length is impact factor associated with stent patency in endoscopic ultrasound-guided hepaticogastrostomy. J Gastroenterol Hepatol. 2015;30:1748–52.
13. Nakai Y, Isayama H, Yamamoto N, Matsubara S, Ito Y, Sasahira N, et al. Safety and effectiveness of a long, partially covered metal stent for endoscopic ultrasound-guided hepaticogastrostomy in patients with malignant biliary obstruction. Endoscopy. 2016;48:1125–8.

EUS-Guided Antegrade Stenting

11

Mouen A. Khashab

11.1 Background

EUS-guided biliary drainage (EUS-BD) covers multiple techniques, all of which have been studied and applied in clinical practice for the last two decades [1–4]. EUS-BD can be performed by one of the three approaches [1]. First, a rendezvous technique may be performed whereby a wire is placed into an intrahepatic or extrahepatic bile duct, advanced through the papilla and is retrieved by a duodenoscope for biliary interventions. Second, direct transluminal stenting using a transgastric or transduodenal approach may be achieved without accessing the papilla. A third approach that has not been expansively reported is EUS-guided antegrade transpapillary (or trans-anastomotic) biliary stent (AGS) placement [5].

11.2 Case History

A 58-year-old man presented with new onset painless jaundice. Abdominal CAT scan revealed a bulky 6 cm pancreatic head mass with biliary obstruction. The mass involved the superior mesenteric artery and the hepatic artery and was deemed unresectable. ERCP with the intent of palliative stenting was attempted and failed due to significant duodenal distortion despite the absence of gastric outlet obstruction. Patient was thus referred for EUS-BD.

Upon careful review of abdominal imaging, the mass resulted in compression of the common bile duct and common hepatic duct and EUS-guided choledochoduodenostomy (EUS-CDS) was clearly not technically possible. Decision was to proceed either with EUS-hepaticogastrostomy (EUS-HGS) or EUS-AGS, especially in view of significant intrahepatic biliary dilation, which simplifies these latter procedures.

11.3 Procedure Plan for EUS-AGS

The EUS-AGS technique involves the following stages [6–10]. The dilated biliary ductal segment is punctured with a fine needle aspiration (FNA) needle and contrast is injected through the needle to obtain a cholangiogram. A hydrophilic 0.025/0.035 inch guidewire is advanced through the needle and manipulated across the hilum towards the bile duct and then across the stricture into the duodenum. The FNA needle is then removed, and the tract/stricture are dilated over the wire. Antegrade stent placement is performed

Supplementary Information The online version contains supplementary material available at [https://doi.org/10.1007/978-981-16-9340-3_11].

M. A. Khashab (✉)
Division of Gastroenterology and Hepatology, Johns Hopkins Hospital, Baltimore, MD, USA
e-mail: mkhasha1@jhmi.edu

A. Y.B. Teoh et al. (eds.), *Atlas of Interventional EUS*, https://doi.org/10.1007/978-981-16-9340-3_11

by advancing the stent through the therapeutic channel of the echoendoscope over the guidewire and the stent is then placed across the stricture in a transpapillary fashion. Some endoscopists perform simultaneous stent placement across the EUS-HGS tract to avoid bile leakage in case of possible antegrade stent occlusion or migration. The simultaneous placement of HGS and AGE appears advantageous because the risk of bile leak is diminished, biliary access is maintained for future intervention, and an additional route for bile drainage is present even with dysfunction of one of the stents [11].

11.3.1 Equipment Needed for EUS-AGS

- Therapeutic linear echoendoscope (oblique or forward viewing).
- 19-gauge FNA needle. Our predilection is for a flexible nitinol needle (Expect 19 Flex, Boston Scientific, Marlborough, MA, USA), although other needles can also be used. An access needle (EchoTip Access Needle, Cook Medical, Winston-Salem, NC, USA) is also commercially available. Once its sharp stylet is removed after puncture of the biliary system, the access needle tip becomes blunt and protects against wire shearing [12]. The main shortcoming of the access needle is its stiffness.
- A hydrophilic guidewire. We prefer a 0.025 inch angled tip wire over a 0.035 inch straight wire. The smaller diameter likely decreases the risk of wire shearing and the angled tip allows wire rotation and manipulation for advancement transhepatically across the hilum and the stricture.
- Dilation catheters. Our ideal catheter is a 4 mm biliary dilation balloon (Hurricane balloon, Boston Scientific, Marlborough, MA, USA) that can be straightforwardly advanced transhepatically without need for cautery. This catheter can be used to dilate the HGS tract and the distal stricture itself. Stricture dilation is not mandatory but is simple to perform and results in smooth stent advancement across the stricture. Oher dilators that can also be utilized include a 6 Fr cystotome and bougie dilators.
- Biliary stents. During EUS-AGS, we favor placing a self-expandable metal stent (covered or uncovered SEMS) across the biliary stricture. If a stent is placed across the HGS tract to ensure direct transgastric access to the biliary system (e.g., patients with surgical anatomy), we favor a fully- or partially-covered SEMS to diminish the risk of leakage across the tract.

11.4 Description of the Current Procedure and Follow-Up

We performed transgastric puncture of a dilated left intrahepatic duct and passed a 0.025 inch guidewire into the duodenum, followed by dilation of the biliary stricture and hepaticogastrostomy fistula using a 4 mm biliary dilation balloon (Fig. 11.1). Antegrade insertion of an uncovered 10 × 80 mm SEMS across the distal biliary stricture and major papilla was carried. A fully covered SEMS (10 × 80 mm) was then placed across the hepaticogastrostomy (Video 11.1). There were no adverse events. The patient was discharged the following day with subsequent resolution of jaundice and treatment with chemo-radiotherapy. Patient expired a year later without any need for further biliary intervention during that period.

11.5 Tips and Tricks

1. Most linear echoendoscopes used during EUS-BD result in oblique endoscopic luminal imaging. Therefore, carrying EUS-BD under the guidance of luminal viewing can be deceptive. After needle access of the biliary system under endosonographic guidance, the wire is pushed into the biliary system and a longitudinal view of the wire should be maintained under endosonographic view throughout the procedure. We accomplish most of the steps subsequently without luminal endoscopic guidance to avoid problematic tract dilation

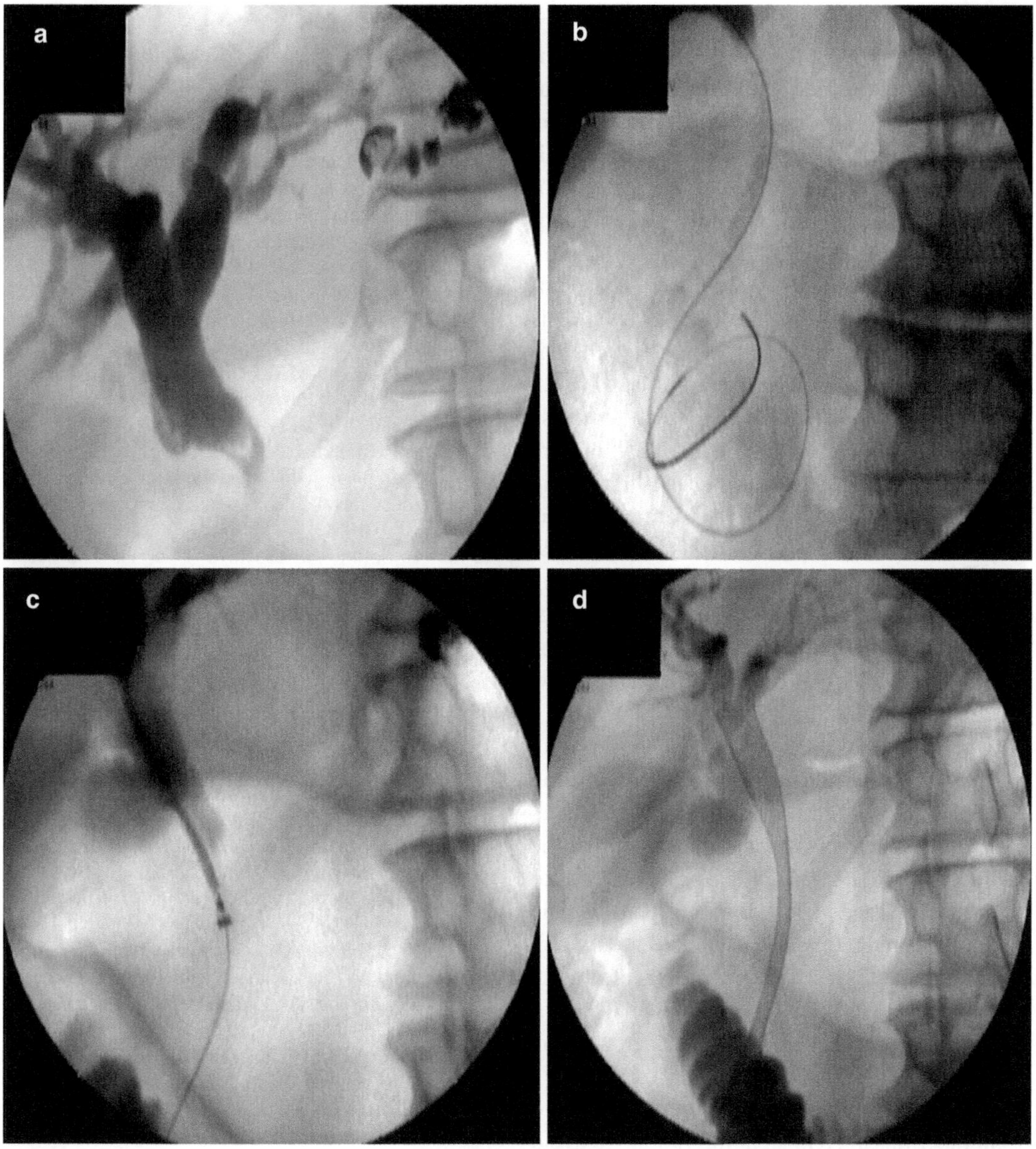

Fig. 11.1 EUS-guided antegrade stenting in a patient with a large mass in the head of the pancreas causing biliary obstruction. (**a**) A left intrahepatic duct was punctured, and antegrade cholangiography revealed a long distal biliary stricture with proximal dilation of the biliary tree. (**b**) A 0.025-inch guidewire was advanced through the stricture and coiled in the duodenum. (**c**) A self-expandable metal stent was advanced antegradely over the guidewire. (**d**) A stent was deployed with 1 end in the duodenum and the other end above the biliary stricture

and loss of wire access [13]. During EUS-AGS, the stent is also positioned under fluoroscopic guidance. It is helpful to acquire an enterogram by injecting contrast initially through the needle and then through the dilating catheter/balloon. This helps in precise placement of the luminal flange and avoids squeezing it against the opposite bowel wall.

2. Fluoroscopy is essential for the performance of EUS-AGS. The tip of the echoendoscope should be pointing towards the hilum. This results in appropriate direction of wire

advancement towards the liver hilum. After biliary access with the FNA needle, a cholangiogram is obtained with detailed interpretation of biliary anatomy, location of obstruction, length of biliary stricture, and degree of biliary dilation. As mentioned above, an enterogram also helps with accurate placement of the stent.

3. Access of the biliary system is best accomplished using a 19-gauge FNA needle. This allows both easy injection of contrast/cholangiography and advancement of either a 0.025 inch or 0.035 inch guidewire. We prefer to use a 0.025 inch wire to diminish the risk of wire shearing. If significant resistance is felt during wire manipulation (usually when the wire is pulled back into the needle), this indicates that the wire coating is jammed against the needle. To avoid wire shearing and retaining of sheared wire within the biliary system, the needle is pulled out of the patient and a new guidewire should be used.
4. Tract dilation is the most intricate step during EUS-AGS. We do not perform tract dilation until satisfactory wire positioning is attained. Failure of stent placement after dilation of the tract may result in biliary leakage. Non-coaxial cautery-assisted tract dilation (e.g., needle knife) should be avoided as it increases the risk of complications. Furthermore, extent of tract dilation should be limited to allow passage of the stent catheter. Large diameter dilation increases the risk of biliary leakage [13].
5. Several mortalities have been reported due to intraperitoneal HGS stent migration. To avoid this disastrous complication, we leave 3–4 cm of the biliary metallic stent in the stomach to account for post-deployment stent shortening and movement of the stomach away from the liver during respiration.

Conflicts of Interest Mouen Khashab is a consultant for BSCI, Olympus, and Medtronic.

References

1. Khashab MA, Levy MJ, Itoi T, et al. EUS-guided biliary drainage. Gastrointest Endosc. 2015;82:993–1001.
2. Khashab MA, Van der Merwe S, Kunda R, et al. Prospective international multicenter study on endoscopic ultrasound-guided biliary drainage for patients with malignant distal biliary obstruction after failed endoscopic retrograde cholangiopancreatography. Endosc Int Open. 2016;4:E487–96.
3. Jovani M, Ichkhanian Y, Vosoughi K, et al. EUS-guided biliary drainage for postsurgical anatomy. Endosc Ultrasound. 2019;8:S57–66.
4. Dhir V, Khashab MA. EUS-guided biliary drainage: moving beyond the cliche of prime time. Endosc Ultrasound. 2019;8:S1–2.
5. Saxena P, Kumbhari V, El Zein M, et al. EUS-guided biliary drainage with antegrade transpapillary placement of a metal biliary stent. Gastrointest Endosc. 2015;81:1010–1.
6. Itoi T, Sofuni A, Tsuchiya T, et al. Endoscopic ultrasonography-guided transhepatic antegrade stone removal in patients with surgically altered anatomy: case series and technical review (with videos). J Hepatobiliary Pancreat Sci. 2014;21:E86–93.
7. Iwashita T, Nakai Y, Hara K, et al. Endoscopic ultrasound-guided antegrade treatment of bile duct stone in patients with surgically altered anatomy: a multicenter retrospective cohort study. J Hepatobiliary Pancreat Sci. 2016;23:227–33.
8. Mukai S, Itoi T, Sofuni A, et al. EUS-guided antegrade intervention for benign biliary diseases in patients with surgically altered anatomy (with videos). Gastrointest Endosc. 2019;89:399–407.
9. Sansak I, Itoi T, Moriyasu F. Endoscopic ultrasonography-guided transhepatic antegrade stone removal in a patient with roux-en-Y anastomosis (with video). J Hepatobiliary Pancreat Sci. 2014;21:719–20.
10. Yamamoto K, Itoi T, Tsuchiya T, et al. EUS-guided antegrade metal stenting with hepaticoenterostomy using a dedicated plastic stent with a review of the literature (with video). Endosc Ultrasound. 2018;7:404–12.
11. Kumbhari V, Tieu AH, Khashab MA. EUS-guided biliary drainage made safer by a combination of hepaticogastrostomy and antegrade transpapillary stenting. Gastrointest Endosc. 2015;81:1015–6.
12. Giovannini M, Bories E. EUS-guided biliary drainage. Gastroenterol Res Pract. 2012;2012:348719.
13. Khashab MA, Giovannini M. How I do therapeutic EUS. Gastrointest Endosc. 2019;90:183–5.

12 EUS-Guided Antegrade Stone Extraction

Takuji Iwashita and Masahito Shimizu

12.1 Background

ERCP is a standard procedure in the management of bile duct stones (BDS) because it is safe, minimally invasive, and has a high success rate. However, ERCP can be challenging in patients with surgically altered anatomy, even with the application of balloon-assisted enteroscopy owing to difficulties in endoscopic insertion into the biliary orifice, restructured maneuverability of the endoscope, and some limitations of device selection. In those patients in whom ERCP failed, PTBD has been performed as an alternative procedure; however, this is usually associated with a lower quality of life due to the need of a percutaneous external drainage tube. Recently, EUS-guided antegrade stone extraction has emerged as a new endoscopic approach [1, 2].

Supplementary Information The online version contains supplementary material available at [https://doi.org/10.1007/978-981-16-9340-3_12].

T. Iwashita (✉) · M. Shimizu
First Department of Internal Medicine, Gifu University Hospital, Gifu, Japan
e-mail: takuji@w7.dion.ne.jp; shimim-gif@umin.ac.jp

12.2 Case History

An 80-year-old man who underwent total gastrectomy with Roux-en-Y reconstruction for gastric cancer had abdominal pain and visited another hospital. His laboratory findings showed elevated liver function, and computed tomography scan revealed BDS. The patient was then referred to us for the management of the BDS. ERCP using double-balloon enteroscopy was initially performed. However, this failed because of technical difficulty in achieving deep biliary cannulation. EUS-guided antegrade stone extraction was planned as a salvage procedure.

12.3 Procedural Plan

In EUS-antegrade stone extraction, the bile duct in the left lobe of the liver, typically B2 or B3, can be accessed from the remnant stomach or the jejunal limb. Biliary access with B2 allows a more rectilinear approach to the common bile duct or the ampulla, which has an advantage in transmitting the pushing force on the retrieval balloon during stone extraction. However, the puncture point is located on the cranial side, which increases the possibility of trans-esophageal puncture, which is considered to have a higher risk of causing adverse complications, such as hemothorax, pneumothorax, mediastinitis, or mediastinal emphysema [3]. At our

A. Y.B. Teoh et al. (eds.), *Atlas of Interventional EUS*, https://doi.org/10.1007/978-981-16-9340-3_12

institution, the B2 approach is the first choice during EUS-guided antegrade stone extraction, and B3 can be selected if there is any chance of trans-esophageal puncture or presence of interposing vessels.

12.4 Description of the Procedure (Video 12.1)

The bile duct in the left lobe was punctured from the jejunal limb using a 19-gauge *FNA needle* primed with a contrast agent. In this case, B3 access was chosen because of the possibility of trans-esophageal puncture. The proper puncture was confirmed by injection of the contrast agent followed by guidewire insertion into the bile duct (Fig. 12.1). The needle tract was dilated with a 7-Fr bougie dilator. After the exchange with the ERCP catheter, an additional cholangiogram was obtained, which showed multiple BDS with a maximum size of 5 mm. The guidewire was further manipulated into the duodenum through the papilla (Fig. 12.2). The ampulla was dilated using a balloon up to 13 mm (Fig. 12.3). The BDS were pushed out from the bile duct into the duodenum using a retrieval balloon (Fig. 12.4). A nasobiliary drainage (NBD) tube was placed for possible residual BDS and to enable future access to the bile duct. Two days later, a cholangiogram of the NBD tube did not show any residual stones, and the NBD tube was removed (Fig. 12.5).

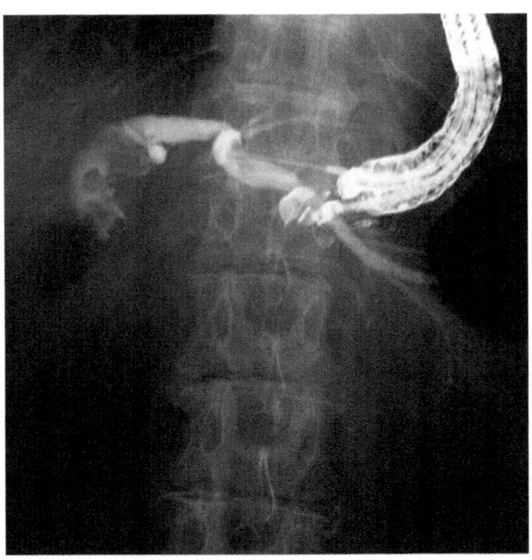

Fig. 12.1 The bile duct was viewed with a cholangiogram to confirm proper puncture

12.5 Post-Procedural Management

At our institution, the patient was managed using the same protocol as ERCP to monitor for possible adverse complications from EUS-guided antegrade stone extraction. Prophylactic antibiot-

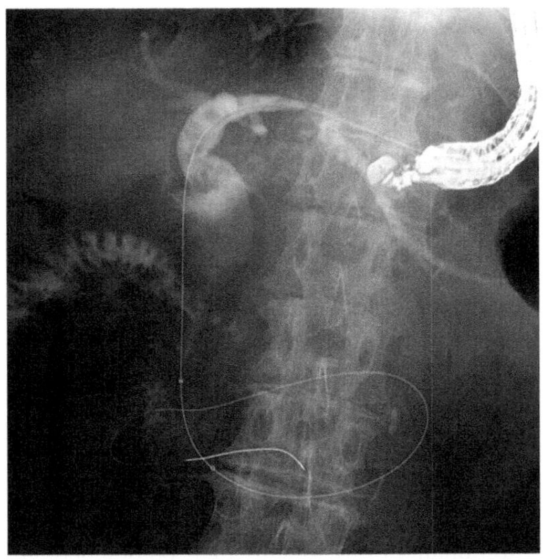

Fig. 12.2 The guidewire was placed into the duodenum

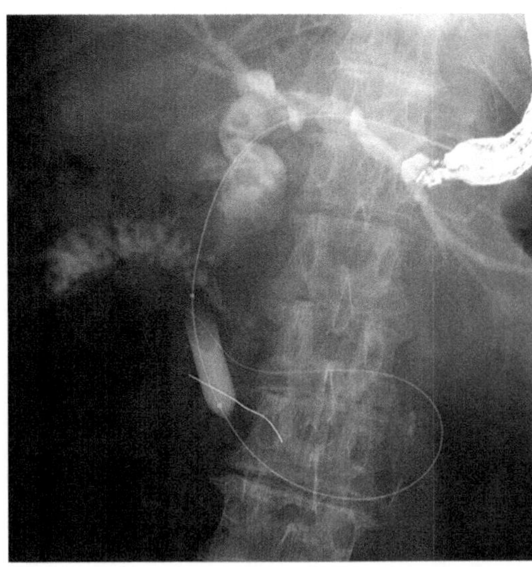

Fig. 12.3 The ampulla was dilated with a large balloon

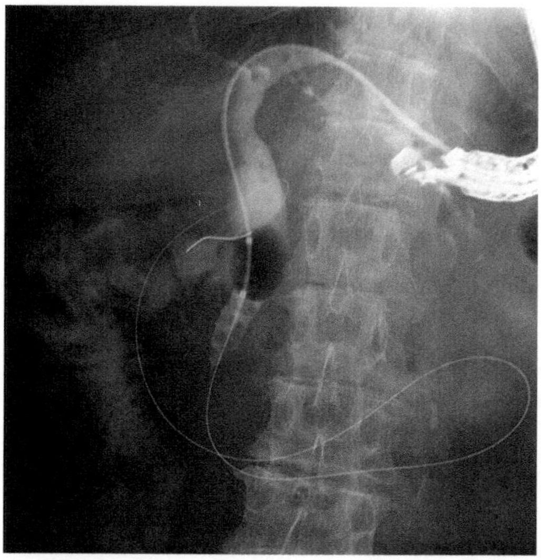

Fig. 12.4 The bile duct stones were extracted using a retrieval balloon

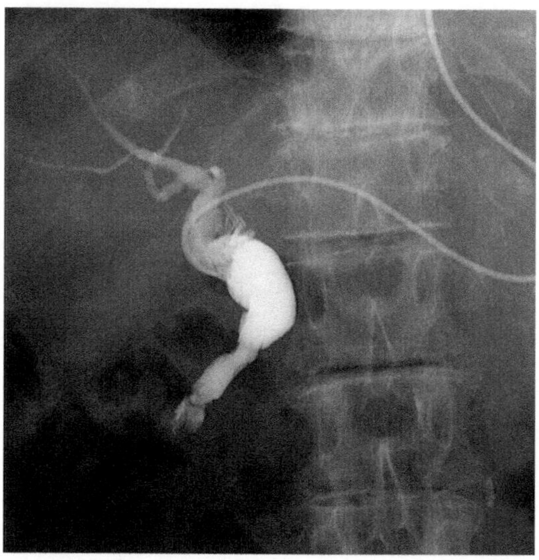

Fig. 12.5 A cholangiogram of the nasobiliary drainage tube did not show any residual stones

ics were used before and after the procedure. The expected adverse events of EUS-BD are perforation, bile peritonitis, bleeding, cholangitis, and pancreatitis [3, 4]. Imaging studies, including computed tomography, are performed if there is any sign of adverse events. Dietary intake can be resumed from the day after the procedure if no adverse events are suspected. A cholangiogram of the NBD tube is obtained to evaluate possible residual stones within a week in cases where an NBD tube is used. A repeat procedure is performed in cases with residual stones. Otherwise, the NBD tube is removed.

12.6 Potential Pitfalls

In EUS-antegrade stone extraction, the BDS are pushed out to the duodenum through the ampulla using a retrieval balloon as the BDS have to be managed through the temporal fistula between the intestine and the bile duct with restriction on the size of the fistula. Due to this, any mismatches, such as a large stone size relative to the size of the dilation balloon or small stones in the large parts of the bile duct, make stone extraction challenging. Recently, a multi-step approach has been reported as a possible strategy to manage BDS with the mismatches mentioned above while keeping the fistula open with a specially designed plastic stent [5]. With the application of the multi-step approach, mechanical lithotripsy or per-oral cholangioscopy with laser or electrohydraulic lithotripsy through the fistula can be used for stone management [6–8]; and EUS-guided antegrade stone extraction may expand its indication to manage BDS in patients with surgically altered anatomy.

References

1. Itoi T, Sofuni A, Tsuchiya T, Ijima M, Iwashita T. Endoscopic ultrasonography-guided transhepatic antegrade stone removal in patients with surgically altered anatomy: case series and technical review (with videos). J Hepatobiliary Pancreat Sci. 2014;21(12):E86–93.
2. Iwashita T, Nakai Y, Hara K, Isayama H, Itoi T, Park do H. Endoscopic ultrasound-guided antegrade treatment of bile duct stone in patients with surgically altered anatomy: a multicenter retrospective cohort study. J Hepatobiliary Pancreat Sci. 2016;23(4):227–33.
3. Isayama H, Nakai Y, Itoi T, Yasuda I, Kawakami H, Ryozawa S, et al. Clinical practice guidelines for safe performance of endoscopic ultrasound/ultrasonography-guided biliary drainage: 2018. J Hepatobiliary Pancreat Sci. 2019;26(7):249–69.
4. Iwashita T, Doi S, Yasuda I. Endoscopic ultrasound-guided biliary drainage: a review. Clin J Gastroenterol. 2014;7(2):94–102.
5. Umeda J, Itoi T, Tsuchiya T, Sofuni A, Itokawa F, Ishii K, et al. A newly designed plastic stent for

EUS-guided hepaticogastrostomy: a prospective preliminary feasibility study (with videos). Gastrointest Endosc. 2015;82(2):390–6 e2.
6. Iwashita T, Uemura S, Shimizu M. Endoscopic ultrasonography-guided antegrade treatment for bile duct stone with multi-step approach in a patient with surgically altered anatomy. Dig Endosc. 2018;30(Suppl 1):77–8.
7. Nakai Y, Isayama H, Koike K. Two-step endoscopic ultrasonography-guided antegrade treatment of a difficult bile duct stone in a surgically altered anatomy patient. Dig Endosc. 2018;30(1):125–7.
8. Ogura T, Okuda A, Higuchi K. Intrahepatic bile duct stone removal using peroral transluminal cholangioscopy (with videos). Endosc Ultrasound. 2019;8(2):131–2.

13 Combined ERCP and EUS Drainage for Hilar Stricture

John Gásdal Karstensen and Peter Vilmann

13.1 Background

In cases with hilar strictures in the liver, sufficient bile duct drainage by conventional ERCP might be challenging or impossible. Traditionally, percutaneous transhepatic cholangiography (PTC) has served as salvage therapy, but the results are often suboptimal and external bile duct drainage decreases the quality of life for patients. Recently, EUS-guided transgastric access to the bile ducts has been introduced as a minimal invasive alternative to PTC [1]. Furthermore, when an EUS-guided access to the bile ducts has been achieved, several possibilities for internal drainage are available including the establishment of a hepaticogastrostomy, antegrade stenting, or rendezvous.

Supplementary Information The online version contains supplementary material available at [https://doi.org/10.1007/978-981-16-9340-3_13].

J. G. Karstensen (✉)
Pancreatitis Centre East (PACE), Gastro Unit, Copenhagen University Hospital - Amager and Hvidovre, Copenhagen, Denmark

Department of Clinical Medicine, University of Copenhagen, Copenhagen, Denmark
e-mail: john.gasdal.karstensen@regionh.dk

P. Vilmann
Department of Surgery, Gastro Unit, Copenhagen University Hospital - Herlev and Gentofte, Hellerup, Denmark

Department of Clinical Medicine, University of Copenhagen, Copenhagen, Denmark
e-mail: Peter.Vilmann@regionh.dk

13.2 Case History

An 80-year-old male patient with a non-resectable colonic carcinoma with liver metastases was admitted due to obstructive jaundice preventing palliative chemotherapy. CT and MRI showed several metastases (Fig. 13.1) including a large hilar mass with dilated intrahepatic bile ducts (Fig. 13.2). An ERCP failed to obtain sufficient drainage and the patient remained jaundiced in particular due to dilated left-sided intrahepatic ducts. Hence, the patient was rescheduled for a combined ERCP and EUS-guided rendezvous drainage procedure aiming at selective drainage of the left liver lobe.

13.3 Procedural Plan

EUS-guided transluminal bile duct drainage can either be performed via a transduodenal route to the common bile duct or a transgastric route aiming at the bile ducts of the left liver lobe. The rate of technical success and risk of adverse events seems similar for the two routes [2]. However, in the present case, the obstruction was localized centrally in the liver; thus, to obtain sufficient drainage, a transgastric approach with puncture of the bile ducts in the left liver lobe was required. After gaining access to the bile duct system, we usually prefer to place a

A. Y.B. Teoh et al. (eds.), *Atlas of Interventional EUS*, https://doi.org/10.1007/978-981-16-9340-3_13

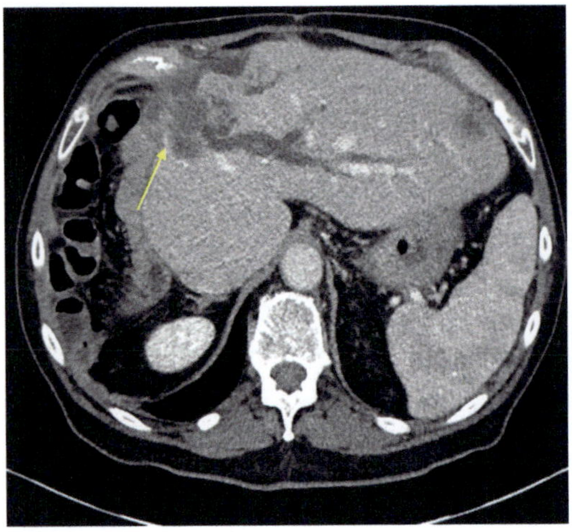

Fig. 13.1 Computed tomography showing an obstructing central metastasis of the liver (*arrow*)

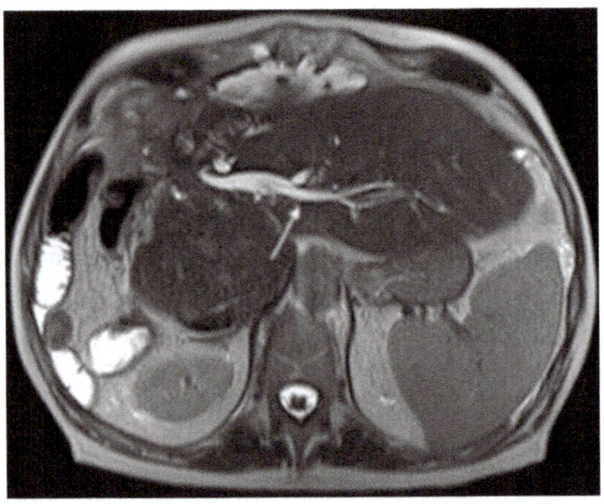

Fig. 13.2 Magnetic resonance imaging demonstrating dilated bile ducts in the left liver lobe (*arrow*)

hepaticogastrostomy with a semi-covered metal stent [3, 4]. In this way, you do not need to pass the obstructing metastasis and the left liver lope is usually sufficiently drained. Alternatively, if a guidewire can pass the metastasis, you can choose antegrade stenting or a rendezvous technique where ERCP and EUS are combined. To avoid reflux of bile, EUS-guided antegrade stenting is preferred in cases where there is either partial or total duodenal obstruction.

In this case, the site of the EUS-guided transgastric puncture was too close to the gastroesophageal junction to insert a hepatogastrostomy stent. Furthermore, as the access to the papilla of Vater was maintained, we decided to apply a rendezvous technique.

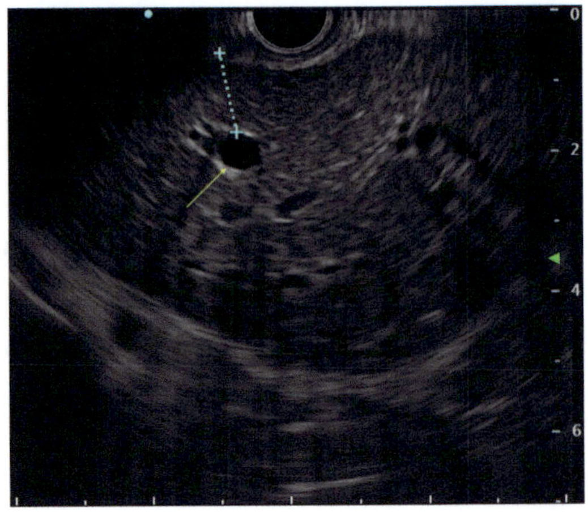

Fig. 13.3 Dilated bile duct (*arrow*) as noted on EUS

13.4 Description of the Procedure (Video 13.1)

With a linear echoendoscope (GF-UTC 180, Olympus Medical Systems Europe, Hamburg, Germany), the left liver lobe with the dilated bile ducts was identified from the stomach and an area without intervening blood vessels was selected for the puncture (Fig. 13.3). The puncture was performed with a 19-gauge access needle, (ECHO-HD-19-A, Cook Medical, Bloomington, IN, USA) followed by a cholangiogram to secure the location during fluoroscopy. A guidewire (VisiGlide 2, Olympus Medical Systems Europe, Hamburg, Germany) was inserted and advanced antegrade into the duodenum (Fig. 13.4). Using an exchange technique, the echoendoscope was then withdrawn, while the guidewire was kept in position. After insertion of a duodenoscope (TJF-Q180V, Olympus Medical Systems Europe, Hamburg, Germany), the wire was captured with a snare thereby gaining retrograde access to the left liver lobe. The malfunctioning plastic stents were removed, and after dilatation up to 7 French, a 16 cm straight plastic stent was inserted over the guidewire, which was then removed (Fig. 13.5).

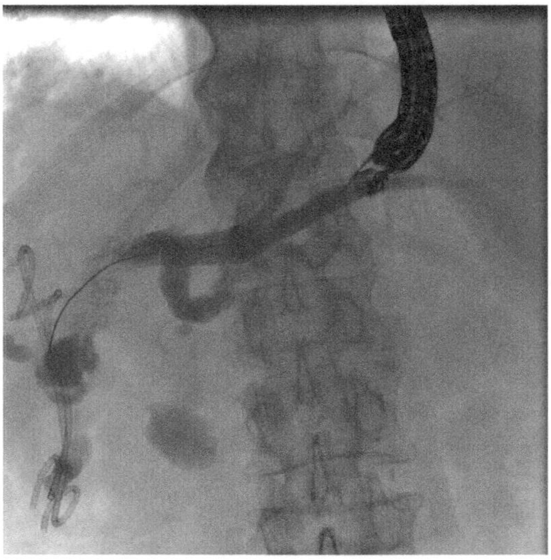

Fig. 13.4 Cholangiogram with antegrade guidewire insertion into the duodenum

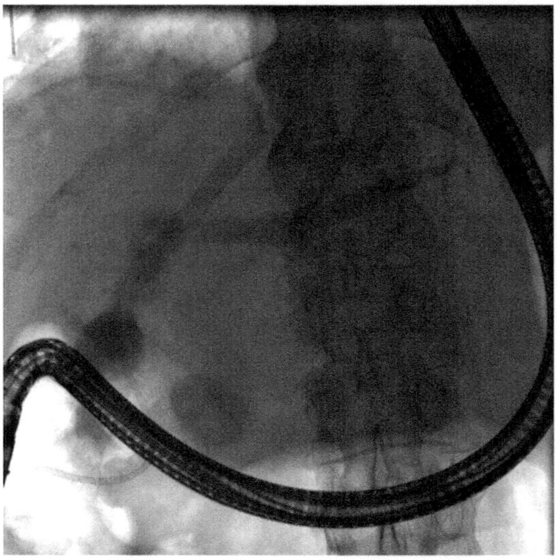

Fig. 13.5 Cholangiogram after retrograde stenting of the left liver lobe

13.5 Post-procedural Management

During the first post-procedural week, the jaundice of the patients dissolved and after 13 days, the patient resumed his palliative chemotherapy. He was scheduled for selective stent replacement after 2 months, where access to the left liver lobe could be accomplished by simply inserting a guidewire alongside the plastic stent. Moreover, the drainage was simultaneously optimized as the stent inserted over the guidewire could be increased to 10 French after dilation.

13.6 Potential Pitfalls

EUS-guided puncture of the intrahepatic bile ducts is quite easy, especially if the ducts are dilated, however, the rendezvous method can be technically challenging. First, you need to secure that there is endoscopic access to the papilla—if this is not the case, you will need to choose antegrade stenting or a hepaticogastrostomy. Second, after the advancement of the guidewire, please take care not to retract the guidewire—during manipulation, you might shear the guidewire at the tip of the EUS needle. This risk can be limited by choosing an access needle, which has a blunt tip or by retracting the needle before the guidewire. Likewise, when the duodenoscope is inserted into the duodenum and the distal end of the guidewire is retracted into the working channel of the duodenoscope, great care should be taken to avoid shearing of the liver parenchyma while feeding the trailing part of the guidewire. Third, to enable rendevous, it is important to choose a long wire (450 cm) for this procedure. Fourth, what is during the EUS procedure the distal part of the guidewire, becomes the trailing part during the ERCP procedure. Thus, to work with the guidewire during the ERCP procedure, you need either to exchange the guidewire over a contrast catheter or better, initially apply a guidewire with soft tips in both ends.

References

1. Guo J, Giovannini M, Sahai AV, Saftoiu A, Dietrich CF, Santo E, et al. A multi-institution consensus on how to perform EUS-guided biliary drainage for malignant biliary obstruction. Endosc Ultrasound. 2018;7(6):356–65.
2. Gupta K, Perez-Miranda M, Kahaleh M, Artifon EL, Itoi T, Freeman ML, et al. Endoscopic ultrasound-assisted bile duct access and drainage: multicenter, long-term analysis of approach, outcomes, and complications of a technique in evolution. J Clin Gastroenterol. 2014;48(1):80–7.
3. Burmester E, Niehaus J, Leineweber T, Huetteroth T. EUS-cholangio-drainage of the bile duct: report of 4 cases. Gastrointest Endosc. 2003;57(2):246–51.
4. Giovannini M. EUS-guided hepaticogastrostomy. Endosc Ultrasound. 2019;8(Suppl 1):S35–S9.

Biliary Interventions after EUS-Biliary Drainage

14

Ramon Sanchez-Ocaña
and Manuel Perez-Miranda

14.1 Background

Biliary intervention following transmural EUS-BD is performed in malignant biliary obstruction to manage stent dysfunction and in complex benign biliary disease as a sequential step of staged treatment.

Stent dysfunction after transmural EUS-BD occurs in around a third of patients in malignant biliary obstruction, most often caused by tissue hyperplasia of partially-covered metal stents [1]. Transmural biliary stent dysfunction is best managed by restoring the patency of the original fistula with a new stent.

EUS-BD replaces PTBD in staged endotherapy of complex benign biliary disease in patients not amenable to ERCP because of surgically altered anatomy (SAA) or disconnected bile ducts requiring combined antegrade and retrograde access [2, 3]. In SAA, the two major indications are heavy stone burden and benign strictures [4, 5], the latter typically located at previous surgical hepaticojejunostomy [6]. Left EUS-guided hepaticoenterotostomy (hepaticogastrostomy or hepaticojejunostomy, depending on the type of prior gastrectomy) serves as a portal to allow iterative antegrade bile duct access for stone clearance, stent replacement, or other interventions, while maintaining biliary drainage until treatment is completed. Interventions can be performed through transmural biliary metal stents or through mature naked fistulas [5]. In either case, peroral transmural (POT) cholangioscopy can be used in addition to cholangiography for diagnosis [7] or therapeutic guidance [2–6].

14.2 Case History

A 76-year-old female with a history of cholecystectomy and biliopancreatic diversion with gastrectomy presented with acute onset pain, fever with chills, and cholestatic liver chemistries. Her total serum bilirubin level was 4.3 mg/dL. Computed tomography showed a dilated common bile duct with a large stone. Intrahepatic bile duct dilation was also present. She improved on intravenous antibiotics and was then scheduled for elective common bile duct stone clearance. Given that her afferent limb was anastomosed to the ileum and that she had prior gastrectomy precluding EUS-directed transgastric access, peroral ERCP was deemed impossible. Bile duct surgery and intraoperative ERCP were undesirable, since the patient already had cholecystectomy. EUS-BD was offered to avoid

Supplementary Information The online version contains supplementary material available at [https://doi.org/10.1007/978-981-16-9340-3_14].

R. Sanchez-Ocaña · M. Perez-Miranda (✉)
Department of Gastroenterology, Hospital Universitario Rio Hortega, Valladolid, Spain
e-mail: mperezmiranda@saludcastillayleon.es

A. Y.B. Teoh et al. (eds.), *Atlas of Interventional EUS*, https://doi.org/10.1007/978-981-16-9340-3_14

external drainage catheters associated with PTBD.

14.3 Procedural Plan

Hepaticogastrostomy with a fully-covered metal stent was chosen to provide initial drainage and to create a portal for elective antegrade stone management in SAA. Transhepatic fully-covered biliary metal stents provide more effective hepaticoenterostomy tract sealing than plastic stents. In contrast to partially-covered biliary metal stents, transhepatic fully-covered metal stents can easily be removed once treatment is completed [4]. The larger diameter of metal stents facilitates through-the-stent interventions, including cholangioscopy for lithotripsy or even just biopsy [7]. Disposable digital baby cholangioscopes are commonly used [4–7]; however, POT cholangioscopy by direct insertion of thin-caliber upper endoscopes is possible, either through mature naked fistulas [2, 4] or through-the-stent. Through-the-stent POT cholangioscopy appears feasible as a single-session procedure [8]. Compared to antegrade stone management alone, adding hepaticoenterostomy reduces leakage risk and allows POT cholangioscopy. Hepaticoenterostomy is thus favored over direct antegrade intervention in complex cases. Staged EUS-BD approaches to benign biliary disease are evolving; however, three incremental variations in technique have been proposed for three possible levels of increasing disease complexity [5]: direct antegrade intervention first, sequential approach after plastic stent hepaticoenterostomy then, and finally, sequential approach after covered metal stent hepaticoenterostomy [5, 6]. According to recent estimates, biliary access procedures through EUS-BD created fistulas may represent 3.6% of overall ERCP volume and up to 8.5% of follow-up procedures [9].

In this case, a second session for stone removal was planned, with cholangioscopy-guided lithotripsy if necessary. Deferred antegrade management takes place through a mature fistula using a standard upper endoscope or a duodenoscope for biliary access, under fluoroscopic guidance. Antegrade guidewire access is obtained through the original fistula after hepatogastric stent removal. Alternatively, cannulation of an indwelling hepatogastric metal stent is possible, as it is done with blocked transmural biliary metal stents [1]. Several interventions can be performed over the wire, including antegrade balloon dilation, stone removal, stent placement, and cholangioscopy [4–7]. Less common interventions such as magnet placement [2, 5] or antegrade sphincterotomy [8] have also been reported.

14.4 Description of the Procedure

EUS-guided puncture of a 0.3 mm left intrahepatic bile duct branch (Fig. 14.1) (Video 14.1) using a linear echoendoscope allowed cholangiography (Fig. 14.2). Hepaticogastrostomy was performed with a 10 × 60 mm fully-covered biliary metal stent with an internal antimigration flap. Two hemoclips and a coaxial 7F double pig-tail stent were placed for additional anchorage. The external end of the stent was left within 1-cm of the gastric wall (Fig. 14.3) to facilitate through-the-stent access. Two months later, antegrade common bile duct stone clearance was attempted. The two transmural stents were sequentially removed through the scope using a polypectomy snare. A thin-caliber upper endoscope was advanced through the naked hepatogastric fistula antegradely into the common bile duct. Saline

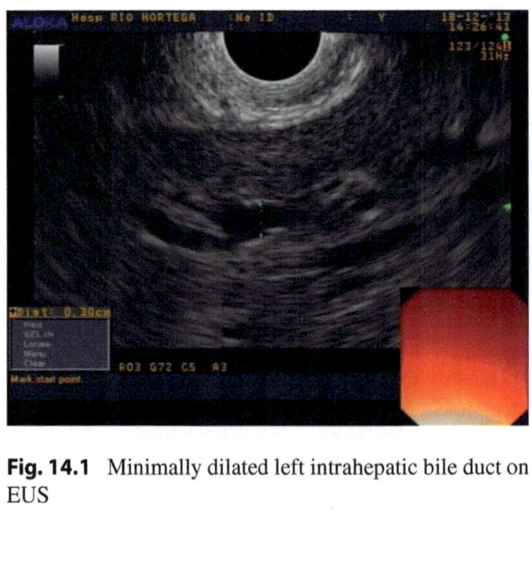

Fig. 14.1 Minimally dilated left intrahepatic bile duct on EUS

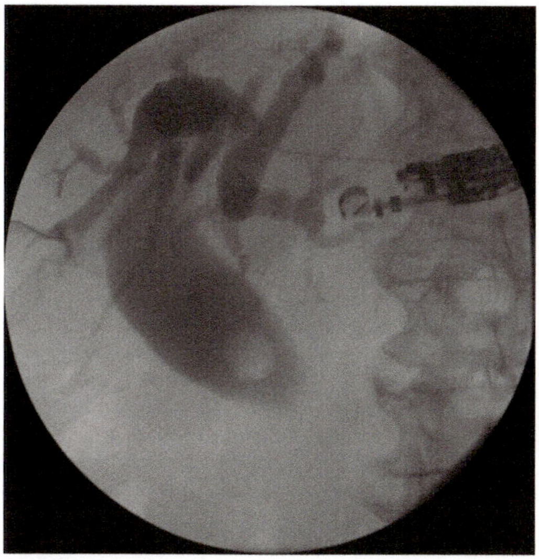

Fig. 14.2 Residual common bile duct stone on transhepatic EUS-cholangiography

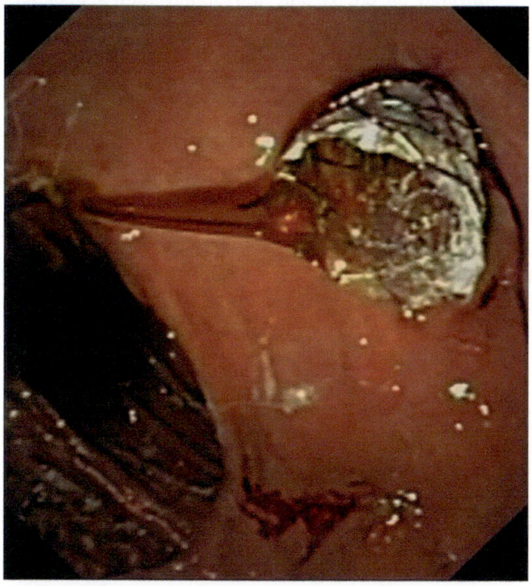

Fig. 14.3 Hepatogastric fully-covered metal stent close to gastric wall before additional anchoring

irrigation and electro-hydraulic lithotripsy were performed under POT cholangioscopy. The upper endoscope was removed leaving a guidewire in place across the papilla and the hepatogastric fistula. Two fully-covered metal stents were placed over the wire through a duodenoscope. One across the papilla to facilitate stone fragment clearance and another across the fistula, with a coaxial double pig-tail, to maintain access. Four months later, all stents were removed. The transmural stents were ensnared and removed through the scope. The transpapillary stent was pulled back into the common bile duct with a stone retrieval balloon catheter, then grasped with a tripod forceps under POT cholangioscopy and removed retrogradely (Fig. 14.4). Direct POT cholangioscopy with antegrade retroflexed duodenoscopy confirmed stone clearance and a patent papilla.

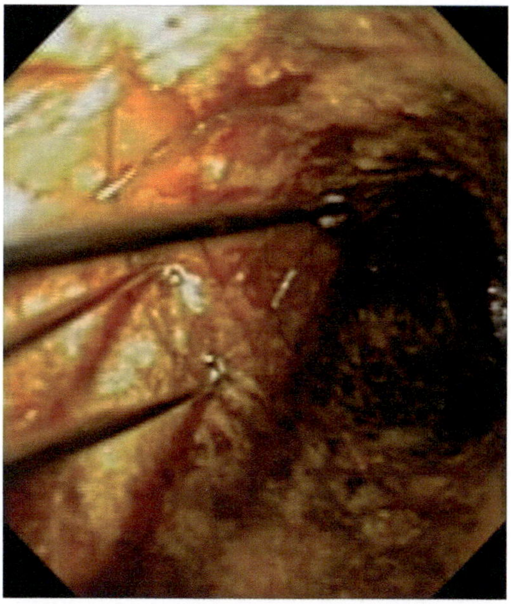

Fig. 14.4 Ultra-slim upper endoscope cholangioscopy image of foreign body forceps grasp of intraductal biliary stent

14.5 Post-procedural Management

Hepaticogastrostomy is usually performed under overnight inpatient observation, with intravenous analgesia if required. Outpatient EUS-BD is also possible [4]. Antibiotics are mandatory if cholangitis is present and are often administered prophylactically. Follow-up sessions for antegrade intervention are typically outpatient procedures. Patients need to be cautioned about stent dysfunction or migration symptoms, and about compliance with follow-up intervals.

14.6 Potential Pitfalls

Transmural biliary intervention is facilitated by the initial placement of a covered metal stent. However, stent migration or side-branch blockage may occur when covered metal stents are placed transhepatically. Antimigration strategies, as described in this case, appear helpful. Standard covered biliary metal stents may migrate in up to 60% of patients when placed transhepatically with hemoclips used as only anchorage [10]. Prolonged transhepatic stent indwell time may incur migration or blockage with relapsing cholangitis. More rarely, metal stents induce arteriobiliary fistulas with severe bleeding requiring angiographic hemostasis. Patient compliance with follow-up sessions is therefore essential. The safety of prolonged treatment intervals is not established. In our practice, sequential sessions are preferentially scheduled 2–8 weeks apart.

Competing Interests Dr. Manuel Perez-Miranda is a consultant for Boston Scientific, Olympus, Medtronic and M.I.Tech.

References

1. Nakai Y, Sato T, Hakuta R, et al. Long-term outcomes of a long, partially covered metal stent for EUS-guided hepaticogastrostomy in patients with malignant biliary obstruction (with video). Gastrointest Endosc. 2020;92:623–31.
2. Perez-Miranda M, Aleman N, de la Serna HC, et al. Magnetic compression anastomosis through EUS-guided choledocho-duodenostomy to repair a disconnected bile duct in orthotopic liver transplantation. Gastrointest Endosc. 2014;80:520–1.
3. Jang SI, Lee KH, Yoon HJ, Lee DK. Treatment of completely obstructed benign biliary strictures with magnetic compression anastomosis: follow-up results after recanalization. Gastrointest Endosc. 2017;85:1057–66.
4. James TW, Fan YC, Baron TH. EUS-guided hepaticoenterostomy as a portal to allow definitive antegrade treatment of benign biliary diseases in patients with surgically altered anatomy. Gastrointest Endosc. 2018;88:547–54.
5. Mukai S, Itoi T, Sofuni A, et al. EUS-guided antegrade intervention for benign biliary diseases in patients with surgically altered anatomy (with videos). Gastrointest Endosc. 2019;89:399–407.
6. Ogura T, Nishioka N, Yamada M et al. Novel transluminal treatment protocol for hepaticojejunostomy stricture using covered self-expandable metal stent. Surg Endosc 2020 Jan 13. https://doi.org/10.1007/s00464-020-07381-2. Online ahead of print.
7. Rosa R, Dioscoridi L, Forti E, et al. Indeterminate biliary stricture treated by antegrade cholangioscopy through an endoscopic ultrasound-guided hepaticojejunostomy. Endoscopy. 2020 Apr 24; https://doi.org/10.1055/a-1149-8684.
8. Sanchez-Ocaña R, Peñas-Herrero I, de la Serna-Higuera C, et al. Peroral transhepatic cholangioscopy and antegrade sphincterotomy via EUS-guided anastomosis. Gastrointest Endosc. 2016;83:466–7.
9. García-Alonso FJ, Peñas I, Sanchez-Ocana R et al. The role of EUS guidance for biliary and pancreatic duct access and drainage to overcome limitations of ERCP: a retrospective evaluation. Endoscopy 2020 Sep 21. https://doi.org/10.1055/a-1266-7592. Online ahead of print.
10. Miranda-García P, Gonzalez JM, Tellechea JI, et al. EUS hepaticogastrostomy for bilioenteric anastomotic strictures: a permanent access for repeated ambulatory dilations? Results from a pilot study. Endosc Int Open. 2016;4:E461–5.

15 EUS-Guided Hepaticogastrostomy to Facilitate Antegrade ERCP for Management of Benign Biliary Obstruction in Roux-en-Y Hepaticojejunostomy Anatomy

Rahman Nakshabendi and Todd H. Baron

15.1 Background

EUS-guided biliary drainage (EUS-BD) can be performed in a variety of ways using transgastric or transduodenal routes using rendezvous or direct drainage methods [1]. EUS-BD is most often performed when traditional ERCP fails and for relief of malignant biliary obstruction. However, EUS-BD can be useful for managing biliary disease, especially in patients with surgically altered anatomy such as Roux-en-Y gastrointestinal or biliary reconstruction an alternative to device-assisted ERCP (DA-ERCP) (e.g., enteroscopy-assisted) or percutaneous transhepatic biliary drainage (PTBD). DA-ERCP is time-consuming and fraught with small caliber working channels and lengths that limit accessories and devices. PTBD is associated with a high morbidity and poor patient quality of life as well as the need for frequent interventions for tube exchanges. EUS-guided hepaticoenterostomy is a broad term as the access point can be gastric, esophageal, jejunal, or even duodenal depending on the best location and patient anatomy. In patients with benign disease, the site of entry is a portal of entry to then allow downstream treatment of disease. This portal of entry can be used to dilate strictures, remove stones, perform cholangioscopy, and place one or more large bore plastic stents [2, 3].

15.2 Case History

A 63-year-old male underwent cholecystectomy one year prior complicated by complete bile duct transection requiring Roux-en-Y hepaticojejunostomy (HJ). He presents now with intermittent fevers and pruritis. Laboratory exam showed normal total bilirubin, AST/ALT 189 and 199 IU/L, respectively, and alkaline phosphatase of 491 IU/L. Abdominal MRI showed dilated intrahepatic ducts, more centrally than peripherally and a stone in the left hepatic duct. EUS-guided hepaticogastrostomy (EUS-HG) was undertaken.

Supplementary Information The online version contains supplementary material available at [https://doi.org/10.1007/978-981-16-9340-3_15].

R. Nakshabendi · T. H. Baron (✉)
Division of Gastroenterology & Hepatology, University of North Carolina, Chapel Hill, NC, USA
e-mail: todd_baron@med.unc.edu

A. Y.B. Teoh et al. (eds.), *Atlas of Interventional EUS*, https://doi.org/10.1007/978-981-16-9340-3_15

15.3 Procedural Plan

EUS-HG is performed via a transgastric approach into the left lobe. We perform EUS-HG using a 19G FNA needle and a standard oblique-viewing echoendoscope. Using Doppler signal, vessels in the needle tract are avoided and the intrahepatic ducts are seen as anechoic structures. The needle is preloaded with contrast. Electrocautery to create the tract is avoided because of the concern for adverse events when non-axial electrocautery is used [4]. In addition, we use a long (450 cm), 0.025″ guidewire that is less likely to shear using the 19G needle. We use fully covered self-expandable metal stents (FCSEMS) of 8 or 10 mm diameters and 6, 8, or 10 cm lengths with antimigration fins and without flanges as they accommodate the relatively smaller intrahepatic ducts. Once access is secured across the gastric wall using the FCSEMS the downstream disease is addressed.

15.4 Description of the Procedure

General anesthesia was administered. Antibiotics were given. The procedure was performed as an outpatient, with the patient in the supine position and CO_2 insufflation and a standard, oblique-viewing linear echoendoscope. A peripheral branch of the left hepatic duct was identified echosonographically. Intrahepatic air within a 5 mm duct was visualized. An area without intervening blood vessels was located (Video 15.1) and the duct of interest was punctured with a standard 19-gauge FNA needle (Fig. 15.1a, Video 15.1). Water-soluble contrast was injected under fluoroscopic guidance to confirm entry and provide cholangiography (Fig. 15.1b) (Video 15.1). The needle was then flushed with sterile saline and a 0.025″ angled guidewire was advanced through the needle into the left hepatic duct. It would not cross the HJ and was coiled in the left hepatic duct. The FNA needle was removed and the tract dilated with a 3–4-5 Fr tapered biliary catheter (Fig. 15.2) to dilate the tract to then allow passage of a 4 mm dilating balloon. The dilation always begins well distal to the echo probe (Fig. 15.3) and the tract dilated sequentially proximally and across the gastric wall. An 8 mm diameter × 8 cm long FCSEMS was deployed across the HG (Video 15.1). Once secured with the SEMS across the HG, the wire was advanced across the HJ, which was then balloon dilated (Fig. 15.4) and a straight 10Fr × 15 cm plastic biliary stent is passed across the HJ to initiate downstream therapy (Fig. 15.5a–b).

15.5 Post-procedural Management

A diet was resumed and the patient was discharged home later the same day. He returned with cholangitis which required a 4-day hospital-

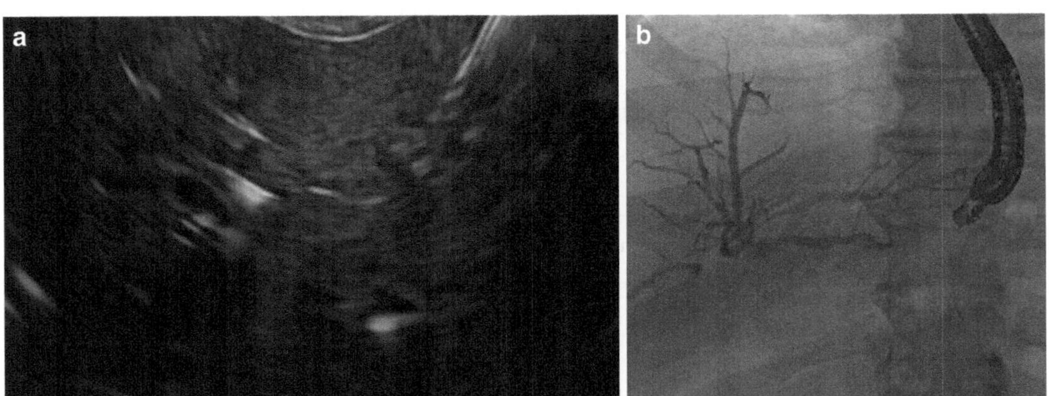

Fig. 15.1 (a) 19G FNA needle is passed into the peripheral hepatic duct and (b) contrast is injected to confirm position

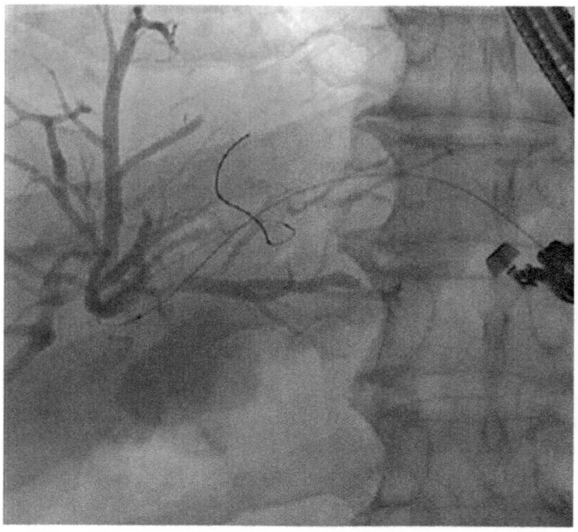

Fig. 15.2 A guidewire is advanced into the left hepatic duct and coiled. A 3–4-5 catheter is passed over the wire and seen in this image near the HJ

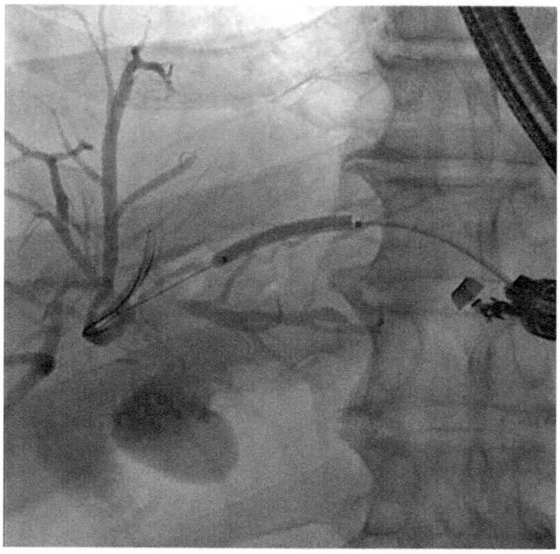

Fig. 15.3 Balloon dilation beginning well distal to the echoscope

ization. He then underwent subsequent outpatient antegrade transgastric cholangiographic procedures using a standard duodenoscope and ERCP accessories for stone removal (Fig. 15.6), additional balloon dilation of the HJ (Fig. 15.7) and placement of multiple side-by-side plastic stents over a 15-month period until follow-up cholangiography showed complete resolution of the HJ stricture (Video 15.1), at which time all stents were removed. The patient remains well without

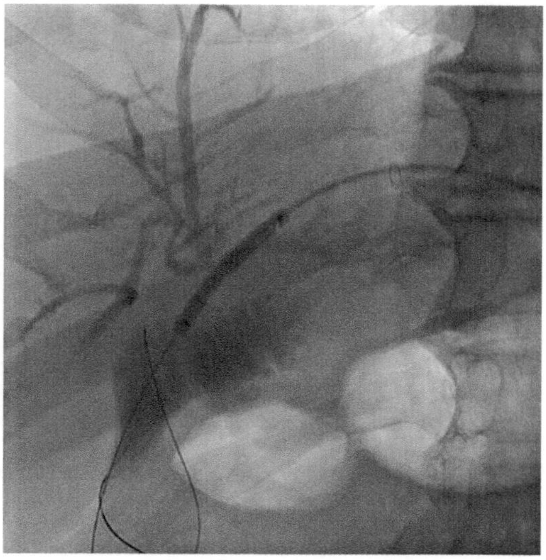

Fig. 15.4 After SEMS deployment a guidewire is passed across the HJ and into the jejunum

symptoms and with normal liver function tests one year after all stents were removed.

15.6 Potential Pitfalls

The potential adverse events after EUS-HG include complete loss of access to the site during device exchange, misdeployment of the stent, internal migration of the stent into the peritoneal space, perforation, bleeding (including intrahepatic hematoma), bile leakage (possibly with peritonitis), liver abscess, biloma, and cholangitis. We have seen cholangitis, particularly in patients with prior instrumentation of the biliary tree because of the rapid hematogenous spread when the biliary tree is accessed through the liver. In the case of stent misdeployment, it usually occurs with the stent too far into the tract on the peritoneal side. If a guidewire is still in place, another stent of the same diameter can be placed in overlapping fashion. If guidewire access is lost at this point, the echoendoscope is used to re-puncture the mouth of the existing stent or the side of the existing stent such that an overlapping stent is placed.

The most feared and dreaded event is complete guidewire loss after dilation of the tract.

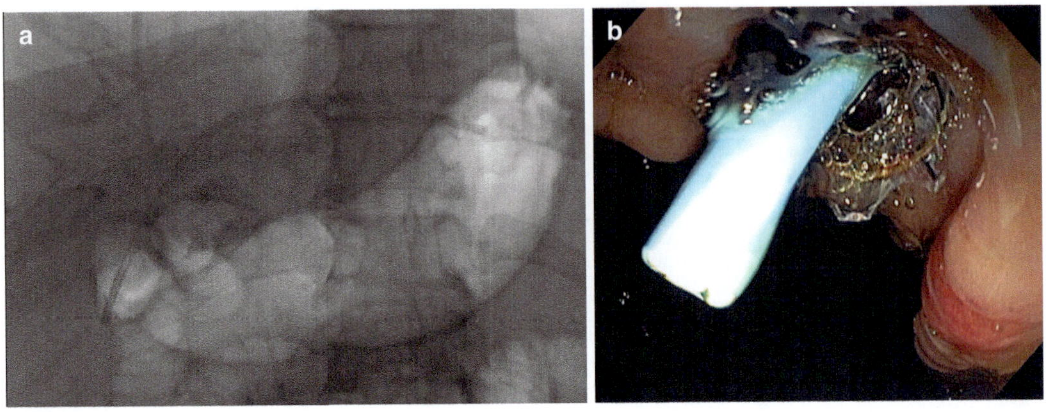

Fig. 15.5 Final images of SEMS across HG and plastic stent within it across the HJ. (**a**) Fluoroscopic and (**b**) Endoscopic

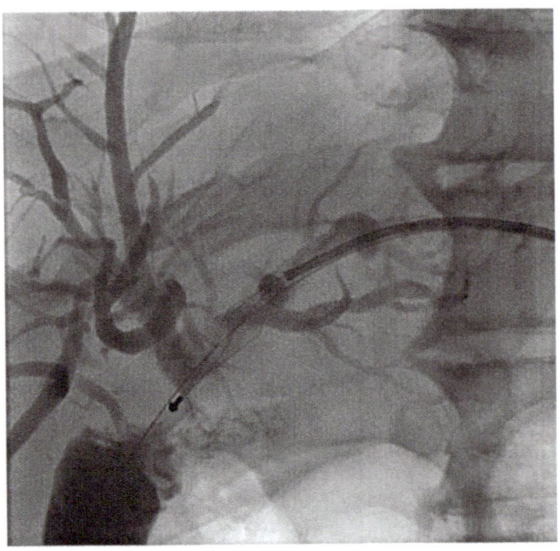

Fig. 15.6 Fluoroscopic image during subsequent antegrade biliary therapy showing lithotripsy basket passed through the endoscopic hepaticogastrostomy into left hepatic duct positioned just above the surgical hepaticojejunostomy

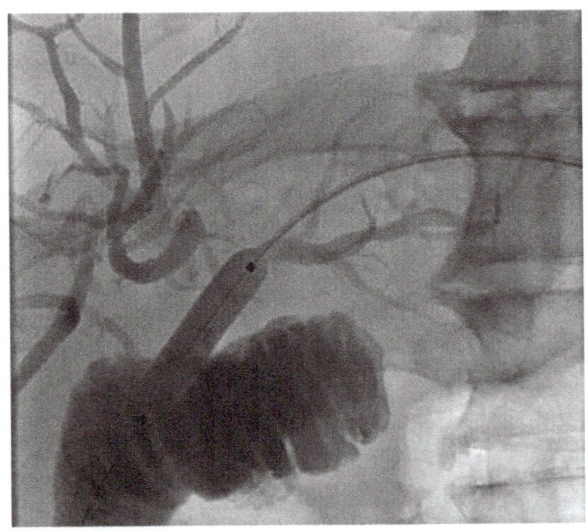

Fig. 15.7 Fluoroscopic image during subsequent antegrade biliary therapy showing 8 mm dilating balloon which was passed through the endoscopic hepaticogastrostomy into left hepatic duct and positioned across the surgical hepaticojejunostomy

This results in bile leakage with decompression of the ducts, a combination that makes re-puncture and regaining access technically difficult. As a last resort, one could try enteroscopy and retrograde cholangiography, assuming the biliary tree can be reached and accessed. Percutaneous drainage or surgery may be required to manage these adverse events, though we have not experienced the need for surgical intervention.

References

1. Canakis A, Baron TH. Relief of biliary obstruction: choosing between endoscopic ultrasound and endoscopic retrograde cholangiopancreatography. BMJ Open Gastroenterol. 2020 Jul;7(1):e000428.
2. Law R, Grimm IS, Baron TH. Endoscopic transhepatic cholangiography with antegrade transanastomotic stent placement in a liver transplantation patient with Roux-en-Y hepaticojejunostomy. Gastrointest Endosc. 2015 Sep;82(3):568–9.
3. James TW, Fan YC, Baron TH. EUS-guided hepaticoenterostomy as a portal to allow definitive antegrade

treatment of benign biliary diseases in patients with surgically altered anatomy. Gastrointest Endosc. 2018 Sep;88(3):547–54.

4. Khashab MA, Messallam AA, Penas I, Nakai Y, Modayil RJ, De la Serna C, Hara K, El Zein M, Stavropoulos SN, Perez-Miranda M, Kumbhari V, Ngamruengphong S, Dhir VK, Park DH. International multicenter comparative trial of transluminal EUS-guided biliary drainage via hepatogastrostomy vs. choledochoduodenostomy approaches. Endosc Int Open. 2016 Feb;4(2):E175–81.

Part III

EUS-Guided Pancreatic Drainage

EUS-Guided Pancreaticogastrostomy

16

Hoonsub So and Do Hyun Park

16.1 Background

For patients with symptomatic obstructive pancreatitis or pancreas ductal stricture/leakage, pancreatic ductal drainage helps relieve pain and reserve pancreas exocrine/endocrine function. For tight anastomotic stricture, obstructing stone, or inaccessible papilla by surgically altered anatomy, or disconnected syndrome, transpapillary drainage is not always possible. Conventionally, they were managed with surgery, percutaneous, or conservative treatment. As surgical or percutaneous approach convey a risk of substantial complications and these procedures are technically challenging, EUS-guided pancreaticogastrostomy (EUS-PG) is a useful option for a rescue for failed transpapillary drainage [1–3]. The downside is relatively low success rate and high risk of adverse events [3].

16.2 Case History

A 66-year-old male was admitted for abdominal pain. He had a history of pylorus-preserving pancreaticoduodenectomy for intraductal papillary mucinous neoplasm of pancreas 4 years ago, and computed tomography (CT) showed pancreatic duct dilatation with an anastomotic stricture. The remnant pancreas showed the feature of acute pancreatitis with main pancreatic ductal dilatation (Fig. 16.1). There was no evidence of tumor recurrence. As it was impossible to find pancreaticojejunostomy (PJ) orifice with deep enteroscopy, we planned to perform PJ stricture dilation via EUS-PG.

16.3 Procedural Plan

EUS-PG can be performed via transgastric approach. Puncture site should be determined in consideration of the distance between stomach and pancreas, location of the stricture, and ductal configuration and size. The direction and optimal access point of the puncture EUS needle are important for a guidewire manipulation, so fluoroscopic examination is necessary before puncturing of EUS needle. For best access point of an

Supplementary Information The online version contains supplementary material available at [https://doi.org/10.1007/978-981-16-9340-3_16].

H. So
Department of Internal Medicine, Ulsan University Hospital, University of Ulsan College of Medicine, Ulsan, South Korea
e-mail: hoon3112@uuh.ulsan.kr

D. H. Park (✉)
Division of Gastroenterology, Department of Internal Medicine, University of Ulsan College of Medicine, Asan Medical Center, Seoul, South Korea
e-mail: dhpark@amc.seoul.kr

A. Y.B. Teoh et al. (eds.), *Atlas of Interventional EUS*, https://doi.org/10.1007/978-981-16-9340-3_16

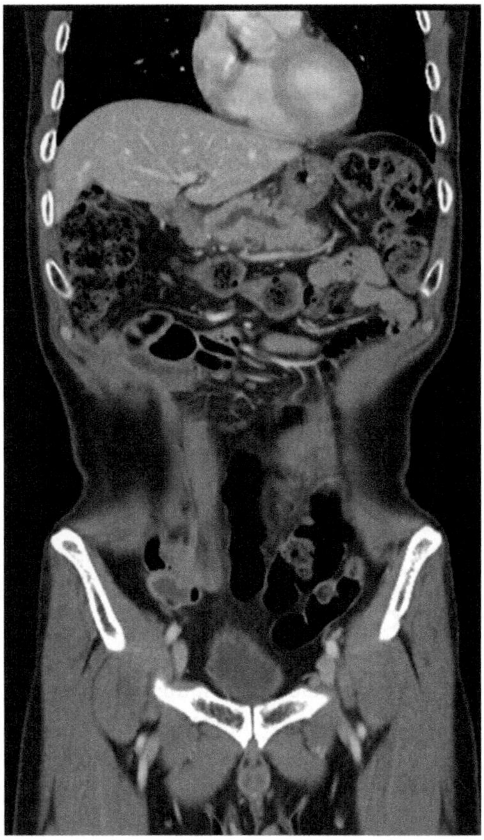

Fig. 16.1 Computed tomography showing pancreaticojejunostomy stricture with dilated main pancreatic duct

EUS needle, endoscopist should try to keep a parallel line between main pancreatic duct and the axis of the EUS needle. If the guidewire manipulation is difficult due to direction of wire or configuration of pancreatic duct, re-puncture in a better access point could be needed. We advise the operator to control the guidewire by oneself as the tactile sensation is important to avoid forced manipulation, which could shear the guidewire or injure the pancreatic duct or parenchyma. Cystotome or needle knife is usually used for a fistula dilation. Soehendra stent retriever (7Fr, Cook Medical, USA) may be a rescue option for difficult fistula dilation. If the guidewire passes the stricture, dilatation and transgastric/transpapillary or transanastomotic stent placement is done just like in other interventions. Generally, 0.025-in guidewire is used because a conventional 0.035-in guidewire may be hard to manipulate in 19-gauge EUS needle, and keeping the line of guidewire in the field of EUS during the procedure including fistula dilation and stent placement is important. If the guidewire could not pass the tight stricture, temporary or permanent EUS-PG with transmural stenting may be considered [4]. Either plastic or self-expanding fully covered metal stent (FCSEMS) could be used. As this various clinical scenario, we proposed an algorithm on EUS-PG according to degree of stricture and passage of guidewire to pancreatic ductal stricture [4]. FCSEMS could be effective for stricture resolution and pain relief with longer placement [5–7]. Especially, our center reported favorable success rate with durable long-term outcome of EUS-PG with an FCSEMS for PJ stricture [4]. FCSEMS also has merits in pushability, shorter procedure time, and prevention of adverse event including the leakage of pancreatic juice in fistula site compared to aplastic stenting in EUS-PG. However, it is known to have a risk of creating de novo stricture in larger diameter of FCSEMS in smaller main pancreatic duct [8]. Therefore, 6 mm or 8 mm as a smaller diameter of an FCSEMS may be more ideal than 10 mm diameter of an FCSEMS in EUS-PG.

16.4 Description of the Procedure

With linear echoendoscope, pancreatic duct at body was measured as 3 mm in diameter. The puncture was done from midbody posterior wall of the stomach to the body of pancreas considering the angle of the 19-gauge needle (EchoTip Ultra, Cook Medical, USA.). Contrast was used to confirm the main pancreatic duct. Then, a guidewire (VisiGlide 2, 0.025 inch in diameter, Olympus, Japan) was inserted but was not able to advance through the stricture (Fig. 16.2) (Video 16.1). We assessed it as a partial PJ stricture (contrast ran off to the jejunum without the passage of the guidewire into jejunum) [4], so decided to perform pancreaticogastrostomy with transmural metal stenting. The tract was dilated with a needle knife and 4 mm balloon (Hurricane RX, Boston Scientific, USA), and FCSEMS (antimigrating flaps in both ends, 6 mm in diameter,

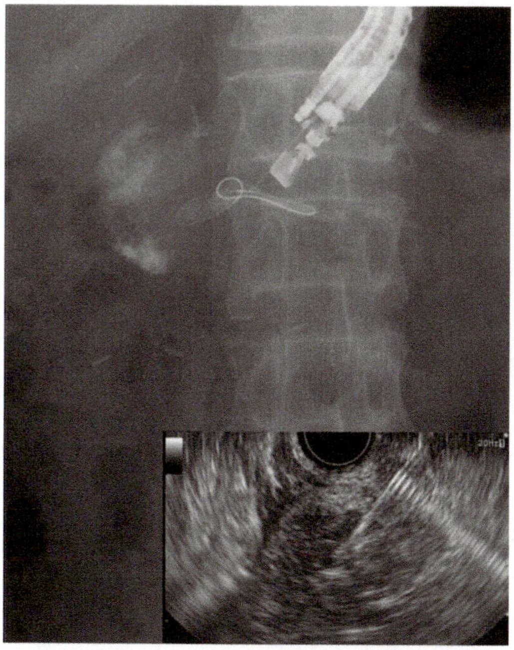

Fig. 16.2 Fluoroscopic image showing partial obstruction of pancreaticojejunostomy. Guidewire was not able to advance through the stricture. Endoscopic ultrasonography image of the puncture of an EUS needle in main pancreatic duct (inset)

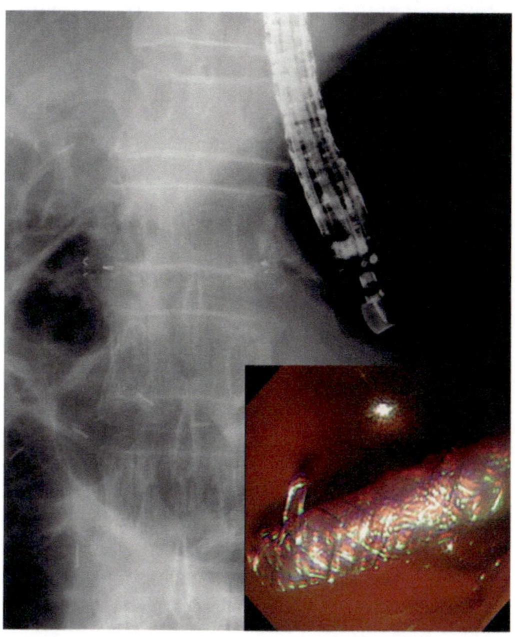

Fig. 16.3 Fluoroscopic image showing a transmural metal stenting through EUS-guided pancreaticogastrostomy. Endoscopic image of placed a transmural metal stent at midbody posterior wall of the stomach (inset)

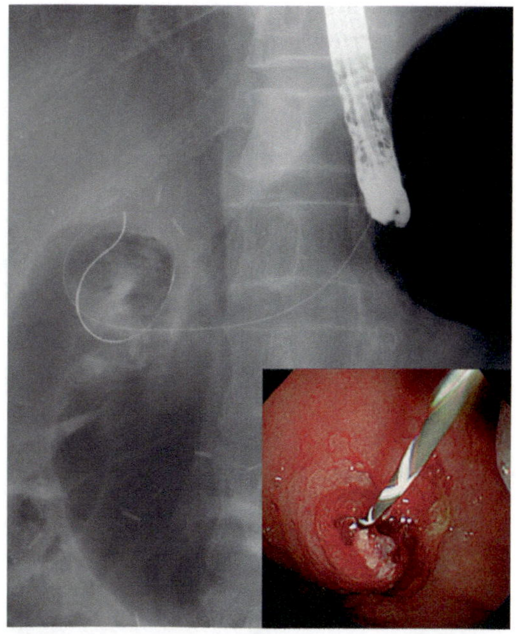

Fig. 16.4a Fluoroscopic image of guidewire passing pancreaticojejunostomy stricture after 3 months of placing metal stent. Endoscopic image of guidewire inserted through the pancreaticogastrostomy fistula (inset)

8 cm in length, MITECH, Korea) was deployed (Fig. 16.3). Pain was relieved and a CT scan showed well decompressed pancreatic duct taken 3 months later. With a duodenoscope, the metal stent was removed with biopsy forceps, and a guidewire was able to across the anastomotic stricture (Fig. 16.4a). The stricture was dilated with an 8 mm balloon (Hurricane RX, Boston Scientific, USA). Then, a double pigtail stent plastic stent could be successfully deployed through the stricture (Fig. 16.4b).

16.5 Post-procedural Management

If the patient has no evidence of post-procedural pancreatitis, diet can be started. The location of the deployed stent can be evaluated either by abdominal x-ray or CT scan. In this patient, the stent was changed 3 months later for retrial of PJ stricture management with transmural and trans-anastomotic plastic stenting. As usual, transpapillary stent removal with resolution of stricture is

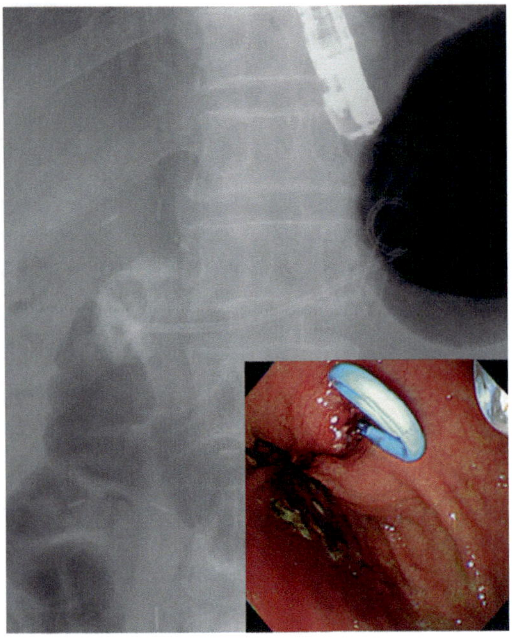

Fig. 16.4b Fluoroscopic image of a double pigtail plastic stent through the pancreaticojejunostomy stricture. Endoscopic image of placed a plastic stent (inset)

the goal of stent therapy for benign PJ stricture. Given difficult endoscopic access in patients with surgically altered anatomy, however, the mainstay of stent therapy for benign PJ stricture may be the continuation of stent placement after EUS-PG [4].

16.6 Potential Pitfalls

EUS-PG requires sufficient EUS interventional experience and the degree of adverse event could be substantial. Therefore, the feasibility of second attempt of ERCP should always be considered before performing EUS-PG. EUS-PG may be possible when pancreatic duct is dilated enough to be punctured. Repeated puncture may result in pancreatitis or pancreatic leakage. Even after successful puncture, fistula dilation may not be possible in fibrotic pancreas parenchyma. If appropriate maintenance of the line of a guidewire on EUS is not feasible during the procedure, a transmural stent placement may not be possible. Other potential adverse events include pancreatic fluid collection, stent migration, perforation and bleeding like in other interventions. Therefore, endoscopist should carefully select candidates for EUS-PG.

References

1. Varadarajulu S, Trevino JM. Review of EUS-guided pancreatic duct drainage (with video). Gastrointest Endosc. 2009;69(2 Suppl):S200–2.
2. Itoi T, Kasuya K, Sofuni A, Itokawa F, Kurihara T, Yasuda I, et al. Endoscopic ultrasonography-guided pancreatic duct access: techniques and literature review of pancreatography, transmural drainage and rendezvous techniques. Dig Endosc. 2013;25(3):241–52.
3. Nakai Y, Kogure H, Isayama H, Koike K. Endoscopic ultrasound-guided pancreatic duct drainage. Saudi J Gastroenterol. 2019;25(4):210–7.
4. Oh D, Park DH, Song TJ, Lee SS, Seo DW, Lee SK, et al. Long-term outcome of endoscopic ultrasound-guided pancreatic duct drainage using a fully covered self-expandable metal stent for pancreaticojejunal anastomosis stricture. J Gastroenterol Hepatol. 2019;
5. Oh D, Lee JH, Song TJ, Park DH, Lee SK, Kim MH, et al. Long-term outcomes of 6-mm diameter fully covered self-expandable metal stents in benign refractory pancreatic ductal stricture. Dig Endosc. 2018;30(4):508–15.
6. Park DH, Kim MH, Moon SH, Lee SS, Seo DW, Lee SK. Feasibility and safety of placement of a newly designed, fully covered self-expandable metal stent for refractory benign pancreatic ductal strictures: a pilot study (with video). Gastrointest Endosc. 2008;68(6):1182–9.
7. Dumonceau JM, Delhaye M, Tringali A, Arvanitakis M, Sanchez-Yague A, Vaysse T, et al. Endoscopic treatment of chronic pancreatitis: European Society of Gastrointestinal Endoscopy (ESGE) guideline—updated august 2018. Endoscopy. 2019;51(2):179–93.
8. Moon SH, Kim MH, Park DH, Song TJ, Eum J, Lee SS, et al. Modified fully covered self-expandable metal stents with antimigration features for benign pancreatic-duct strictures in advanced chronic pancreatitis, with a focus on the safety profile and reducing migration. Gastrointest Endosc. 2010;72(1):86–91.

17 Pancreaticojejunostomy with Forward-Viewing Echoendoscope

Mitsuhiro Kida, Tomohisa Iwai, Rikiya Hasegawa, Toru Kaneko, and Kosuke Okuwaki

17.1 Background

EUS-guided pancreatic duct drainage (EUS-PD) is a new therapeutic technique which introduces as an alternative to endoscopic retrograde cholangio-pancreatographic approach, when ERCP failed [1, 2]. After the introduction of balloon enteroscopy, balloon enteroscopy assisted ERCP(BAE-ERCP) started in patients with surgically altered anatomy in 2005 [3, 4]. In general, anastomotic stenosis can be observed in approximately 30% of pancreatoduodenectomy patients in Japan [5]. Therefore, it is difficult to find an anastomosis site and complete the procedures in many patients. As a result, half of the cases who had pancreatoduodenectomy in our department were failed in the treatment with BAE-ERCP [6]. On the other hand, EUS-PD was firstly reported by Francois et al. and Bataille et al. in 2002 [1, 2]. Asian EUS Group (AEG) guideline for EUS-PD was published [7]. There are several ways of EUS-PD such as Pancreato-gastrostomy, Antegrade stenting, and Rendezvous stenting. Then, EUS-PD, specially rendezvous stenting, has become popular in the treatment of anastomotic stenosis in cases of pancreatoduodenectomy. However, EUS-PD which was reported 77% in clinical success and 21% in adverse event rate by a recent meta-analysis has been still a difficult technique [8]. In this situation, forward-viewing echoendoscope-guided hepaticojejunostomy (FV-EUS-HJS) or pancreaticojejunostomy (FV-EUS-PJS) has developed in EUS-PD and EUS-BD [6, 9, 10].

This procedure has been shown to be completed, even in difficult cases by EUS-PD (transmural drainage: TMD). I have believed this is an alternative to EUS-PD (TMD) in the future.

17.2 Case History

A 48-year-old man who had pancreatoduodenectomy (Child's operation) because of papillary tumor was admitted for abdominal pain. Physical examination showed upper quadrant tenderness and elevation of serum amylase and lipase. Computed tomography showed dilatation of the main pancreatic duct (Fig. 17.1). The features are compatible with obstructive pancreatitis. BAE-ERCP failed 1 year ago and EUS-rendezvous PD was not completed because the guidewire slipped out because of not passing through the

Supplementary Information The online version contains supplementary material available at [https://doi.org/10.1007/978-981-16-9340-3_17].

M. Kida (✉) · T. Iwai · R. Hasegawa · T. Kaneko · K. Okuwaki
Department of Gastroenterology, Kitasato university, School of Medicine, Sagamihara, Kanagawa, Japan
e-mail: m-kida@kitasato-u.ac.jp; t-iwai@kitasato-u.ac.jp; k-r.h@kitasato-u.ac.jp; t.kaneko@kitasato-u.ac.jp; kokuwaki@kitasato-u.ac.jp

A. Y.B. Teoh et al. (eds.), *Atlas of Interventional EUS*, https://doi.org/10.1007/978-981-16-9340-3_17

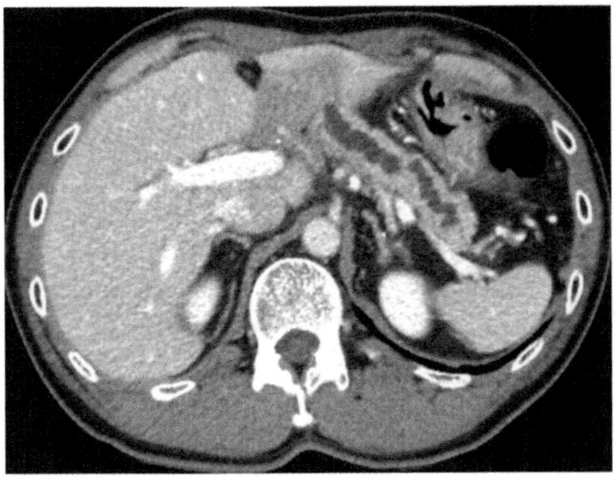

Fig. 17.1 Computed tomography demonstrating obstructive pancreatitis before FV-EUS-PJS

anastomotic site. Then, FV-EUS-PJS was offered to the patient.

17.3 Procedural Plan

There are several endoscopic techniques to treat this patient such as stenting pass through the anastomotic site with BEA-ERCP, EUS-rendezvous PD, and FV-EUS-PJS.

We would like to create pancreaticojejunostomy through the anastomotic site, not from the stomach. It seems to be practicable to create pancreaticojejunostomy with a stent from the stomach, but not to be stent-free. Otherwise, we have to exchange the stent every several months forever. At first, we have failed to treat this case with BEA-ERCP last time. And using EUS-rendezvous PD, guidewire also could not pass through the anastomotic site last time. In general, the success rate of EUS-rendezvous PD is around 55.6%, compared to 93.8% in EUS-PD (TMD) [6]. Optimally, we would like to pass through the original anastomotic lumen; however, we could not last time. Using forward-viewing echoendoscope, we could puncture the nearest point to dilated pancreatic duct in the scarring area of the anastomotic site with 19G and dilate with electrocautery. Probably, we could create a new traversable route that seems to be close to original anastomotic lumen. Then we decided to perform FV-EUS-PJS in this case. Our aim is to create pancreaticojejunostomy, to dilate the anastomotic site with a stent or balloon, and finally to be stent-free. According to the paper concerning the long-term follow-up outcome of 7 Fr plastic stent, 36% (9/25) patients had complete stent removal without symptom [10]. Of course, further follow-up studies of multiple plastic stent or metallic stent with large subjects are needed to evaluate the evidence.

17.4 Description of the Procedure (Video 17.1)

At first, the forward-viewing echoendoscope was inserted carefully to the anastomotic site to the main pancreatic duct after Child's operation (Fig. 17.2). Because the forward-viewing echoendoscope was thick and stiff, compared to balloon enteroscope. Then we looked for the nearest point to the dilated pancreatic duct in the scarring area of anastomotic site (Fig. 17.3, Videoclip). After confirming these findings, we punctured the dilated pancreatic duct with a 19G needle and filled the contrast or inserted a guidewire, in order to confirm whether the needle was in the pancreatic duct or not. The next step was to dilate the punctured route with 6.5 Fr electrocautery. Finally, we deployed a 7 Fr plastic pancreatic stent (Fig. 17.4). 10Fr plastic stent, or multiple plastic stents, or metallic stent could be inserted in the followed-up session, if necessary.

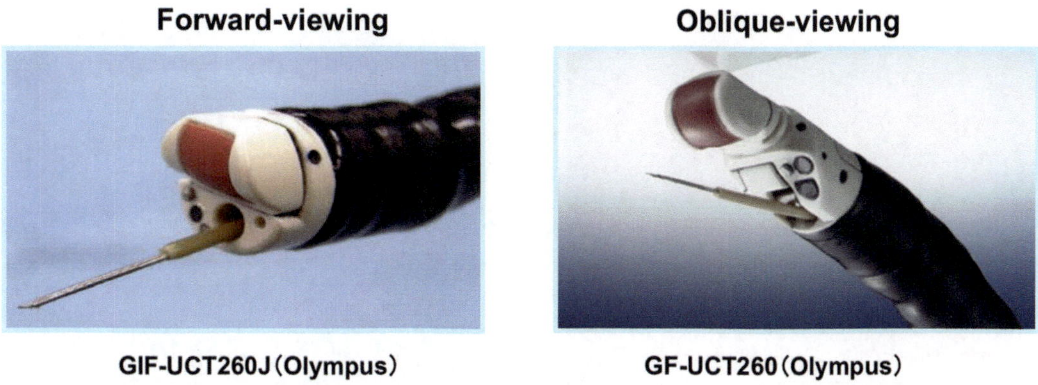

		GIF-UCT260J	GF-UCT260
Direction		0° (forward-view)	55° (Oblique-view)
Size of Channel		φ3.7mm	φ3.7mm
Elevator		×	O
Second water channel		O	×
US Function	View	90°	180°
	Balloon	×	O

Fig. 17.2 Equipment for EUS-PD

17.5 Post-procedural Management

Non per oral intake and antibiotics are continued up to the next day. Diets can be resumed when fever or pain is settled and laboratory data do not show pancreatitis and severe inflammation. If fever does not settle and pancreatitis is suspected, then a computed tomography should be arranged to assess the cause. Post-procedurally, the patients are scheduled for a follow-up session for dilation of anastomotic stenosis with large or multiple plastic stent or metallic stent. In general, these stents should be exchanged every 3–6 months up to 1 year. Most EUS-PD indications are benign including in this case, we have to think about the next strategy such as operation. Otherwise, long-term stent exchange is needed because of being benign.

17.6 Potential Pitfalls

The adverse events of EUS-PD include stent migration, fluid collection, pancreatitis, pneumoperitoneum, peritonitis and bleeding, etc. occurred in 21.8% [11]. There are few reports of FV-EUS-PJS; its potential adverse events seem to be almost the same as EUS-PD, even though not enough evidence at the moment. Fluid collection, pneumoperitoneum, local peritonitis, and pancreatitis can be treated with conservative therapy of antibiotics and intravenous infusion, if pancreatic stent is deployed correctly. Stent migration can be treated by balloon enteroscopic ERCP approach with basket etc. Bleeding can be also treated by electrocoagration or injection of 1/10000 epinephrine etc. Angiography approach can be employed, if these therapies failed.

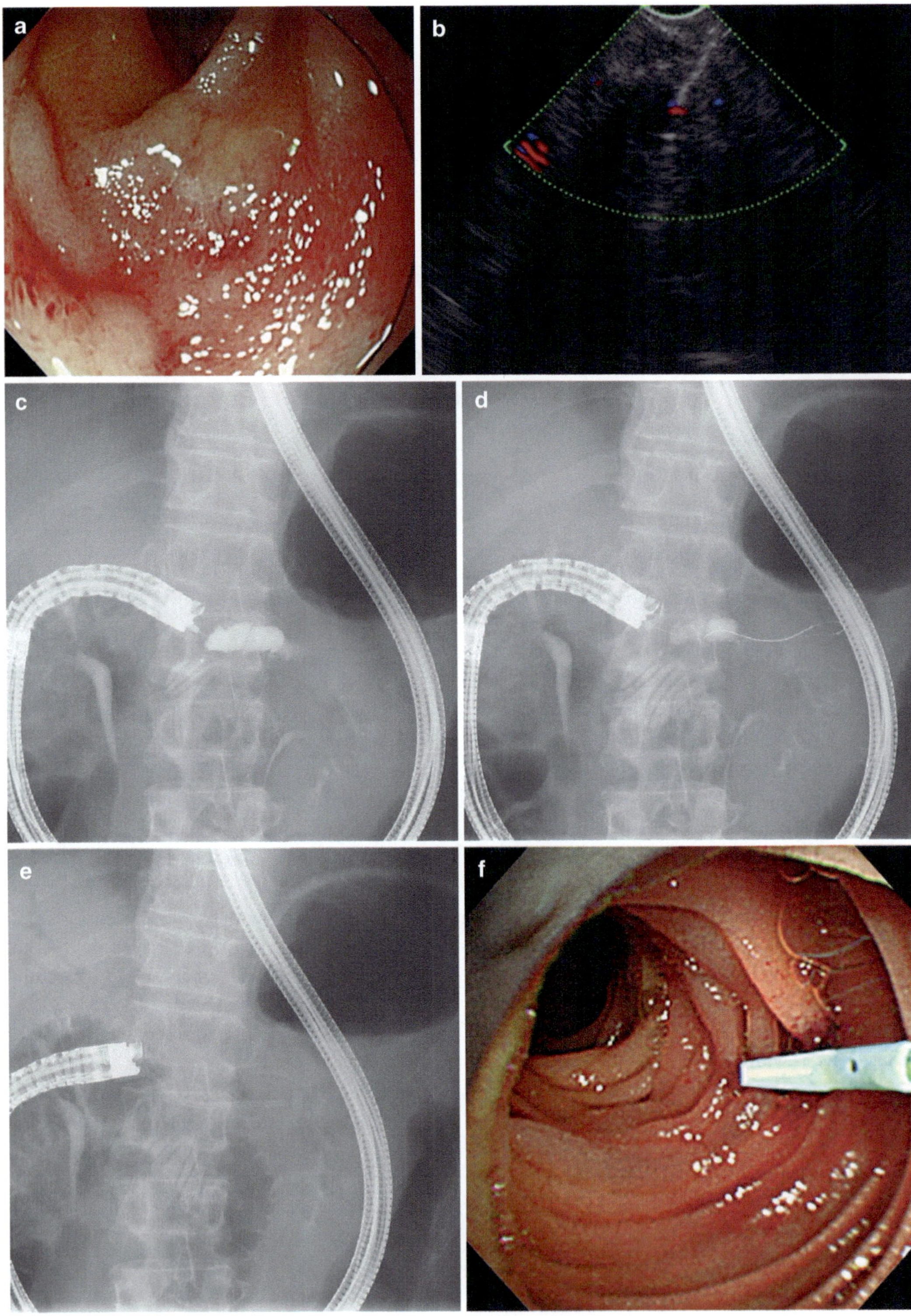

Fig. 17.3 FV-EUS-guided pancreaticojejunostomy for severe anastomotic stricture. (**a**) The endoscopic image shows the complete stricture of pancreatojejunostomy. (**b**) EUS image shows a 19-gauge needle passed into a dilated main pancreatic duct. (**c**) The fluoroscopic image shows the injection of the contrast medium into the main pancreatic duct. (**d**) Advancement of a guidewire into the main pancreatic duct. (**e**) Deployment of a 7-French pancreatic stent (allow) after dilatation with an electrocautery dilator. (**f**) The endoscopic image depicts a plastic stent at the anastomosis

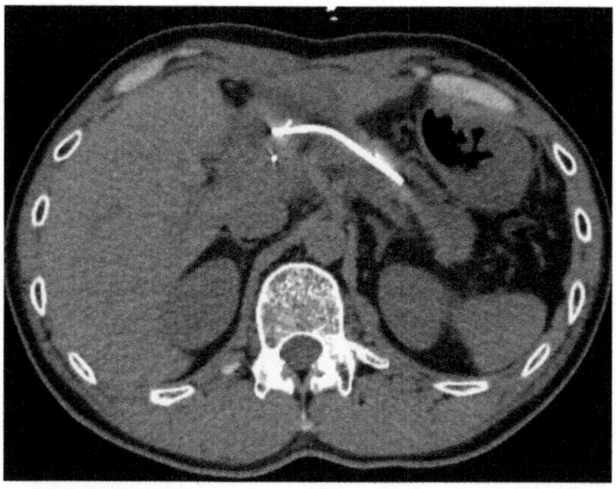

Fig. 17.4 Computed tomography demonstrating deployed stent after FV-EUS-PJS

References

1. Francois E, Kahaleh M, Giovannini M, et al. EUS-guided pancreatico -gastrostomy. Gastrointest Endosc. 2002;56:128–33.
2. Bataille L, Deprez P. A new application for therapeutic EUS: main pancreatic duct drainage with a "pancreatic rendezvous technique". Gastrointest Endosc. 2002;55:740–3.
3. Haruta H, Yamamoto H, Mizuta K, et al. A case of successful enteroscopic balloon dilation for late anastomotic stricture of choledochojejunostomy after living donor liver transplantation. Liver Transpl. 2005;11:1608–10.
4. Yamauchi H, Kida M, Imaizumi H, et al. Innovations and techniques for balloon-enteroscopeassisted endoscopic retrograde cholangiopancreatography in patients with altered gastrointestinal anatomy. WJG. 2015 June;7(21):6460–9.
5. Tanaka S, Ito Y, Oishi H, et al. A retrospective analysis of 88 patients with pancreaticogastrostomy after pancreaticoduodenectomy. Hepato-Gastroenterology. 2000;47:1454–7.
6. Iwai T, Kida M, Yamauchi H, et al. EUS-guided trans-anastomotic drainage for severe bilio-pasncreatic anastomotic stricture using forward-viewing echoendoscope in patients with surgically altered anatomy. Endoscopic Ultrasound. Endoscopic Ultrasound 2021;10: January-February.
7. Teoh A, Dhir V, Kida M, et al. Consensus guidelines on the optimal management in interventional EUS procedures: results from the Asian EUS group RAND/UCLA expert panel. Gut. 2018;67:1209–28.
8. Nakai Y, Kogure T, Isayama H, et al. Endoscopic ultrasound-guided pancreatic duct drainage. Saudi J Gastroenterol. 2019;25:210–7.
9. Kida M, Yamauchi OK, et al. Endoscopic ultrasound-guided choledocho-jejunostomy with a forward-viewing echoendoscope for severe benign bilioenteric stricture in a patient with Child's resection. Endoscopy. 2015;47:E303–4.
10. Nakaji S, Hirata N, Shiratori T, et al. Endoscopic ultrasound-guided pancreatico-jejunal anastomosis. Endoscopy. 2015;47:E41–2.
11. Matsunami Y, Itoi T, Sofuni A, et al. Evaluation of a new stent for EUS-guided pancreatic duct drainage: long term follow-up outcome. Endosc Int open. 2018;06:E505–12.

EUS-Guided Pancreatic Rendezvous

18

Rafael Mejuto Fernandez, Marina Kim, and Michel Kahaleh

18.1 Background

EUS-guided pancreatic drainage (EUS-PD) arose as a minimally invasive alternative to surgery or percutaneous drainage in altered anatomy (previous Whipple surgery) or simply the failure of conventional ERCP approach [1–4]. The procedure is divided into two main techniques: EUS-guided rendezvous (EUS-RV) and pancreatic transmural stenting (EUS-PTS); in this chapter, we will focus on the first.

18.2 Case History

A 69-year-old patient with known chronic pancreatitis and multiple co-morbidities was admitted for high fever, severe pain, and failure to thrive. Physical examination showed epigastric pain, fever with mild jaundice. Blood culture grew *E. coli*. Computed tomography showed a distended biliary tree with prior biliary stent in place. EUS revealed a 3 cm abnormal area in the pancreatic head suspicious for a mass and biopsies were obtained with a 22G needle. A dilated CBD and dilated PD up to 7 mm in the head were noted with multiple cysts throughout the pancreas up to 5 mm in size. Conventional PD access was not feasible due to the severe inflammation of the duodenum. EUS-RV was offered.

18.3 Procedural Plan

EUS-RV can be performed using a transgastric or transduodenal approach. We prefer the transgastric approach since the risk of perforation is limited and permit an appropriate decompression of the dilated main pancreatic duct in case the rendezvous is not feasible. Some endoscopists prefer a transduodenal drainage as the duct is in theory easier to puncture; however, the duodenal location does not permit as much maneuverability and is less forgiven in case of perforation or bleeding.

We prefer to puncture the main pancreatic duct with a 19 gauge needle since it permits the use of 0.035 inches guidewire after injection. The 19 gauge needle offers more leverage for wire manipulation in order to facilitate access into the duodenum followed by removal of the echoendoscope over the wire placed across the ampulla. Our favorite wires are the Terumo guidewire (Terumo, Somerset, NJ, USA) or the Visiglide (Olympus, Center Valley, PA, USA).

Supplementary Information The online version contains supplementary material available at [https://doi.org/10.1007/978-981-16-9340-3_18].

R. M. Fernandez · M. Kim · M. Kahaleh (✉)
Division of Gastroenterology, Rutgers Robert Wood Johnson Medical School, Robert Wood Johnson University Hospital, New Brunswick, NJ, USA
e-mail: Rafael.Mejuto.Fernandez@sergas.es

A. Y.B. Teoh et al. (eds.), *Atlas of Interventional EUS*, https://doi.org/10.1007/978-981-16-9340-3_18

18.4 Description of the Procedure (Video 18.1)

EUS-RV was performed with a GF-UCT180 linear array echoendoscope (Olympus America) using a transgastric approach. The pancreatic duct was first identified and an area without intervening blood vessels was located (Fig. 18.1) (Video 18.1). The pancreatic duct was punctured with a 19 gauge needle (USN-19-T; Cook Endoscopy, Winston-Salem, North Carolina, USA). A Visiglide guidewire was then passed into the pancreatic duct (Fig. 18.2) and advanced across the distal pancreatic stricture into the duodenum (Fig. 18.3). The echoendoscope was then removed over the wire (Fig. 18.4). The duodenoscope was then advanced facing the wire (Fig. 18.5). We do not routinely attempt to retrieve the wire through the working channel of the endoscope. We prefer, to pull the wire crossing the ampulla to the mouth before retrieving it through the working channel of the duodenoscope.

18.5 Post-procedural Management

The patient is typically kept NPO post procedure and resumed on a clear diet the next day. Antibiotics are continued for up to one week. Cross-sectional imaging is ordered in case of severe pain or fever. All patients are scheduled for a follow-up visit at one month with repeat cross-sectional imaging. Repeat ERCP with PD stent revision is typically performed at 3 months intervals.

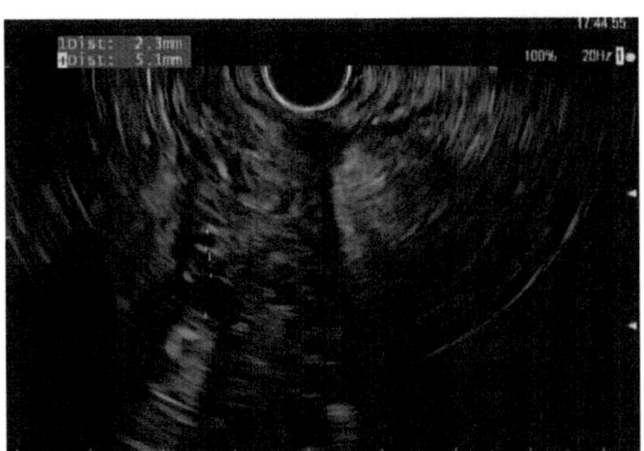

Fig. 18.1 Dilated main pancreatic duct on ultrasonography

18.6 Potential Pitfalls

The potential adverse events after EUS-PD techniques include perforation and bleeding. In the case of bleeding, failure to locate a deep vessel endoscopically will typically lead to emergent embolization by interventional radiology.

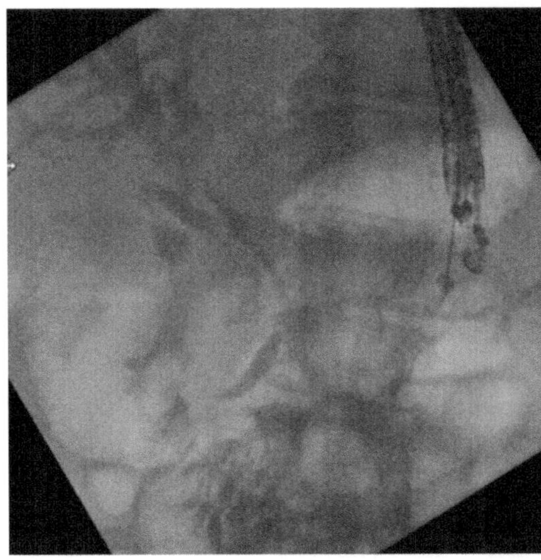

Fig. 18.2 Opacification of the pancreatic duct after contrast injection

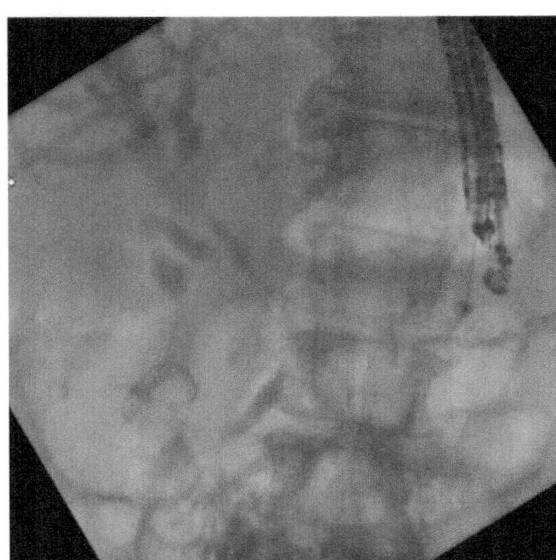

Fig. 18.3 Advancement of the guidewire across the ampulla in an antegrade fashion

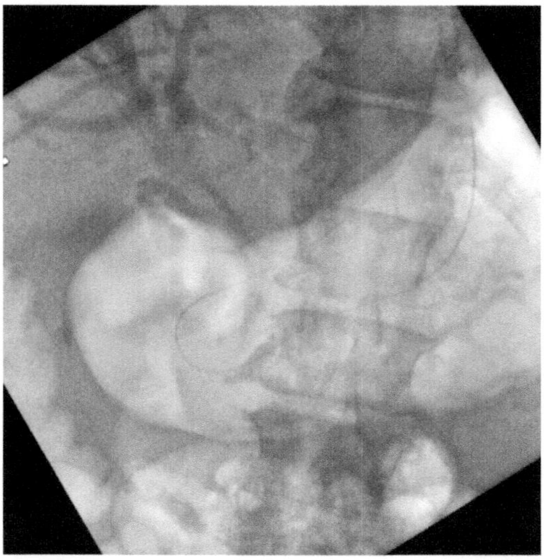

Fig. 18.4 Removal of the echoendoscope leaving the wire placed for the rendezvous

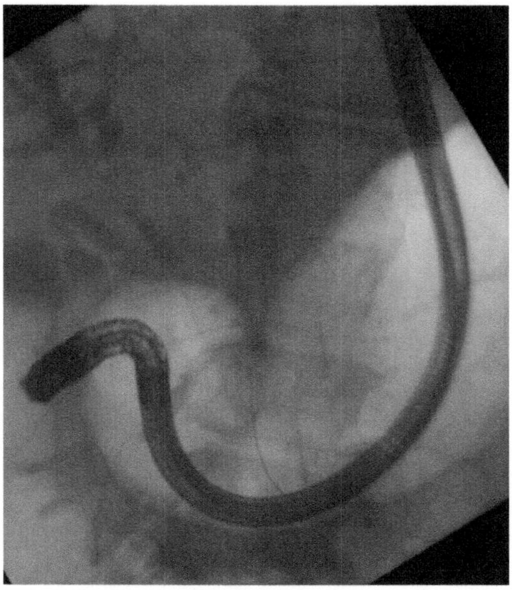

Fig. 18.5 Insertion of the duodenoscope facing the wire

Perforation in the stomach can be more easily managed than in the duodenum and typically include the placement of hemoclips or ovesco clip. Inability to perform a rendezvous can be seen in up to a third of the patients and is related either to a severe periampullary or anastomotic stricture. If a guidewire is still in the pancreatic duct during the procedure, we recommend decompressing the main pancreatic duct using a transgastric approach. In case a patient has severe calcified stone in the distal pancreatic duct, we always recommend ESWL before attempting a two-steps procedure which includes transgastric stent placement followed by laser lithotripsy [5].

References

1. Itoi T, Kasuya K, Sofuni A, et al. Endoscopic ultrasonography-guided pancreatic duct access: techniques and literature review of pancreatography, transmural drainage and rendezvous techniques. Dig Endosc. 2013;25(3):241–52. https://doi.org/10.1111/den.12048.
2. Harada N, Kouzu T, Arima M, Asano T, Kikuchi T, Isono K. Endoscopic ultrasound-guided pancreatography: a case report. Endoscopy. 1995;27(8):612–5. https://doi.org/10.1055/s-2007-1005769.
3. Shawn LS, Tyberg A. Endoscopic ultrasound-guided pancreatic duct drainage (EUS-PD). Springer nature Switzerland AG 2019 45 D. G. Adler (ed.). Interventional Endoscopic Ultrasound. https://doi.org/10.1007/978-3-319-97376-0_5.
4. Oh D, Park DH, Cho MK, et al. Feasibility and safety of a fully covered self-expandable metal stent with antimigration properties for EUS-guided pancreatic duct drainage: early and midterm outcomes (with video). Gastrointest Endosc. 2016;83(2):366–73.e2. https://doi.org/10.1016/j.gie.2015.07.015.
5. Novikov A, Kumta NA, Samstein B, Kahaleh M. Endoscopic ultrasound-guided transhepatic biliary drainage in altered anatomy: a two-step approach. Endoscopy. 2016;48(Suppl 1):E287. Epub 2016 Sep 14

EUS-PD for Pancreaticojejunostomy Stricture

19

Yukitoshi Matsunami and Takao Itoi

19.1 Background

For patients with a surgically altered anatomy (SAA), such as for those who have undergone pancreaticoduodenectomy, pancreatic duct drainage by endoscopic retrograde cholangiopancreatography (ERCP) for pancreaticojejunostomy stricture (PJS) is technically challenging. Recently, the short-type single- and the double-balloon enteroscopes have become available for pancreaticobiliary diseases. Despite the use of balloon enteroscope, there are still some hurdles. The difficulty of balloon enteroscopy-assisted ERCP (BE-ERCP) is dependent on the length of the afferent limb and the extent of the adhesion of the intestinal tract. Moreover, identification of the pancreatic ductal orifice may be challenging. One review demonstrated that the technical success rate of BE-ERCP for PJS was less than 30%, which was not a satisfactory outcome [1]. More recently, endoscopic ultrasonography-guided pancreatic duct drainage (EUS-PD) has been advocated as an alternative therapy for PJS [2]. EUS-PD is useful as a salvage therapy of PJS in patients who are not candidates for surgery or in those in whom BE-ERCP was unsuccessful. Herein, we describe a case of EUS-PD for PJS.

Supplementary Information The online version contains supplementary material available at [https://doi.org/10.1007/978-981-16-9340-3_19].

Y. Matsunami · T. Itoi (✉)
Department of Gastroenterology and Hepatology, Tokyo Medical University, Tokyo, Japan
e-mail: itoi@tokyo-med.ac.jp

19.2 Case History

A 52-year-old female, who had a past history of pylorus-preserving pancreaticoduodenectomy for pancreatic cystic lesion 7 years ago, was admitted for upper left abdominal and back pain. Since the surgery, the patient has had about five recurrences of pancreatitis. Physical examination showed upper left quadrant tenderness. Computed tomography (CT) showed that pancreatic duct dilation with peri-pancreatic inflammation of the remnant pancreas [Fig. 19.1a]. The features were compatible with acute recurrent pancreatitis owing to the PJS, and there was no evidence of tumor recurrence. Firstly BE-ERCP was attempted for drainage of dilated pancreatic duct; however, the identification of the pancreatic ductal orifice was unsuccessful. Therefore, the patient was referred to our institution to undergo the EUS-PD.

19.3 Procedural Plan

To understand the anatomy and the extent of pancreatic duct dilation in each patient, magnetic resonance cholangiopancreatography and/or

A. Y.B. Teoh et al. (eds.), *Atlas of Interventional EUS*, https://doi.org/10.1007/978-981-16-9340-3_19

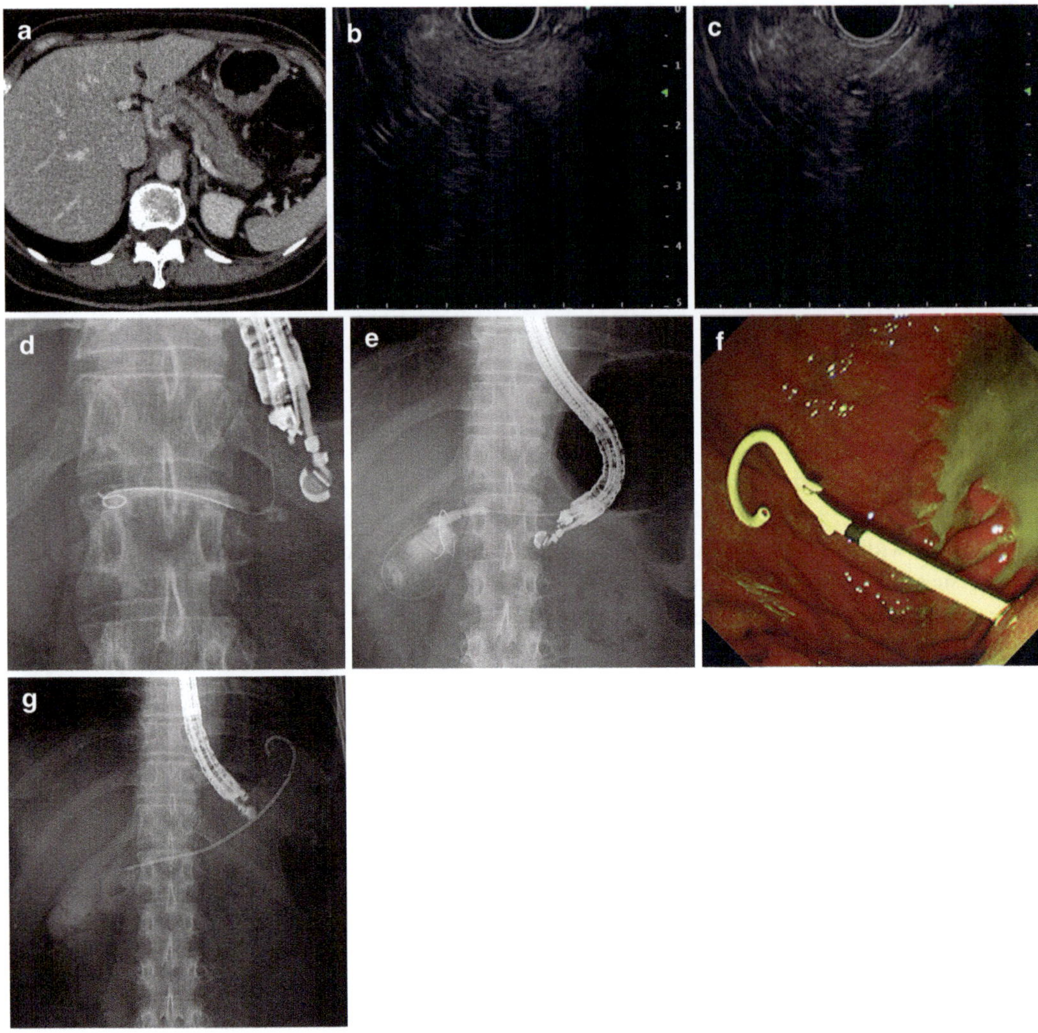

Fig. 19.1 Images of the EUS-PD procedure. (**a**) CT shows PJS with pancreatic duct dilation in whom patients with recurrent pancreatitis after pancreaticoduodenectomy. (**b**) EUS shows a fibrotic pancreatic parenchyma and dilated pancreatic duct. (**c**) A 22-gauge needle is advanced into the pancreatic duct. (**d**) A 0.018-inch guidewire is advanced into the pancreatic duct through the needle. (**e**) Bougie of anastomotic stricture is carried out using a 6 mm balloon dilator. (**f**) Pancreaticogastrostomy is completed using a 7Fr plastic stent (Through & Pass® Type IT; Gadelius Medical, Tokyo, Japan). An endoscopic view of stent placement. (**g**) A fluoroscopic view of stent placement

contrast-enhanced CT should be performed before the procedure. EUS-PD can be divided into two main categories, i.e., the rendezvous technique and transmural drainage. In the rendezvous technique, access to the pancreatic duct and passage of the guidewire is performed by EUS. Then, after exchanging the scope, retrieval of the guidewire and sequential ERCP with pancreatic duct stenting via anastomotic site is performed. Rendezvous pancreatic duct stenting is one option in case of guidewire passage into the anastomotic site. However, it takes time to change the scope and the procedure is more complicated than transmural drainage, especially in patients whose anatomy is surgically altered. In fact, most of the previously reported data showed that the indication of this technique is limited to patients with a normal anatomy and an accessible papilla

[3]. On the other hand, transmural EUS-guided pancreatic duct drainage, "EUS-PD" in a narrow sense, involves transmural needle puncture, guidewire passage, creation of a fistula, and transmural stenting, which is a more simple procedure than rendezvous technique [4, 5]. In the case of PJS, not a rendezvous technique, but an EUS-PD is more recommended for the following reasons. One is that the rendezvous technique requires longer procedural time owing to the balloon enteroscope insertion, which can lead to pancreatic juice leakage. Second is the ease of re-intervention. As most PJS are refractory and sustained, long-term follow-up with stent exchange is needed [6]. Once a fistula between the pancreatic duct and stomach is created by EUS-PD, it is not difficult to perform stent exchange. Re-access of the pancreatic duct is feasible from the created anastomotic hole or along the placed stent with using a therapeutic duodenoscope. On the other hand, once a stent is placed by rendezvous technique, insertion of balloon enteroscope is required in every single stent exchange procedure. Re-intervention after EUS-PD might be less time-consuming and technically easier than that of rendezvous technique. Owing to the above reasons, the patient was to be offered an EUS-PD.

19.4 Description of the Procedure

A therapeutic curved linear array echoendoscope was used under carbon dioxide. After confirming no intervening vessels using the Doppler mode, the pancreatic duct was punctured transgastrically [Fig. 19.1b, c] [Video 19.1]. In patients with a dilated pancreatic duct, a 19-gauge conventional sharp tip needle (SonoTip® Pro Control; Medi-Globe, Tokyo, Japan or EZ shot 3 Plus; Olympus Medical Systems, Tokyo, Japan) may be suitable for the puncture, as it enables the insertion of a 0.035-inch stiff guidewire. However, use of a 0.025-inch guidewire Visiglide2® (Olympus Medical Systems) is preferable, because it features a soft, highly flexible tip with outstanding radiopacity, sufficient stiffness at the guidewire shaft, and high seeking ability. In contrast, if the pancreatic duct is not dilated or if the parenchyma of the pancreas is fibrotic, a 22-gauge needle is preferable because it enables easy puncture. The patient's diameter of main pancreatic duct was 2.3 mm, and 22-gauge needle with a 0.018-inch guidewire was used [Fig. 19.1d]. After the guidewire placement, dilation of the needle tract was performed prior to stenting. An electrocautery dilator, a mechanical dilator, and a balloon dilator are available for bougieing the needle tract. In this case, ES dilator (7Fr, Zeon Medical, Tokyo, Japan), which is a plastic mechanical dilator whose tip is extremely tapered up to 2.5Fr, enables easy penetration, smooth insertion, and is less likely to cause bleeding and pancreatitis than an electrocautery dilator, was used for tract dilation [7]. However, if the pancreatic parenchyma is too hard to penetrate by mechanical dilator, an electrocautery dilator may be useful. The use of a coaxial electrocautery dilator, Cyst-gastro set (6.5Fr, Endoflex, Voerde, Germany) may be preferable to a precut papillotome, as the direction of cutting is along the axis of the tract. The anastomotic stricture was dilated by using a 6 mm REN (Kaneka Medix Corp, Osaka, Japan) balloon dilator [Fig. 19.1e]. This balloon dilator is designed for use with a 0.025-inch guidewire, and whose tip is more tapered and has high insertability and passability. After enough tract dilation, 7fr dedicated straight plastic stent with a proximal pigtail anchor was placed as pancreaticogastrostomy [Fig. 19.1f, g].

19.5 Post-procedural Management

Periprocedural antibiotics is recommended, as in other interventional EUS procedures [8]. A liquid diet is begun 1 or 2 days after the procedure after confirmation of the absence of pancreatitis. Then, the diet is advanced as tolerated by the patient, to a full diet. Stent exchange is planned every 3 to 4 months during the year after initial stent placement unless spontaneous stent dislodgement occurs. One year later, if the pancreatography shows no stricture with an improvement of pancreatic duct dilation, the stent is removed completely.

19.6 Potential Pitfalls

In the case of PJS, not all pancreatic duct dilations are an indication of EUS-PD, as asymptomatic pancreatic duct dilations with remnant gland atrophy are frequently observed in patients after pancreaticoduodenectomy [9]. In terms of patient symptoms, pancreatic pain with ductal dilation owing to PJS and/or obstructive stones causing recurrent pancreatitis is the agreeable indication. Regarding technical aspects, difficulty in accessing the site of PJS or unsuccessful ERCP are good indications. Contraindications of EUS-PD include an invisible or non-dilated pancreatic duct, a long distance from the stomach to the pancreatic duct, an intervening large vessel in the puncture route, marked thrombocytopenia, and anticoagulation therapy [10]. One literature review stated that technical success and adverse event (AEs) rates of EUS-PD were 78.7% and 21.8%, respectively [11]. Although most of the data were from tertiary referral centers and were performed by an expert, the technical success rate of EUS-PD was lower than that of other interventional EUS [8]. Possible reasons for this are that the targeted pancreatic duct is smaller than that of other interventional EUS, the stomach is anatomically not adhered to the pancreas and hence a change in breathing may cause difficulty in needle puncture, the fibrotic pancreatic parenchyma is technically difficult to puncture correctly even using a thin needle, and occasionally an optimum puncture angle cannot be obtained and a perpendicular puncture makes the sequential wire manipulation more difficult. The puncture point is recommended in more tail side of the remnant pancreatic duct, as far from anastomotic site as possible, to obtain sufficient length of the pancreatic duct for stent placement in case of inability to advance the guidewire across the anastomotic site, as the length of the remnant pancreatic duct is short. To prevent kinking and peeling of the guidewire at the tip of the needle, gentle wire manipulation is mandatory. Ideally, the guidewire should be advanced as long as possible in preparation for subsequent stenting. If the guidewire passes through the anastomotic stricture site, this stricture should also be dilated before stenting. Stents for drainage can be either plastic or metal; however, a plastic stent is more preferable than a metal stent, as the self-expandable metal stent has a higher risk of blockage of side branches of the pancreatic duct, leading to obstructive pancreatitis. A 7Fr straight plastic stent without a side hole in the middle part of the stent is most commonly used. Compared to a distal side pigtail stent, the straight stent has higher pushability and lower risk of slipping into the peritoneal cavity. However, the straight stent has a higher possibility of stent migration into the pancreatic duct [12]. Once a stent has migrated into the pancreatic duct, its retrieval by endoscopy is technically difficult and surgical stent removal may be required. From these viewpoints, ideal stent is thought to be a straight plastic stent with a proximal pigtail anchor, which has high pushability with preventing stent migration into the pancreatic duct [6, 13]. AEs associated with EUS-PD include pancreatitis, perforation, bleeding, peripancreatic pseudocyst/abscess formation, abdominal pain, pancreatic juice leakage, pneumoperitoneum, pseudoaneurysm, and shearing of the guidewire [12]. These adverse events lead to serious conditions, and therefore EUS-PD should be performed by experts of both interventional EUS and ERCP with highly experienced assistants in the setting of multidisciplinary support, which include endoscopist, surgeon, and radiologist [14]. In addition, the indication should be carefully discussed before the procedure.

References

1. Zarzavadjian Le Bian A, Cesaretti M, Tabchouri N, et al. Late pancreatic anastomosis stricture following pancreaticoduodenectomy: a systematic review. J Gastrointest Surg. 2018;22(11):2021–8.
2. Chen YI, Levy MJ, Moreels TG, et al. An international multicenter study comparing EUS-guided pancreatic duct drainage with enteroscopy-assisted endoscopic retrograde pancreatography after Whipple surgery. Gastrointest Endosc. 2017;85:170–7.
3. Ergun M, Aouattah T, Gillain C, et al. Endoscopic ultrasound-guided transluminal drainage of pancre-

atic duct obstruction: long-term outcome. Endoscopy. 2011;43(6):518–25.
4. Will U, Reichel A, Fueldner F, et al. Endoscopic ultrasonography-guided drainage for patients with symptomatic obstruction and enlargement of the pancreatic duct. World J Gastroenterol. 2015;21:13140–51.
5. Tyberg A, Sharaiha RZ, Kedia P, et al. EUS-guided pancreatic drainage for pancreatic strictures after failed ERCP: a multicenter international collaborative study. Gastrointest Endosc. 2017;65:164–9.
6. Mastunami Y, Itoi T, Sofuni A, et al. Evaluation of a new stent for EUS-guided pancreatic duct drainage: long-term follow-up outcome. Endos Int Open. 2018;06:E505–12.
7. Honjyo M, Itoi T, Tsuchiya T, et al. Safety and efficacy of ultra-tapered mechanical dilator for EUS-guided hepaticogastrostomy and pancreatic duct drainage compared with electrocautery dilator (with video) endoscopic. Ultrasound. 2018;7:376–82.
8. Dhir V, Isayama H, Itoi T, Almadi M, Siripun A, Teoh AY, et al. Endoscopic ultrasonography-guided biliary and pancreatic duct interventions. Dig Endosc. 2017;29:472–85.
9. Cioffi JL, McDuffie LA, Roch AM, et al. Pancreaticojejunostomy stricture after Pancreatoduodenetomy: outcomes after operative revision. J Gastrointest Surg. 2016;20:293–9.
10. Itoi T, Kasuya K, Sofuni A, et al. Endoscopic ultrasonography-guided pancreatic duct access: technique and literature review of pancreatography, transmural drainage and rendezvous techniques. Dig Endosc. 2013;25:241–52.
11. Nakai Y, Kogure H, Isayama H, et al. Endoscopic ultrasound guided pancreatic duct drainage. Saudi J Gastroenterol. 2019;25(4):210–7.
12. Fujii LL, Topazian MD, Abu Dayyeh BK, et al. EUS-guided pancreatic duct intervention: outcomes of a single tertiary-care referral center experience. Gastrointest Endosc. 2013;78(6):854–64.
13. Itoi T, Sofuni A, Tsuchiya T, et al. Initial evaluation of a new plastic pancreatic duct stent for endoscopic ultrasonography-guided placement. Endoscopy. 2015;47:462–5.
14. Teoh AY, Dhir V, Kida M, Yasuda I, Jin ZD, Seo DW, et al. Consensus guidelines on the optimal management in interventional EUS procedures: results from the Asian EUS group RAND/UCLA expert panel. Gut. 2018;67:1209–28.

Part IV

EUS-Guided Celiac Plexus Ablation

EUS-Guided Celiac Plexus Neurolysis

20

Neil Marya, Tarek Sawas, and Michael J. Levy

20.1 Background

Endoscopic ultrasound-guided celiac plexus neurolysis (EUS-CPN) is an endoscopic procedure performed to manage the debilitating and refractory chronic pain caused by pancreatic cancer [1] and chronic pancreatitis [2]. Although CPN could be performed percutaneously under ultrasound or computed tomography (CT) guidance [3], EUS has the advantage of easily identifying and getting in close proximity to the celiac plexus, which enhances needle localization and the spread of the injected material and potentially minimizes adverse events and improves pain response [4]. Under EUS guidance, the celiac plexus is injected with a mixture of bupivacaine (0.25%) and dehydrated alcohol (99%) for neurolysis. When EUS-CPN is used for chronic pancreatitis, alcohol is substituted by steroid (Triamcinolone 80 mg) for what is referred to as celiac plexus block.

Supplementary Information The online version contains supplementary material available at [https://doi.org/10.1007/978-981-16-9340-3_20].

N. Marya
Division of Gastroenterology, University of Massachusetts, Worcester, MA, USA

T. Sawas
Digestive and Liver Diseases Division, University of Texas Southwestern, Dallas, TX, USA

M. J. Levy (✉)
Division of Gastroenterology and Hepatology, Mayo Clinic, Rochester, MN, USA
e-mail: levy.michael@mayo.edu

20.2 Case History

An 80-year-old male with type 2 diabetes, coronary artery disease, and atrial fibrillation was referred to our clinic with severe abdominal pain, after a newly diagnosed metastatic pancreatic cancer. He reported 12 months history of left flank pain, which progressed and formed a band around his upper abdomen. Alongside his pain, he lost 25 lb. CT abdomen showed a poorly defined 2.6 × 2.4 × 2 cm pancreatic body mass abutting the spleno-portal confluence with a 1.5 cm metastatic lesion in segment 5 of the liver (Fig. 20.1). EUS with fine-needle aspiration (FNA) from the pancreatic mass revealed adenocarcinoma. The severity of the abdominal and back pain caused insomnia despite multiple narcotics use including Hydrocodone-Acetaminophen 10–325 mg as needed and Oxycodone 10 mg every 8 h as needed. The patient was offered palliative chemotherapy but he refused given his poor expected survival and other comorbidities. He expressed his interest in palliative therapy with the goal of getting his pain under control. Therefore, EUS-CPN was offered since his pain had been difficult to control with oral pain medications.

A. Y.B. Teoh et al. (eds.), *Atlas of Interventional EUS*, https://doi.org/10.1007/978-981-16-9340-3_20

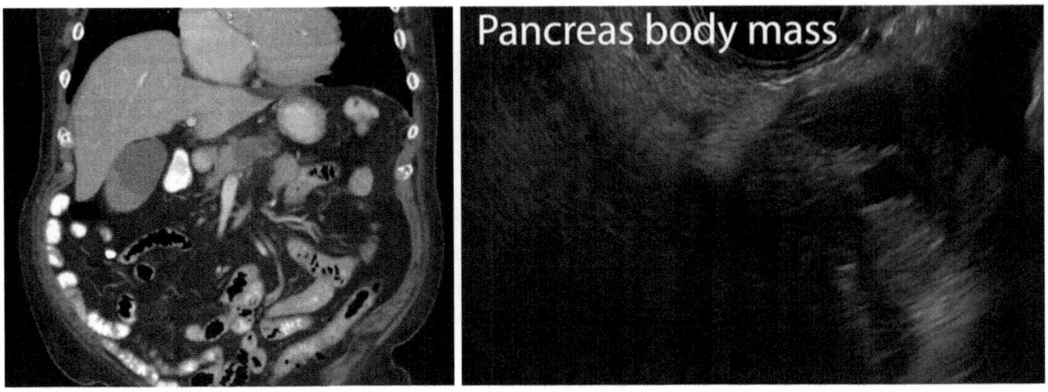

Fig. 20.1 Poorly defined 2.6 × 2.4 × 2 cm pancreatic body mass abutting the spleno-portal confluence on CT (*left*) and EUS (*right*)

20.3 Procedural Plan

CPN can be performed percutaneously or EUS guided via a transgastric approach. However, EUS-CPN is the preferred method and has been shown to be a safer and more effective option. There are two main methods of performing EUS-CPN. The conventional EUS-CPN is performed by diffusely injecting throughout the celiac plexus region after identifying the celiac artery origin from the aorta. The second method is performed by directly injecting into the celiac ganglia.

In a meta-analysis of 8 studies including 283 patients with pancreatic cancer-related pain who underwent EUS-CPN, 80% of patients witnessed pain relief [5]. In the same meta-analysis, patients who received bilateral injections on both sides of the celiac artery had better pain relief (85%) compared to those who received an injection on one side only (46%). In a randomized controlled trial of 96 patients with unresectable pancreatic adenocarcinoma comparing early EUS-CPN to conventional pharmacological pain management, patients managed with early EUS-CPN had significantly higher pain relief with no difference in quality of life scores or survival [6]. A special 20-gauge spray needle with side holes (EUSN-20-CPN: Cook Endoscopy, Winston-Salem, NC) is available for the purpose of spreading the injected material. However, the traditional 22-gauge EUS-FNA needle is sufficient for the purpose of this procedure.

The second technique is performed by directly injecting the celiac ganglia (CGN). Although initially there was a misconception that the celiac plexus could not be identified as a distinct structure, it is now known that celiac plexus can be identified directly with the EUS [7]. This recognition allowed direct injection into the celiac ganglia [8]. This is technique is similar to the first method with few modifications. This approach targets as many ganglia as possible. We target and inject the center point of the ganglia smaller than 1 cm. Whereas in ganglia larger than 1 cm, we start injecting at the deepest point then we slowly withdraw the needle and inject alongside the needle tract. Direct injection is typically associated with the immediate onset of pain. This is usually recognized by altered vital signs (pulse and respiration), increased movement, and attempted verbalization. This acute pain usually lasts few seconds only. In a study including 17 patients with pancreatic cancer who underwent CGN, pain relief was reported by 94% of patients [8].

We usually avoid CPN when the tumor infiltrates the celiac artery or the celiac plexus. Data have demonstrated a lack of response when the celiac plexus is involved. Another consideration before performing CPN is tumor resectability. EUS-CPN creates inflammation and fibrosis and makes surgical resection more difficult and therefore it should be reserved for patients who are not surgical candidates [9]. Finally, we assure correction of coagulopathy and thrombocytopenia before proceeding with the procedure. We recommend international normalize ratio (INR) <1.5 and Platelets >50,000/L.

20.4 Description of the Procedure

The procedure was performed in the outpatient setting under deep conscious sedation. The linear EUS scope was positioned in the stomach. The celiac artery origin from the aorta was then identified from the posterior lesser curvature of the proximal stomach. The celiac artery is the first branch originating from the aorta under the diaphragm. The celiac ganglia were visualized directly to the left of the celiac artery and appeared as a hypoechoic, oval-shaped structure (Fig. 20.2, Video 20.1). A 22-gauge needle was primed with normal saline to remove air from the needle. The needle was advanced through the working channel of the EUS scope and fixed in place. Color Doppler was used to assure the absence of any vascular structure along the anticipated needle tract. The celiac ganglion was then punctured directly under EUS guidance using a 22-gauge needle. The needle is then flushed with 3 cc of normal saline to remove any tissue that could have entered the needle during the insertion part. Aspiration was performed to rule out penetration of an adjacent vascular structure. The celiac ganglion was then injected with 20 ml of 99% dehydrated alcohol and 4 ml of bupivacaine for CPN. The injected alcohol created an echogenic cloud. The needle was flushed with 3 cc of normal saline before withdrawal to avoid alcohol seeding along the needle tract, which could result in severe post-procedural pain.

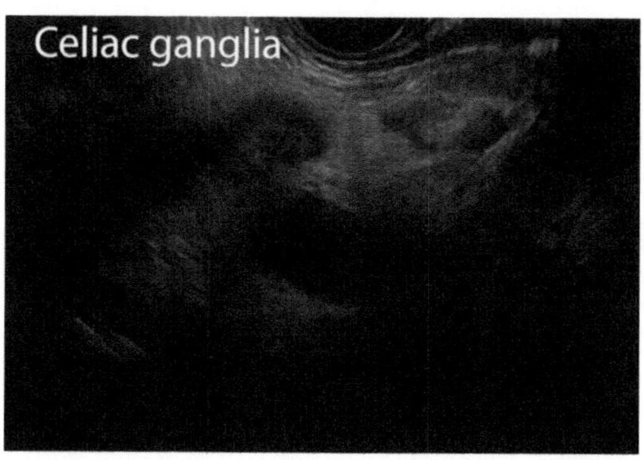

Fig. 20.2 The celiac ganglia visualized on endoscopic ultrasound (EUS) directly to the left of the celiac artery

20.5 Post-procedural Management

Blood pressure and orthostatic blood pressure are monitored closely in the post-operative area for 2 hours after the procedure. Diet as tolerated can be resumed immediately after the procedure. There is no need for antibiotics. Initial pain exacerbation can also occur and usually predict a better response to CPN [8]. Transient diarrhea and hypotension are common manifestations as a result of sympathetic blockade and unopposed parasympathetic activity.

20.6 Potential Pitfalls

Patients with unresectable pancreatic cancer and abdominal pain requiring opioid analgesics are potential candidates for CPN. CPN was more effective when performed early after pain onset rather than late in its course. Patients with chronic pancreatitis and refractor pain on high opiates doses are other potential candidates. Avoid CPN if the tumor is invading the celiac artery or the celiac plexus. The potential risks and adverse events should be properly discussed with the patient including transient and self-limited diarrhea, hypotension, constipation, nausea, vomiting, and lethargy. Initial hydration with 500–1000 cc of normal saline can ameliorate the severity of hypotension. While extremely rare, patients should be made aware of the potential of neurologic adverse events such as lower extremities paralysis, weakness, and bilateral diaphragmatic paralysis [10].

References

1. Eisenberg E, Carr DB, Chalmers TC. Neurolytic celiac plexus block for treatment of cancer pain: a meta-analysis. Anesth Analg. 1995;80:290–5.
2. Kaufman M, Singh G, Das S, et al. Efficacy of endoscopic ultrasound-guided celiac plexus block and

celiac plexus neurolysis for managing abdominal pain associated with chronic pancreatitis and pancreatic cancer. J Clin Gastroenterol. 2010;44:127–34.
3. Wang PJ, Shang MY, Qian Z, et al. CT-guided percutaneous neurolytic celiac plexus block technique. Abdom Imaging. 2006;31:710–8.
4. Gress F, Schmitt C, Sherman S, et al. A prospective randomized comparison of endoscopic ultrasound- and computed tomography-guided celiac plexus block for managing chronic pancreatitis pain. Am J Gastroenterol. 1999;94:900–5.
5. Puli SR, Reddy JB, Bechtold ML, et al. EUS-guided celiac plexus neurolysis for pain due to chronic pancreatitis or pancreatic cancer pain: a meta-analysis and systematic review. Dig Dis Sci. 2009;54: 2330–7.
6. Wyse JM, Carone M, Paquin SC, et al. Randomized, double-blind, controlled trial of early endoscopic ultrasound-guided celiac plexus neurolysis to prevent pain progression in patients with newly diagnosed, painful, inoperable pancreatic cancer. J Clin Oncol. 2011;29:3541–6.
7. Levy M, Rajan E, Keeney G, et al. Neural ganglia visualized by endoscopic ultrasound. Am J Gastroenterol. 2006;101:1787–91.
8. Levy MJ, Topazian MD, Wiersema MJ, et al. Initial evaluation of the efficacy and safety of endoscopic ultrasound-guided direct ganglia neurolysis and block. Am J Gastroenterol. 2008;103:98–103.
9. Wyse JM, Battat R, Sun S, et al. Practice guidelines for endoscopic ultrasound-guided celiac plexus neurolysis. Endosc Ultrasound. 2017;6:369–75.
10. Mulhall AM, Rashkin MC, Pina EM. Bilateral diaphragmatic paralysis: a rare complication related to endoscopic ultrasound-guided celiac plexus neurolysis. Ann Am Thorac Soc. 2016;13:1660–2.

21 EUS-Guided Celiac Ganglia Neurolysis

Ichiro Yasuda and Shinpei Doi

21.1 Background

EUS-guided celiac ganglia neurolysis (EUS-CGN) is a modified technique of EUS-guided celiac plexus neurolysis (EUS-CPN). In this technique, the celiac ganglia (CG) are punctured and a neurolytic agent is directly injected into them, whereas the agent is injected at the base (the central technique) or on both sides (the bilateral technique) of the celiac axis in EUS-CPN. EUS-CPN and EUS-CGN can be performed for alleviating pain originating from the upper abdominal organs. In particular, their most prominent indication is pancreatic cancer pain, because pain is a common symptom reported in approximately 80% of patients with advanced pancreatic cancer, representing a major issue in the management of patients [1].

Supplementary Information The online version contains supplementary material available at [https://doi.org/10.1007/978-981-16-9340-3_21].

I. Yasuda (✉)
Third Department of Internal Medicine, University of Toyama, Toyama, Japan
e-mail: yasudaic@med.u-toyama.ac.jp

S. Doi
Department of Gastroenterology, Teikyo University Mizonokuchi Hospital, Kawasaki, Japan

21.2 Case History

A 66-year-old man was admitted for epigastric and back pain. Computed tomography revealed a hypovascular mass with a diameter of 5 cm in the body of the pancreas, with dilation of the upstream main pancreatic duct and multiple liver masses (Fig. 21.1). After pathological confirmation of pancreatic cancer with multiple liver metastases by EUS-FNA, chemotherapy was commenced. Additionally, pain medication was attempted, starting with nonsteroidal anti-inflammatory drugs (NSAIDs) and progression to incremental doses of opioid analgesics. However, the pain management was inadequate, and increasing the opioid dose was difficult because of adverse effects such as nausea, constipation, and somnolence. Therefore, EUS-CGN was suggested.

21.3 Procedural Plan

In cases such as the current one, the central or bilateral technique of CPN as well as EUS-CGN can be performed. However, in our previous randomized controlled trial, the response rate for pain relief was demonstrated to be significantly higher with EUS-CGN than with the central technique of EUS-CPN [2]. Another retrospective comparative study suggested that EUS-CGN was more effective than the bilateral technique of

A. Y.B. Teoh et al. (eds.), *Atlas of Interventional EUS*, https://doi.org/10.1007/978-981-16-9340-3_21

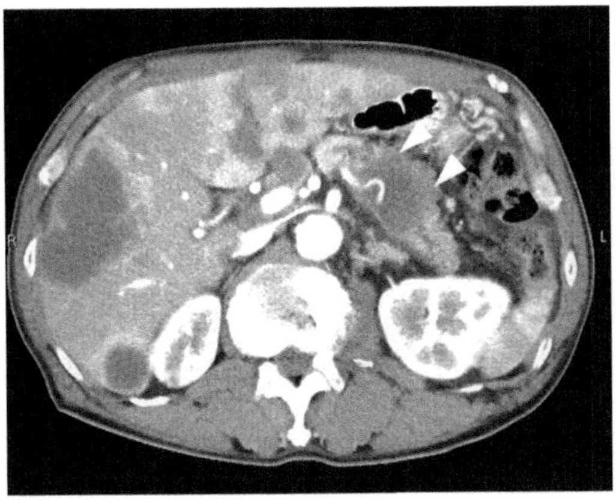

Fig. 21.1 Computed tomography showing a hypovascular mass in the body of the pancreas with dilation of the upstream main pancreatic duct and multiple liver masses

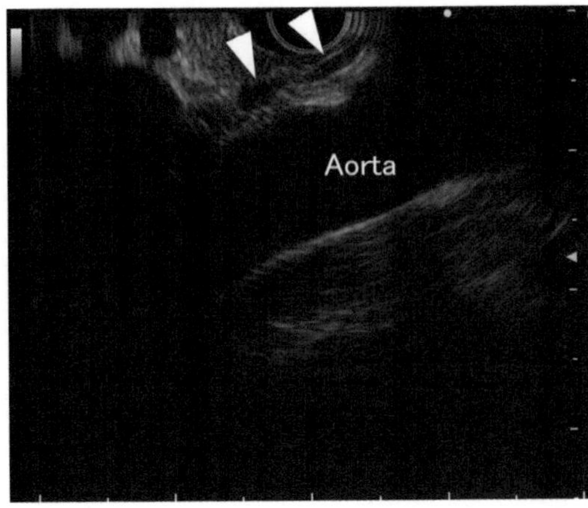

Fig. 21.2 Celiac ganglia observed on EUS

EUS-CPN [3]. Furthermore, the puncture target is clearer in EUS-CGN than in bilateral EUS-CPN if the CG is visible. Therefore, we prefer EUS-CGN in our clinical practice [4]. In terms of the puncture needle, a 22-gauge or 25-gauge needle is used, although it is easier to puncture the target with a 25-gauge needle than with a 22-gauge needle because of its sharpness. However, the use of a 22-gauge needle is preferred because higher resistance is observed and greater effort is required for pushing the syringe's piston while injecting the neurolytic agent when a 25-gauge needle is used [2, 5].

21.4 Description of the Procedure

In most patients, by repeated gradual clockwise and counterclockwise rotation of the echoendoscope between the aorta and left adrenal gland, CG can be observed in this region, at the level between the celiac and left renal arteries (Fig. 21.2). Additionally, they may be located cephalad to the origin of the celiac axis [4]. After identification of the CG, each ganglion is punctured and the neurolytic agent, namely, absolute ethanol, is injected into it (Video 21.1). The punctures are usually made in an order corresponding to the distance from the EUS probe. The farthest ganglion is punctured first, such that the visualization of other CG at the proximal side can be hindered after the agent is injected. A needle is advanced to puncture the target ganglion (Fig. 21.3), and absolute ethanol is injected. The volume of injected ethanol was, previously, 1 mL for small CG (smaller than 5 mm in diameter) and 3–5 mL for relatively large CG. However, recently, we have injected more ethanol (more than 3 mL) even in small CG, which helps in wider distribution of the agent. The agent may thus reach unidentified CG, which might result in a better effect [6]. However, we do not inject bupivacaine prior to ethanol injection in this technique because the neurolytic effect of ethanol can be weakened by dilution.

21.5 Post-procedural Management

Diets can be resumed following the day of the procedure. Prophylactic antibiotics are not required. Pain is evaluated after the operation. In case of inadequate pain relief, secondary interventional therapies (repeated EUS-CGN, EUS-CPN, initiation of narcotic therapy, or increase in the dose of narcotic agents) are considered. According to our data, complete and partial pain relief was obtained in 50.0% and 73.5% of the patients, respectively. A positive response was retained for 8 months in approximately 70% of the patients [2].

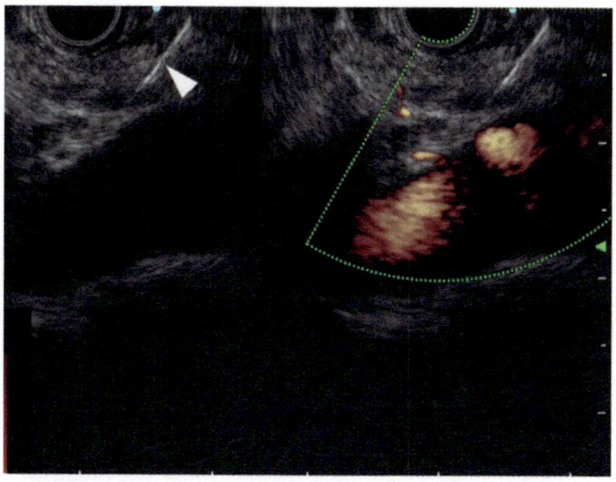

Fig. 21.3 A needle puncturing the celiac ganglion

21.6 Potential Pitfalls

The potential adverse events during and after EUS-CGN include transient hypotension, pain exacerbation, and diarrhea and inebriation. However, these are generally minor and do not require specific treatment [4]. This technique has a technical limitation. CG visualization may not always be possible, suggesting that there is a learning curve for their detection, although according to our experience, CG can be visualized in all cases. However, when the ganglia cannot be identified, EUS-CPN is performed [2, 4].

References

1. Koulouris AI, Banim P, Hart AR. Pain in patients with pancreatic cancer: prevalence, mechanisms, management and future developments. Dig Dis Sci. 2017;62(4):861–70.
2. Doi S, Yasuda I, Kawakami H, Hayashi T, Hisai H, Irisawa A, et al. Endoscopic ultrasound-guided celiac ganglia neurolysis vs. celiac plexus neurolysis: a randomized multicenter trial. Endoscopy. 2013;45(5):362–9.
3. Ascunce G, Ribeiro A, Reis I, Rocha-Lima C, Sleeman D, Merchan J, et al. EUS visualization and direct celiac ganglia neurolysis predicts better pain relief in patients with pancreatic malignancy (with video). Gastrointest Endosc. 2011;73(2):267–74.
4. Teoh AYB, Dhir V, Kida M, Yasuda I, Jin ZD, Seo DW, et al. Consensus guidelines on the optimal management in interventional EUS procedures: results from the Asian EUS group RAND/UCLA expert panel. Gut. 2018;67(7):1209–28.
5. Yasuda I, Wang HP. Endoscopic ultrasound-guided celiac plexus block and neurolysis. Dig Endosc. 2017;29(4):455–62.
6. Kappelle WFW, Bleys R, van Wijck AJM, Siersema PD, Vleggaar FP. EUS-guided celiac ganglia neurolysis: a clinical and human cadaver study (with video). Gastrointest Endosc. 2017;86(4):655–63.

EUS-Guided Broad Plexus Neurolysis

22

Masayuki Kitano, Keiichi Hatamaru, and Kosuke Minaga

22.1 Background

Since it was initially described in 1996 [1], endoscopic ultrasound-guided celiac plexus neurolysis (EUS-CPN) has been widely applied as a minimally invasive approach to block abdominal visceral nerves and relieve chronic cancer pain caused by upper abdominal malignancies. In EUS-CPN, a local anesthetic and a neurolytic agent are injected into and around the celiac plexus via the transgastric anterior approach under EUS guidance.

Two meta-analyses reported the pain-alleviation rates for unresectable pancreatic cancer to be 73–80%, with a treatment duration of approximately 1–2 months [2, 3]. To improve the efficacy of this EUS-guided technique, two new modified EUS-CPN approaches have been developed: EUS-guided celiac ganglia neurolysis (EUS-CGN) [4] and EUS-guided broad plexus neurolysis (EUS-BPN) [5]. EUS-BPN is a technique in which a needle is advanced deeply into the plexus around the origin of the superior mesenteric artery (SMA) to produce a wide distribution of the neurolytic agent. EUS-BPN has been shown to provide significantly better pain relief than conventional EUS-CPN in patients whose tumors have extended beyond the SMA [5]. Furthermore, EUS-BPN in combination with EUS-CGN was reported to be a predictor of good pain-relief response for pancreatic cancer-associated pain [6].

22.2 Case History

A 72-year-old woman with advanced pancreatic cancer was admitted for pain control. The patient suffered from chronic abdomen and back pain. Computed tomography (CT) showed widespread pancreatic body cancer extending from the periphery of the celiac artery and the SMA. The imaging findings revealed that her pain was caused by neuropathic pain from cancer invasion of the splanchnic nerves. Therefore, we provided her with EUS-BPN.

Supplementary Information The online version contains supplementary material available at [https://doi.org/10.1007/978-981-16-9340-3_22].

M. Kitano (✉) · K. Hatamaru
Second Department of Internal Medicine, Wakayama Medical University, Wakayama, Japan
e-mail: kitano@wakayama-med.ac.jp; papepo51@wakayama-med.ac.jp

K. Minaga
Departement of Gastroenterology and Hepatology, Kindai University Faculty of Medicine, Osaka, Japan

A. Y.B. Teoh et al. (eds.), *Atlas of Interventional EUS*, https://doi.org/10.1007/978-981-16-9340-3_22

22.3 Procedural Plan

Among the different EUS-guided approaches, we prefer to perform EUS-BPN with the belief that widespread drug distribution contributes to better pain relief. During EUS-guided neurolysis, it is recommended to locate the injection target at the shortest distance from the stomach while confirming the tip of the puncture needle under real-time EUS guidance. Real-time observation with high-resolution EUS allows for safer treatment and fewer complications than CPN guided by conventional transabdominal ultrasound or CT [6–8].

In EUS-BPN, the puncture needle is advanced beyond the level of the celiac trunk, and the drugs are injected around the SMA trunk. It has been reported that this results in more effective pain relief in patients with extensive tumor extension [5]. To ensure safety and flexibility while advancing the puncture needle deeply into the target area, the use of a small-diameter 25-gauge aspiration needle is preferable. Before the needle puncture, we prepare a syringe filled with 3 ml of 1% Lidocaine and another syringe filled with anhydrous ethanol mixed with a water-soluble contrast medium.

22.4 Description of the Procedure (Video 22.1)

EUS-BPN is a recently developed variation of EUS-guided neurolysis that was first described in 2010 [5]. EUS-BPN was performed using a convex array echoendoscope (GF-UCT 260; Olympus Medical Systems, Tokyo, Japan) together with an image analysis processor (ALOKA ProSound SSD α10; Hitachi Aloka Medical, Ltd., Tokyo, Japan).

When the echoendoscope was advanced into the stomach, the echoendoscope tip was deflected upward so that the US probe made contact with the gastric wall. Subsequently, the echoendoscope was rotated so that a longitudinal image of the aorta could be seen, and it was then advanced until the celiac trunk could be seen branching anteriorly and inferiorly from the aorta (Fig. 22.1). At a point 1–2 cm inferior to the celiac trunk, the SMA trunk branching from the aorta could be similarly visualized (Fig. 22.1). These vascular landmarks were confirmed by color Doppler imaging. At the SMA level, the probe was gradually rotated clockwise toward the patient's left side until the SMA origin could no longer be visualized but the aorta could still be seen. A 25-gauge needle filled with normal saline solution was advanced adjacent and anterior to the lateral aspect of the aorta at a level next to the SMA trunk under direct EUS visualization (Fig. 22.2). An aspiration test was then performed. To prevent transient neurolytic agent-induced pain, 3 ml of local anesthetic agent consisting of 1% lidocaine was first injected. Subsequently, a neurolytic agent consisting of a mixed solution of 9 ml absolute alcohol and 1 ml contrast medium was injected up to a maximum

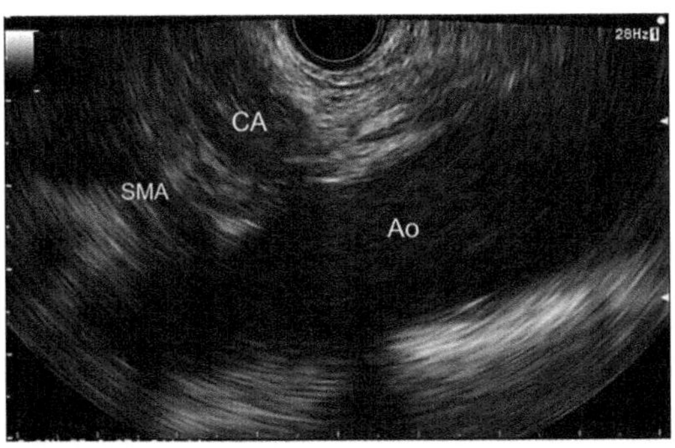

Fig. 22.1 EUS image of EUS-guided broad plexus neurolysis (BPN) before needle puncture. The celiac artery (CA), superior mesenteric artery (SMA), and aorta (Ao) were visualized on EUS

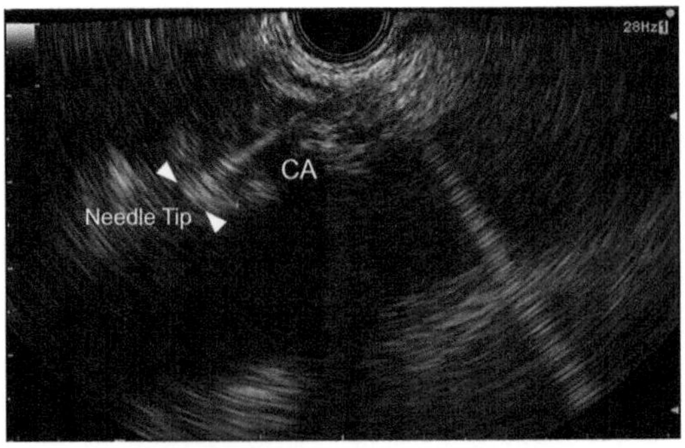

Fig. 22.2 EUS image of EUS-BPN during needle puncture. A 25-gauge needle was advanced adjacent to the SMA trunk. The needle tip is shown by arrowheads

volume of 10 ml. The needle was then withdrawn from the patient, flushed with saline solution.

22.5 Post-procedural Management

Immediately after the treatment, CT was performed to assess the spread of the mixture of neurolytic agents and contrast medium around the celiac, superior, and inferior mesenteric areas, and to evaluate the relationship between pain relief and contrast-bearing areas (Fig. 22.3). To evaluate the spread pattern, the region examined on CT, including the celiac artery and SMA, was divided into six areas: upper right and left (above the celiac artery), middle right and left (between the celiac artery and SMA), and lower right and left (below the SMA) (Fig. 22.3). In this case, neurolytic/contrast agents were spread over all six areas on post-procedural CT obtained immediately after EUS-BPN (Fig. 22.3). Previous studies showed that the pain-alleviation rate correlated with the number of neurolytic/contrast agent-bearing areas [5, 6]. If sufficient spread of the neurolytic/contrast agent across the areas is not observed on CT, a repeat EUS-guided neurolysis may be an option [9].

Although EUS-guided neurolysis has been shown to be a safe procedure, side effects and complications can occur during and after the procedure. Most of the side effects and complications associated with EUS-guided neurolysis are not severe and are self-limiting, usually lasting less than 2 days [10]. Frequent complications associated with EUS-guided neurolysis include diarrhea, hypotension, drunkenness, and a transient increase in pain [5, 10, 11]. Although serious complications are as low as about 0.2% [11], some severe hemorrhagic and ischemic complications, which can be fatal, have been reported [12–14]. To date, four cases of paraplegia due to spinal cord infarction [15–18] and one case of acute respiratory failure due to bilateral diaphragmatic paralysis [19] have been reported. Therefore, postoperative management should be performed with intensive care, considering the possibility of serious complications.

22.6 Potential Pitfalls

There are a few pitfalls to the EUS approach for broad plexus neurolysis if the procedure is performed carefully. Although rare, it may sometimes not be possible to visualize anatomical landmarks to ensure correct needle-tip placement because of postoperative change or a large tumor mass. In addition, cachexia can cause a loss of soft tissue space between the gastric wall and aorta, leaving little space for the tip of the needle to be placed, and dilation or anomaly of the arteries can also cause technical difficulties. Therefore, a detailed preoperative simulation should be performed with 3D-CT angiography, if available. As EUS-BPN has only been reported from a single University Hospital at the time of writing [5, 6], a multicenter study with a larger cohort is required to confirm its efficacy and safety.

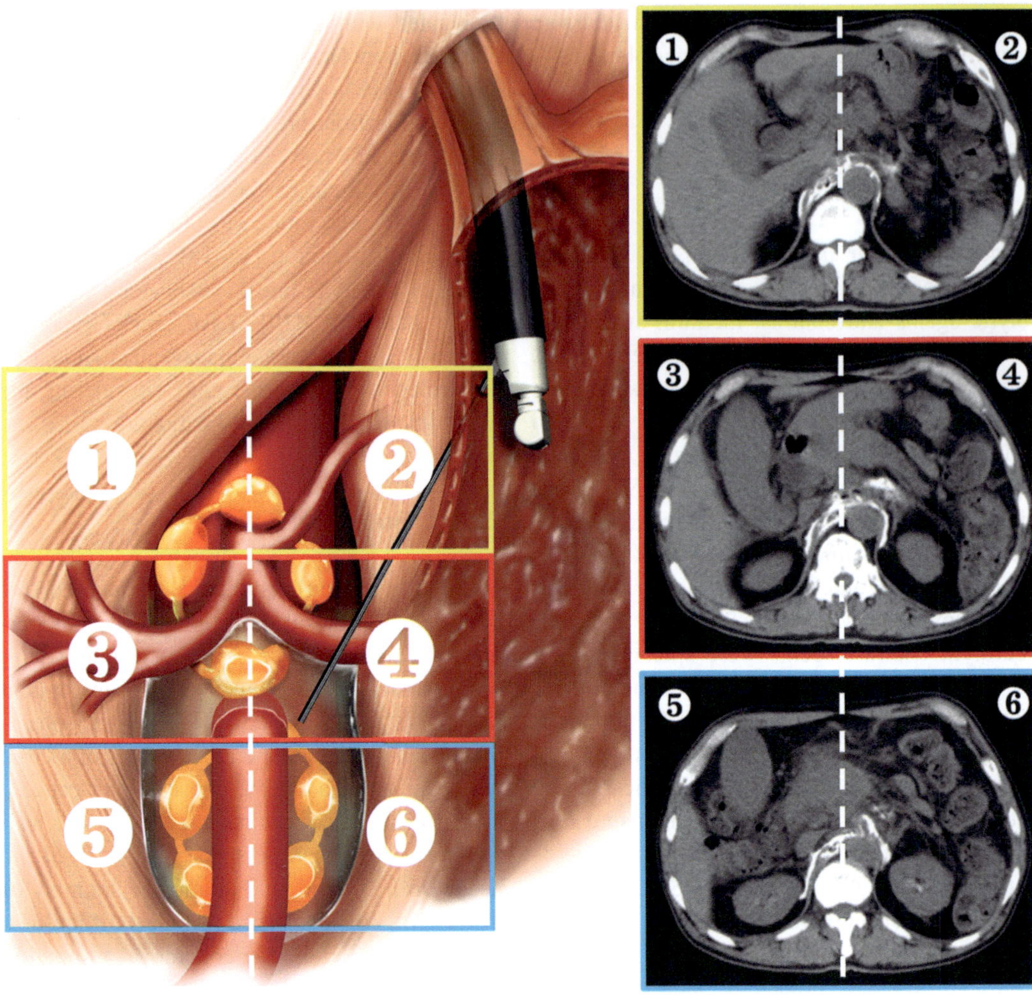

Fig. 22.3 Left (reproduced with permission from Therap Adv Gastroenterol. 2016;9:483–94). Division of the celiac, superior mesenteric, and inferior mesenteric regions into six areas: two upper areas (❶, upper right; ❷, upper left), two middle areas, (❸, middle right; ❹, middle left), and two lower areas (❺, lower right; ❻, lower left). Right. Post-procedural distribution of neurolytic/contrast agents on computed tomography (CT). Neurolytic/contrast agents were spread over all six areas

References

1. Wiersema MJ, Wiersema LM. Endosonography—guided celiac plexus neurolysis. Gastrointest Endosc. 1996;44:656–62.
2. Puli SR, Reddy JB, Bechtold ML, Antillon MR, Brugge WR. EUS-guided celiac plexus neurolysis for pain due to chronic pancreatitis or pancreatic cancer pain: a meta-analysis and systematic review. Dig Dis Sci. 2009;54:2330–7.
3. Kaufman M, Singh G, Das S, Concha-Parra R, Erber J, Micames C, Gress F. Efficacy of endoscopic ultrasound-guided celiac plexus block and celiac plexus neurolysis for managing abdominal pain associated with chronic pancreatitis and pancreatic cancer. J Clin Gastroenterol. 2010;44:127–34.
4. Levy MJ, Topazian MD, Wiersema MJ, Clain JE, Rajan E, Wang KK, et al. Initial evaluation of the efficacy and safety of endoscopic ultrasound-guided direct Ganglia neurolysis and block. Am J Gastroenterol. 2008;103:98–103.
5. Sakamoto H, Kitano M, Kamata K, Komaki T, Imai H, Chikugo T, et al. EUS-guided broad plexus neurolysis over the superior mesenteric artery using a 25-gauge needle. Am J Gastroenterol. 2010;105:2599–606.
6. Minaga K, Kitano M, Sakamoto H, Miyata T, Imai H, Yamao K, et al. Predictors of pain response in patients

undergoing endoscopic ultrasound-guided neurolysis for abdominal pain caused by pancreatic cancer. Therap Adv Gastroenterol. 2016;9:483–94.
7. Santosh D, Lakhtakia S, Gupta R, Reddy DN, Rao GV, Tandan M, et al. Clinical trial: a randomized trial comparing fluoroscopy guided percutaneous technique vs. endoscopic ultrasound guided technique of coeliac plexus block for treatment of pain in chronic pancreatitis. Aliment Pharmacol Ther. 2009;29:979–84.
8. Gress F, Schmitt C, Sherman S, Ikenberry S, Lehman G. A prospective randomized comparison of endoscopic ultrasound- and computed tomography-guided celiac plexus block for managing chronic pancreatitis pain. Am J Gastroenterol. 1999;94:900–5.
9. Facciorusso A, Del Prete V, Antonino M, Buccino VR, Muscatiello N. Response to repeat echoendoscopic celiac plexus neurolysis in pancreatic cancer patients: A machine learning approach. Pancreatology. 2019;19:866–72.
10. O'Toole TM, Schmulewitz N. Complication rates of EUS-guided celiac plexus blockade and neurolysis: Results of a large case series. Endoscopy. 2009;41:593–7.
11. Alvarez-Sánchez MV, Jenssen C, Faiss S, Napoléon B. Interventional endoscopic ultrasonography: an overview of safety and complications. Surg Endosc. 2014;28:712–34.
12. Minaga K, Takenaka M, Kamata K, Yoshikawa T, Nakai A, Omoto S, et al. Alleviating pancreatic cancer-associated pain using endoscopic ultrasound-guided neurolysis. Cancers (Basel). 2018;10:50.
13. Gleeson FC, Levy MJ, Papachristou GI, Pelaez-Luna M, Rajan E, Clain JE, et al. Frequency of visualization of presumed celiac ganglia by endoscopic ultrasound. Endoscopy. 2007;39:620–4.
14. Sahai AV, Lemelin V, Lam E, Paquin SC. Central vs. bilateral endoscopic ultrasound-guided celiac plexus block or neurolysis: a comparative study of short-term effectiveness. Am J Gastroenterol. 2009;104:326–9.
15. Fujii L, Clain J, Morris J, Levy M. Anterior spinal cord infarction with permanent paralysis following endoscopic ultrasound-guided celiac plexus neurolysis. Endoscopy. 2012;44:E265–6.
16. Mittal M, Rabinstein A, Wijdicks E. Acute spinal cord infarction following endoscopic ultrasound-guided celiac plexus neurolysis. Neurology. 2012;78:e57–9.
17. Minaga K, Kitano M, Imai H, Miyata T, Kudo M. Acute spinal cord infarction after EUS-guided celiac plexus neurolysis. Gastrointest Endosc. 2016;83:1039–40.
18. Köker IH, Aralaşmak A, Ünver N, Asil T, Şentürk H. Spinal cord ischemia after endoscopic ultrasound guided celiac plexus neurolysis: Case report and review of the literature. Scand J Gastroenterol. 2017;52:1158–61.
19. Mulhall AM, Rashkin MC, Pina EM. Bilateral diaphragmatic paralysis: A rare complication related to endoscopic ultrasound-guided celiac plexus neurolysis. Ann Am Thorac Soc. 2016;13:1660–2.

Part V

EUS-Guided Gallbladder Drainage

23 EUS-Guided Gallbladder Drainage for Acute Cholecystitis

Anthony Y.B. Teoh

23.1 Background

EUS-guided gallbladder drainage (EUS-GBD) is gaining popularity as an alternative to percutaneous cholecystostomy in the management of patients suffering from acute cholecystitis but are at very high risk for cholecystectomy [1–4]. The procedure has been shown to be associated with fewer adverse events, shorter hospital stays, fewer reinterventions, and unplanned readmissions [5]. Apart from acute cholecystitis, EUS-GBD is also indicated in patients who are on long-term cholecystostomy or suffering from malignant biliary obstruction with failed ERCP or EUS-guided biliary drainage [6].

23.2 Case History

An 80-year-old uncommunicable lady with multiple co-morbidities was admitted for high fever. Physical examination showed right upper quadrant tenderness with a positive Murphy's sign. Blood culture showed Klebsiella species. Computed tomography showed a distended gallbladder with surrounding inflammation and gallstones (Fig. 23.1). The features are compatible with acute cholecystitis. EUS-guided gallbladder drainage (EUS-GBD) was offered to the patient.

23.3 Procedural Plan

EUS-GBD can be performed via a transgastric or transduodenal approach. We prefer to drain the gallbladder via a transduodenal approach as the risk of food residue entering the gallbladder and buried stent syndrome is lower. Furthermore, when draining through the stomach, the proximal flange of the stent may be very close or even partially obstruct the pylorus. On the other hand, the condition of some patients may improve after drainage and cholecystectomy may be contemplated. Some surgeons may prefer transgastric drainage as the opening in the stomach is in theory easier to close. Nevertheless, despite the above considerations, the results of a prior study did not show any difference in outcomes between the transgastric and transduodenal approaches [7]. In addition, another study showed no difference in outcomes of cholecystectomies after PT-GBD and EUS-GBD [8].

We prefer to drain the gallbladder using lumen apposing metallic stents (LAMS). This is because the gallbladder is a mobile organ and

Supplementary Information The online version contains supplementary material available at [https://doi.org/10.1007/978-981-16-9340-3_23].

A. Y.B. Teoh (✉)
Department of Surgery, The Prince of Wales Hospital, The Chinese University of Hong Kong, Shatin, Hong Kong SAR, China
e-mail: anthonyteoh@surgery.cuhk.edu.hk

A. Y.B. Teoh et al. (eds.), *Atlas of Interventional EUS*, https://doi.org/10.1007/978-981-16-9340-3_23

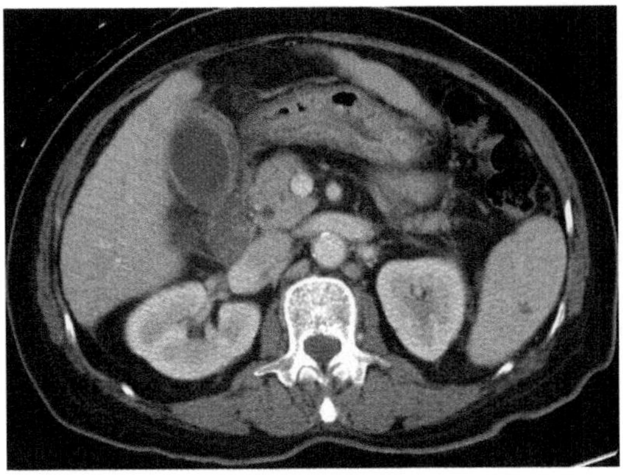

Fig. 23.1 Computed tomography demonstrating acute cholecystitis

the use of LAMS can in theory reduce the chance of leakage and stent migration. A cautery enhanced system can allow direct puncture of the gallbladder and reduces the procedural time and the need for exchange of devices. Some operators may perform a hybrid procedure with insertion of guidewire after direct puncture with the cautery enhanced delivery system. Alternatively, the procedure can be performed by the conventional method with a 19-gauge needle, followed by guidewire insertion and stent insertion.

23.4 Description of the Procedure

EUS-GBD was performed with a cautery enhanced LAMS via the transduodenal approach using a linear echoendoscope. The gallbladder was first identified and an area without intervening blood vessels was located (Video 23.1). Since the gallbladder was partially obscured by gallstones, the gallbladder was first punctured with a 19-gauge needle. A guidewire was then passed into the gallbladder and the cautery enhanced delivery system was inserted (Fig. 23.2). The distal flange was opened under EUS guidance (Fig. 23.3). The stent was then pulled back to appose the two organs. The proximal flange was then opened in the instrument channel and pushed out (Fig. 23.4). We do not routinely dilate the stent after deployment as it

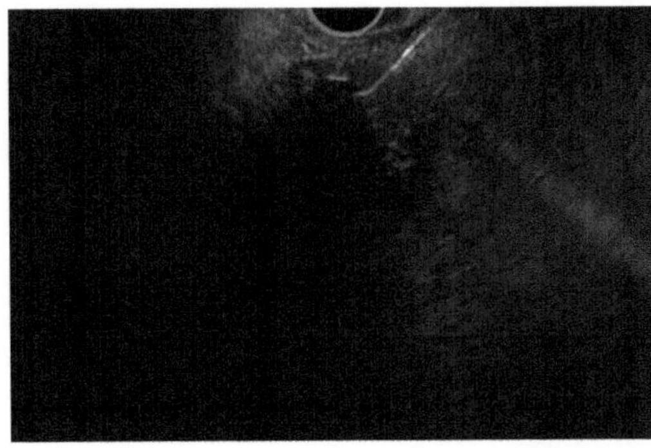

Fig. 23.2 Insertion of the cautery enhanced delivery system on a guidewire

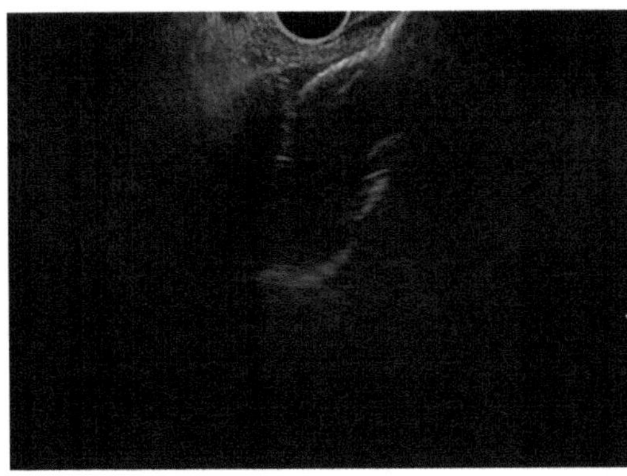

Fig. 23.3 Distal flanged deployed under EUS guidance

should be completely opened the next day. A double pigtail plastic stent was inserted to prevent large stones from obstructing the lumen of the stent (Fig. 23.5).

23.5 Post-procedural Management

Diets can be resumed when fever or pain is settled. Antibiotics are continued for up to one week. If fever does not settle then a computed tomography should be arranged to assess the cause. Post procedurally, the patients are scheduled for a follow-up cholecystoscopy for stone removal and a complete stone clearance rate could be achieved in up to 88% of the patients [9]. Alternatively, in frail patients that do not want to undergo a second procedure, long-term stenting is another option and up to 96.4% of the patients do not experience recurrent cholecystitis although stent-related complications are a potential concern [10].

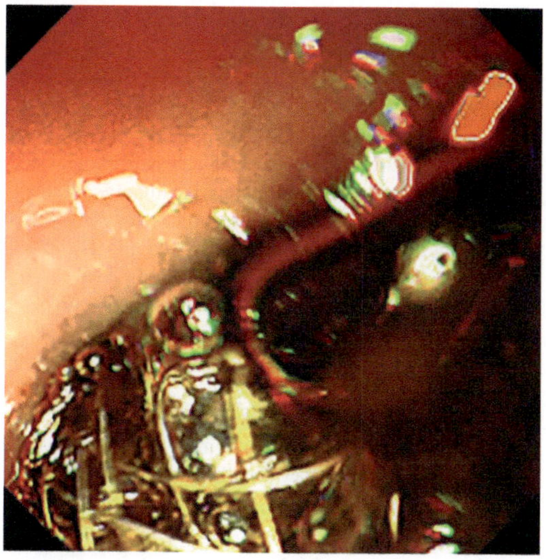

Fig. 23.4 Proximal flange deployed in the channel of the echoendoscope and pushed out of the endoscope

23.6 Potential Pitfalls

The potential adverse events after EUS-GBD include misdeployment of the stent, migration, buried stent syndrome, perforation, and bleeding. In the case of stent misdeployment, management depends on which flange is misdeployed and whether a guidewire is still in situ. If a guidewire is still in situ, then a bridging tubular metal stent or LAMS can be inserted to bridge the two lumens. If there is no access, then an experienced interventional endosnographer should be consulted for management of the condition. Percutaneous drainage may be required. If stent migration occurs and the patient suffers from recurrent acute cholecystitis, endoscopy can be performed to assess if a fistula tract is still present. If present, then it can be used to insert another plastic or metal stent. If absent, then EUS-GBD can be repeated. Buried stent syndrome usually occurs when the gallbladder is drained from the stomach. In this case, the LAMS can usually be removed and exchanged for a double pigtail plastic stent.

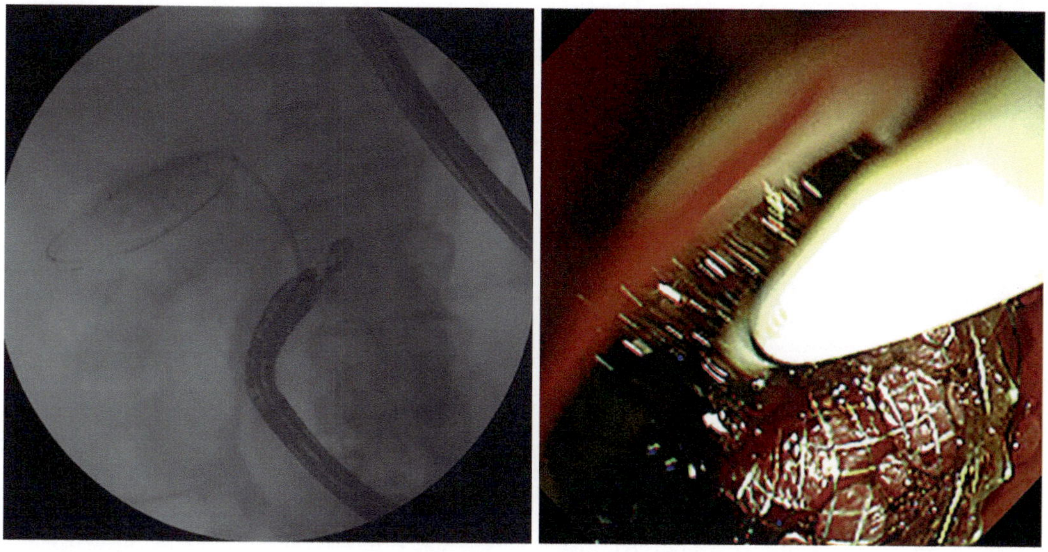

Fig. 23.5 Insertion of additional double pigtail plastic stent through the LAMS

References

1. Teoh AYB, Serna C, Penas I, Chong CCN, Perez-Miranda M, Ng EKW, et al. Endoscopic ultrasound-guided gallbladder drainage reduces adverse events compared with percutaneous cholecystostomy in patients who are unfit for cholecystectomy. Endoscopy. 2017;49(2):130–8.
2. Tyberg A, Saumoy M, Sequeiros EV, Giovannini M, Artifon E, Teoh A, et al. EUS-guided versus percutaneous gallbladder drainage: Isn't it time to convert? J Clin Gastroenterol. 2018;52(1):79–84.
3. Irani S, Ngamruengphong S, Teoh A, Will U, Nieto J, Abu Dayyeh BK, et al. Similar efficacies of endoscopic ultrasound gallbladder drainage with a lumen-apposing metal stent versus percutaneous transhepatic gallbladder drainage for acute cholecystitis. Clin Gastroenterol H. 2017;15(5):738–45.
4. Choi JH, Kim HW, Lee JC, Paik KH, Seong NJ, Yoon CJ, et al. Percutaneous transhepatic versus EUS-guided gallbladder drainage for malignant cystic duct obstruction. Gastrointest Endosc. 2017;85(2):357–64.
5. Luk SW, Irani S, Krishnamoorthi R, Wong Lau JY, Wai Ng EK, Teoh AY. Endoscopic ultrasound-guided gallbladder drainage versus percutaneous cholecystostomy for high risk surgical patients with acute cholecystitis: a systematic review and meta-analysis. Endoscopy. 2019;
6. Teoh AYB. ERCP failure: EUS gallbladder drainage as first alternative? Endosc Int Open. 2019;7(5):E662–E3.
7. Teoh AY, Serna C, Penas I, Chong CC, Perez-Miranda M, Ng EK, et al. Endoscopic ultrasound-guided gallbladder drainage reduces adverse events compared with percutaneous cholecystostomy in patients who are unfit for cholecystectomy. Endoscopy. 2017;49(2):130–8.
8. Saumoy M, Tyberg A, Brown E, Eachempati SR, Lieberman M, Afaneh C, et al. Successful cholecystectomy after endoscopic ultrasound gallbladder drainage compared with percutaneous cholecystostomy, can it be done? J Clin Gastroenterol. 2019;53(3):231–5.
9. Chan SM, Teoh AYB, Yip HC, Wong VWY, Chiu PWY, Ng EKW. Feasibility of per-oral cholecystoscopy and advanced gallbladder interventions after EUS-guided gallbladder stenting (with video). Gastrointest Endosc. 2017;85(6):1225–32.
10. Choi JH, Lee SS, Choi JH, Park DH, Seo DW, Lee SK, et al. Long-term outcomes after endoscopic ultrasonography-guided gallbladder drainage for acute cholecystitis. Endoscopy. 2014;46(8):656–61.

EUS-Guided Gallbladder Drainage for Malignant Cystic Duct Obstruction

24

Sang-Soo Lee

24.1 Background

Although gallstones account for 90–95% of acute cholecystitis causes, acute acalculous cholecystitis accounts for 3.7–14% of acute cholecystitis [1]. Risk factors include surgery, trauma, long-term intensive care unit stay, infection, thermal burn, and parenteral nutrition. Malignant cystic duct obstruction also frequently causes acute cholecystitis, especially after metallic stent placement in the bile duct. The main pathophysiology is similar to that of acute calculous cholecystitis. That is, cystic duct obstruction and cholestasis within the gallbladder might be occurred due to cancer involved cystic duct or self-expandable metallic stent overlying placed the cystic duct opening into the common bile duct. This situation is not uncommon in patients with hilar cholangiocarcinoma, extrahepatic bile duct cancer, and pancreatic head cancer. Percutaneous drainage can serve as a bridge to future cholecystectomy. However, many patients have comorbid medical conditions or prior abdominal surgeries that preclude safe surgical intervention, thus committing many patients to long-term external gallbladder drainage. Most cases cannot be removed external tubes due to the high recurrence of cholecystitis after tube removal. Therefore continuous care of the cholecystostomy tube is required. EUS-GBD has been used to overcome these limitations [2, 3]. Since EUS-GBD provides continuous internal drain, the recurrence rate of cholecystitis caused by cystic duct obstruction can be lowered.

24.2 Case History

A 72-year-old gentleman was admitted to our department with right upper quadrant pain and mild fever. Physical examination showed right upper quadrant tenderness with a positive Murphy's sign. Past medical history, he was diagnosed with an unresectable Klatskin tumor. He had undergone biliary metal stenting and Concurrent chemo-radiotherapy. Laboratory findings showed leukocytosis but normal liver function tests. C-reactive protein was also markedly elevated. Computed tomography showed a distended gallbladder with surrounding inflammation, and gallstones were not noted (Fig. 24.1a). The features are compatible with acute cholecystitis. He underwent emergency percutaneous gallbladder drainage (p-GBD)

Supplementary Information The online version contains supplementary material available at [https://doi.org/10.1007/978-981-16-9340-3_24].

S.-S. Lee (✉)
Department of Gastroenterology, University of Ulsan College of Medicine, Asan Medical Center, Seoul, Korea
e-mail: ssleedr@amc.seoul.kr

A. Y.B. Teoh et al. (eds.), *Atlas of Interventional EUS*, https://doi.org/10.1007/978-981-16-9340-3_24

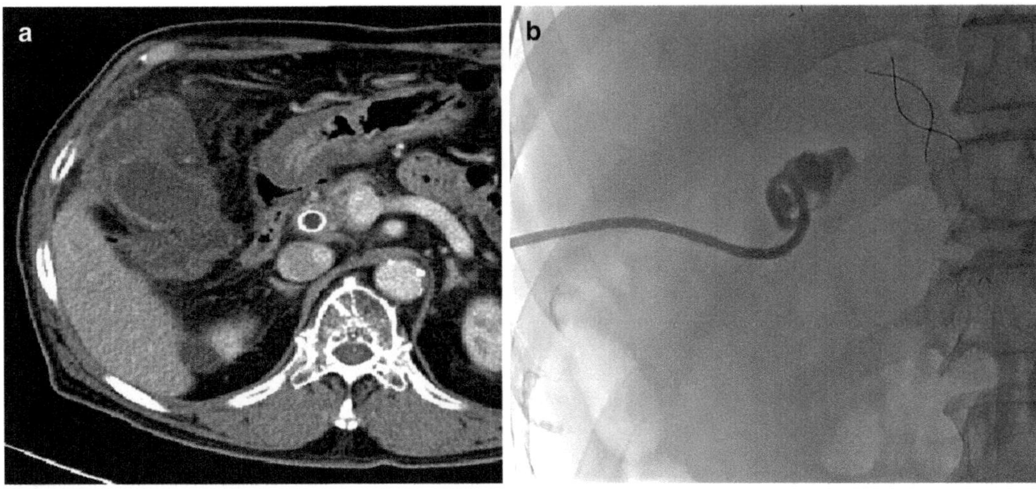

Fig. 24.1 A 72-year-old gentleman was admitted to our department with right upper quadrant pain and mild fever. (**a**) CT shows a distended gallbladder with surrounding inflammation, and gallstones were not noted. (**b**) He underwent emergency percutaneous transhepatic gallbladder drainage

(Fig. 24.1b). This case expected higher recurrence of cholecystitis after PTGBD tube removal. We decided to perform EUS-GB stenting.

24.3 Procedural Plan

In this case, we can consider several treatment options for the treatment of cholecystitis. First, it is laparoscopic cholecystectomy. However, this patient had been diagnosed as an unresectable Klatskin tumor and was undergoing systemic chemotherapy. Considering the morbidity of surgery and the patient's systemic condition (limited life expectancy) would be a physical burden to the patient. Second, maintaining the PTGBD tube. However, the external tube is associated with patient discomfort, pain, and accidental tube dislodgement, and continuous care of the cholecystostomy tube is required. As a result, the patient's quality of life deteriorates. Third, another option is removing the PTGBD tube after the improvement of acute cholecystitis. After removing the tube, however, there is a risk of high recurrence of cholecystitis and the risk of biloma or bile peritonitis through the PTGBD tube tract. Considering this situation, EUS-GBD was considered a good treatment option. EUS-GBD is known to have a recurrence rate of less than 5% of cholecystitis, moreover, it can be performed under conscious sedation, and therefore, the physical burden on the patient is significantly less than that of cholecystectomy [4].

We decided to use antimigrating tubular SEMS (AT-SEMS) (Fig. 24.2). AT-SEMS has the advantage that the diameter of the delivery system is 8Fr, which is thinner than the existing LAMS. The delicate delivery system may provide easy maneuverability in gallbladder drainage even in a long scope position, and the 8Fr delivery system needs only 6Fr cystotome without additional balloon dilatation [5].

24.4 Description of the Procedure (Video 24.1)

Before performing EUS-GBD, obtain a cholecystogram through a P-GBD tube. It is necessary to check whether the cystic duct is patent on the cholecystogram (Fig. 24.3a). In this case, cystic duct obstruction was observed on the cholecystogram. After acquiring the cholecystogram through the P-GBD tube, an additional 50–100cc of saline is injected into the gallbladder for sufficient distension of the gallbladder. Afterward, the endosonographer finds the ideal puncture site while delineating the gallbladder under EUS.

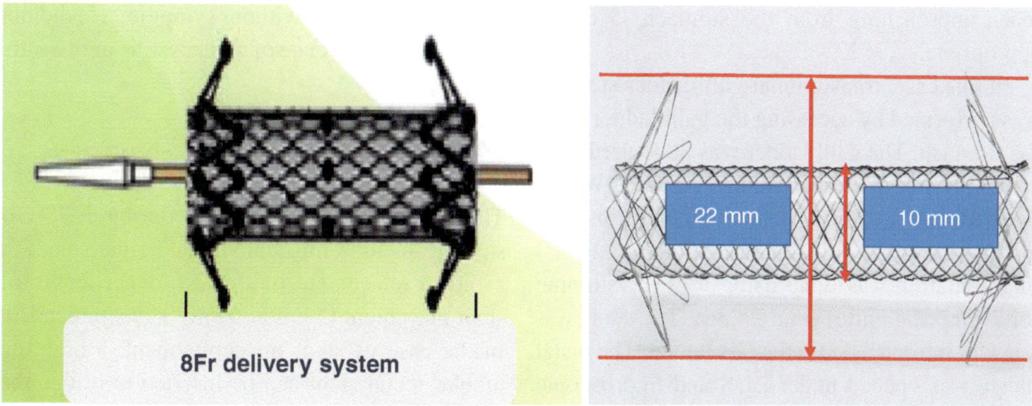

Fig. 24.2 The stent has large flanges at both ends to prevent stent migration. The outer diameter of delivery system is 8Fr

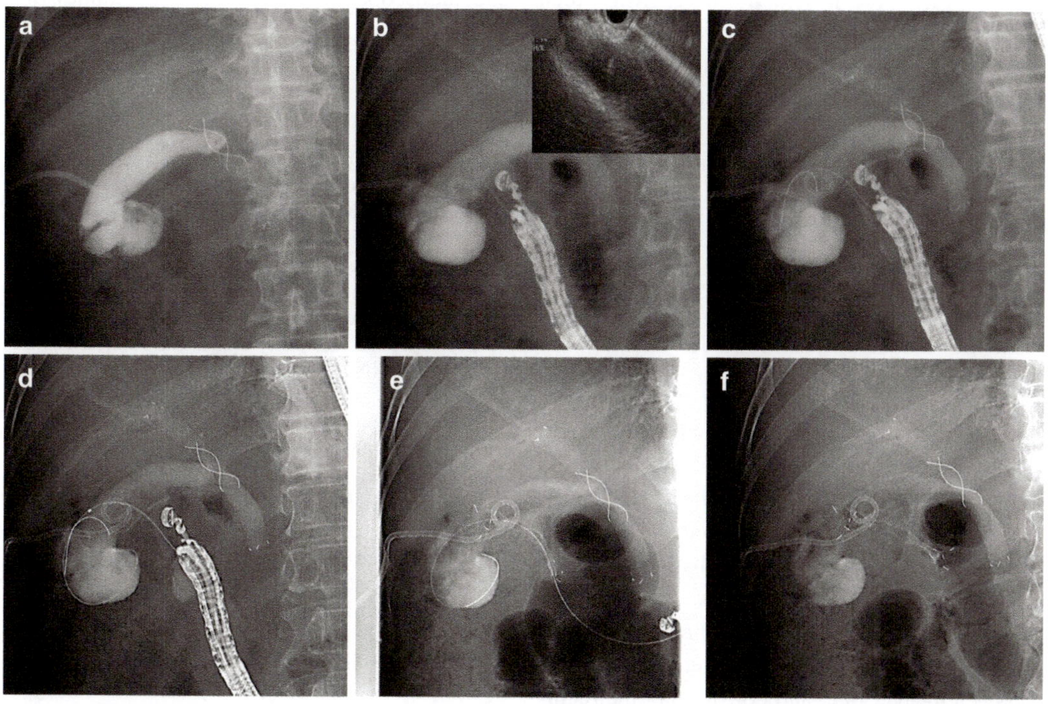

Fig. 24.3 The process of EUS-GB stenting. (**a**) Before EUS-GB stenting, check the cystic duct patency on cholecystogram via PTGBD tube. In this case, cystic duct obstruction was observed on the cholecystogram. After acquiring the cholecystogram through the P-GBD tube, an additional 50–100cc of saline is injected into the gallbladder for sufficient distension of the gallbladder. (**b**) The gallbladder is punctured under EUS-guidance by using a 19G FNA needle. (**c**) The guidewire is introduced through the FNA needle and coiled in the gallbladder. (**d**) The fistula is dilated by using a 6 Fr cystotome. (**e**) The stent is deployed under EUS and fluoroscopic guidance. (**f**) The distal end is inside of the gallbladder, and the distal end of the stent is stomach lumen

In the case of LAMS, there is a risk of buried LAMS syndrome [6], but in the case of AT-SEMS, there is no lumen apposing function, so buried LAMS syndrome does not occur. Therefore, it does not cause any problem even if it brings a stent between the stomach and the gallbladder. When approaching from the duodenum to the gallbladder, the length of the stent is 4 cm, and when approaching from the stomach, 5 cm is appropriate.

In this case, transluminal gallbladder stenting was performed by accessing the gallbladder from the stomach. The gallbladder was punctured with a 19G FNA needle (Fig. 24.3b). A 0.025 GW was inserted into the gallbladder and coiled into the gallbladder lumen (Fig. 24.3c). After that, the fistula dilatation was done using a 6Fr cystotome (or 7Fr needle knife) (Fig. 24.3d). The stent system was introduced into the GB lumen. The distal flange was opened under EUS and fluoroscopic guidance. The stent was then pulled back slightly to achieve a secure length of the stent and prevent inward migration of the proximal flange after deployment. The proximal flange was then opened in the working channel and pushed out (Fig. 24.3e, f). We did not routinely dilate the stent after deployment as it should be completely opened the next day and did not additional double pigtail stent through the AT-SEMS (Video 24.1).

24.5 Post-Procedural Management

Post procedurally, the patients are scheduled for a follow-up cholecystogram to confirm the stent function. The contrast was well-drained into the stomach lumen via the stent. The P-GBD tube removal was done after percutaneous tract maturation. The tract maturation usually takes about a week.

In the case of AT-SEMS, stent-related adverse events occurred in 3.6% of long-term follow-ups. This is a meager rate, and considering the recurrence rate of cholecystitis due to cystic duct obstruction, it is better to follow up without removing the stent.

He survived for more than five years after EUS-GB stenting. The stent was spontaneously migrated in 3 years without symptom. He did not experience recurrence of cholecystitis until death.

24.6 Potential Pitfalls

The potential adverse events during EUS-GB stenting include misdeployment of the stent. To avoid misplacement of stent, a longer length of stent placement (5 cm or 6 cm) is recommended. In the case of stent misdeployment, a bridging tubular metal stent can be inserted to bridge the two lumens. Therefore keeping guidewire is very important after deployment of the stent. After confirming the stent location with fluoroscopy and endoscope, carefully remove the guidewire.

References

1. Miyayama S, Yamashiro M, Takeda T, et al. Acute cholecystitis caused by malignant cystic duct obstruction: treatment with metallic stent placement. Cardiovasc Intervent Radiol. 2008;31(Suppl 2):S221–6.
2. Lee SS, Park DH, Hwang CY, et al. EUS-guided transmural cholecystostomy as rescue management for acute cholecystitis in elderly or high-risk patients: a prospective feasibility study. Gastrointest Endosc. 2007;66:1008–12.
3. Jang JW, Lee SS, Song TJ, et al. Endoscopic ultrasound-guided transmural and percutaneous transhepatic gallbladder drainage are comparable for acute cholecystitis. Gastroenterology. 2012;142:805–11.
4. Choi JH, Lee SS, Choi JH, et al. Long-term outcomes after endoscopic ultrasonography-guided gallbladder drainage for acute cholecystitis. Endoscopy. 2014;46:656–61.
5. Cho SH, Oh D, Song TJ, et al. Comparison of the effectiveness and safety of lumen-apposing metal stents and anti-migrating tubular self-expandable metal stents for EUS-guided gallbladder drainage in high surgical risk patients with acute cholecystitis. Gastrointest Endosc. 2020;91:543–50.
6. Peñas-Herrero I, de la Serna-Higuera C, Perez-Miranda M. Endoscopic ultrasound-guided gallbladder drainage for the management of acute cholecystitis (with video). J Hepatobiliary Pancreat Sci. 2015;22:35–43.

25 EUS-Guided Gallbladder Drainage in a Case with Malignant Biliary Obstruction

Yousuke Nakai

25.1 Background

Endoscopic transpapillary metal stent placement is the standard of care for unresectable malignant biliary obstruction (MBO) but cholecystitis can be encountered in 5 to 10% after metal stent placement. Although its risk factors have been investigated i.e. tumor involvement to the orifice of cystic duct and metal stents with high axial force [1, 2], there are no definite methods to prevent cholecystitis. Since patients with unresectable MBO are not good candidates for cholecystectomy, EUS-guided gallbladder drainage (EUS-GBD) [3] is increasingly utilized in those patients. Percutaneous transhepatic gallbladder drainage (PTGBD), which is not technically difficult, often needs permanent external drainage tube placement and impairs the quality of life, and endoscopic transpapillary gallbladder drainage is often technically impossible since the orifice of cystic duct is covered by the indwelling biliary metal stent. EUS-GBD can be also performed as a biliary drainage technique in cases with failed ERCP or EUS-guided biliary drainage (EUS-BD) [4]. EUS-GBD using a lumen apposing metal stent (LAMS) with electric cautery system can be a quick and safe procedure [5]. However, LAMS is expensive and not yet available for cholecystitis in some countries including Japan, and EUS-GBD using a plastic stent can be an option.

25.2 Case History

An 82-year old female was admitted for MBO due to unresectable pancreatic cancer. ERCP revealed distal biliary stricture with tumor involvement to the orifice of cystic duct and a fully covered stent placement was placed across the papilla. Two weeks later the patient developed fever with right upper quadrant pain and transabdominal ultrasound revealed distended gallbladder and percutaneous transhepatic gallbladder aspiration (PTGBA) was performed. The aspirated bile juice was positive for Enterobacter aerogenes. Abdominal pain did not resolve and a decision was made to perform EUS-GBD because of the lack of pain control.

Supplementary Information The online version contains supplementary material available at [https://doi.org/10.1007/978-981-16-9340-3_25].

Y. Nakai (✉)
Department of Endoscopy and Endoscopic Surgery, Graduate School of Medicine, The University of Tokyo, Tokyo, Japan
e-mail: ynakai-tky@umin.ac.jp

A. Y.B. Teoh et al. (eds.), *Atlas of Interventional EUS*, https://doi.org/10.1007/978-981-16-9340-3_25

25.3 Procedural Plan

There are some procedure options during EUS-GBD using a plastic stent: Approach route (transduodenal or transgastric), drainage method (internal, external, or its combination), and tract dilation (cautery, non-cautery or its combination).

We prefer a transduodenal approach, non-cautery dilation, and a combined internal and temporary external drainage placement in cases with moderate/severe cholecystitis. The use of a cautery dilator has a potential risk of delayed bleeding due to its burning effects especially when a covered metal stent is not placed. A balloon dilator with a tapered tip is our first choice but we do not hesitate to use a cautery dilator in cases with difficult device insertion because prolonged procedure time will increase a chance of intra-procedure bile leakage. A single double pigtail stent is often enough to resolve cholecystitis but in cases with severe infection, we prefer a combination of internal and external drainage using a double guidewire technique. External naso-gallbladder drainage tube can be used for aspiration or irrigation if necessary and be easily removed after resolution of cholecystitis. Double guidewire technique can also help stabilize the scope and keep the plane of EUS image, which is essential for the success of all types of EUS-guided intervention.

25.4 Description of the Procedure (Video 25.1)

EUS-GBD was performed via the transduodenal approach using a combination of a double pigtail plastic stent and a pigtail naso-gallbladder drainage. After insertion of a linear echoendoscope, the distended gallbladder was visualized in a U-shape, long position with the echo probe facing the right side of the patient. The puncture site was located where the duodenum and gallbladder were close to each other and there was no intervening vessel on EUS. After gallbladder puncture using a 19-gauge FNA needle without a stylet, a small amount of bile was aspirated, followed by contrast injection (Fig. 25.1). Then, a 0.025-inch guidewire was inserted through the needle and coiled in the gallbladder. The fistula was dilated with a 4-mm tapered tip balloon [6] to facilitate the subsequent devise insertion (Fig. 25.2). A double guidewire technique was achieved by adding a 0.035-inch guidewire, using an uneven double lumen catheter [7] (Fig. 25.3). First, a 7 Fr double pigtail stent was inserted. Once the proximal pigtail end was inserted, the guidewire was pulled into the stent to make a pigtail shape in the gallbladder. Then, the EUS scope was slowly pulled back while pushing the stent into the duodenum and the distal end of the pigtail was fully deployed under both fluoroscopic

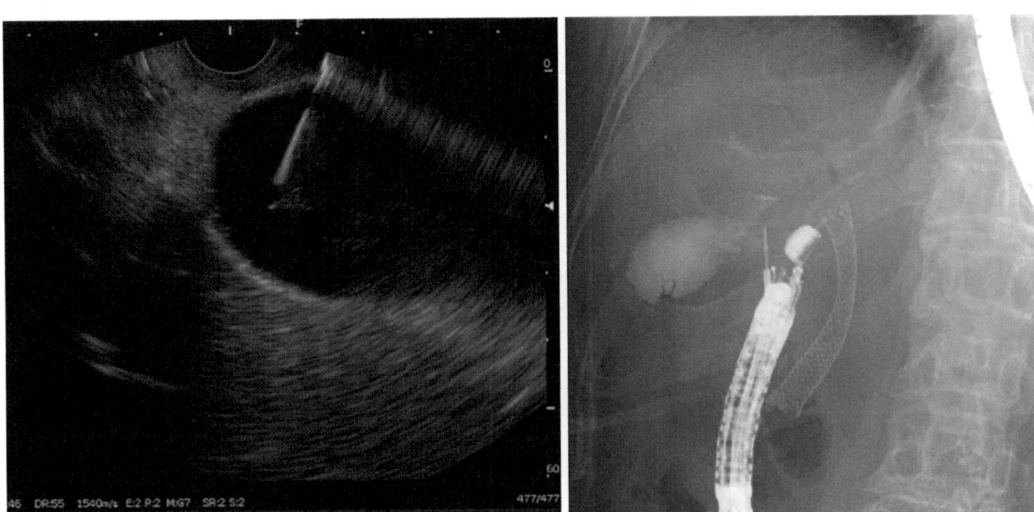

Fig. 25.1 Distended gallbladder punctured from the duodenal bulb under EUS and fluoroscopy guidance

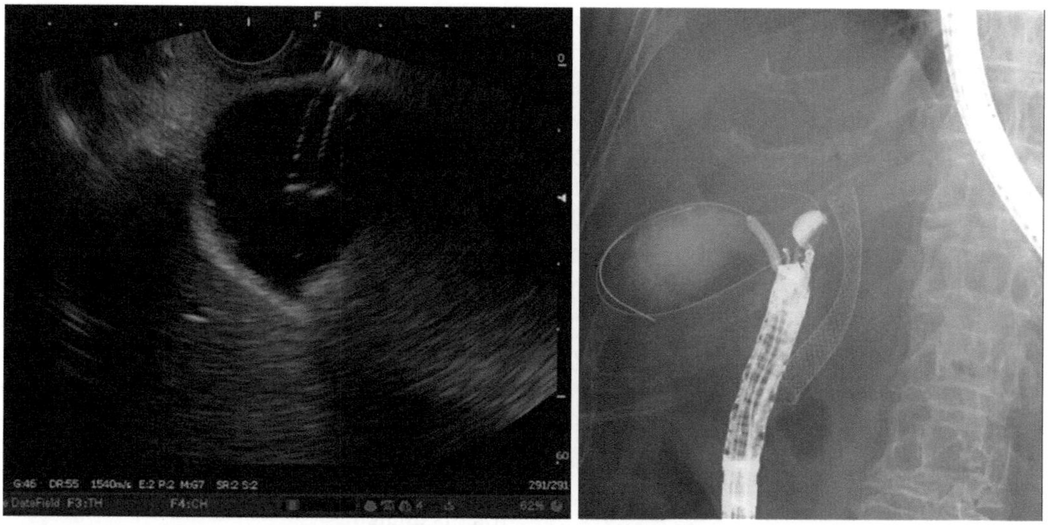

Fig. 25.2 Tract dilation using a 4 mm balloon was performed under EUS and fluoroscopy guidance

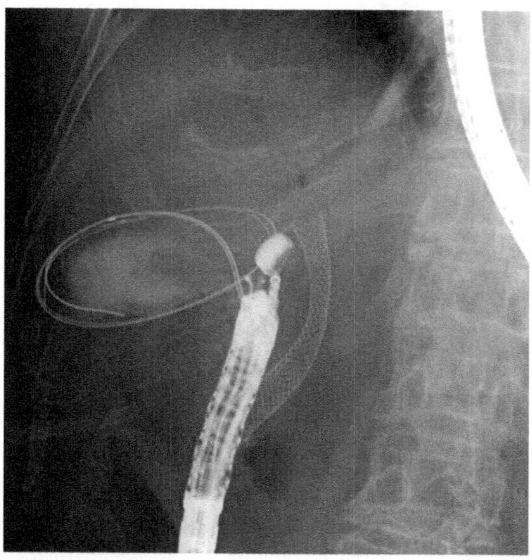

Fig. 25.3 Double guidewire placement using a double lumen catheter

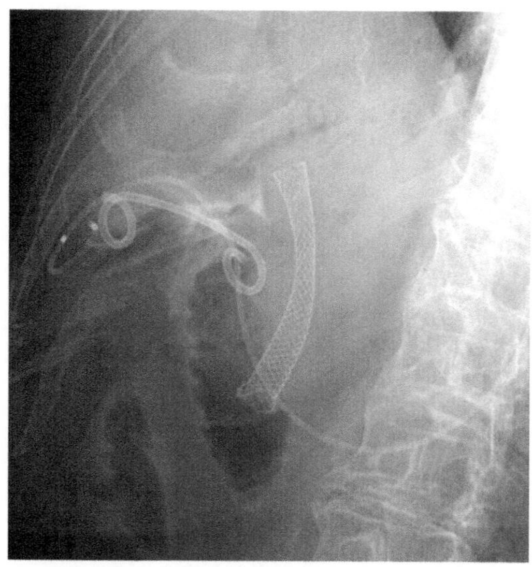

Fig. 25.4 A double pigtail stent and a naso-gallbladder drainage tube placed as internal and external drainage

and endoscopic guidance to prevent stent misplacement outside the duodenum. The EUS scope was pushed back into the bulb while the remaining guidewire left coiled in the gallbladder. The scope position was confirmed on EUS and fluoroscopy; the guidewire along the stent was visualized on EUS once the appropriate plane was obtained. A 5 Fr naso-gallbladder drainage tube was then inserted into the gallbladder (Fig. 25.4) and the procedure was completed.

25.5 Post-procedural Management

Physical examination, blood tests, and X-ray should be performed on the next day. CT is recommended if there is a concern. Diets can be resumed when fever or pain is settled. In cases with a combination of internal and external drainage, external drainage can be removed once cholecystitis is resolved. The duration of antibiotics varies depending on the severity of cholecystitis. We do not recommend scheduled stent exchange due to the limited life expectancy in cases with unresectable MBO. In addition, stent patency of EUS-GBD is longer than that of plastic stent in the bile duct. At the time of recurrent cholecystitis, stent exchange can be easily performed through the matured deudeno-cholecysto fistula. In cases with stent migration, stent placement can be performed if the fistula is present. Otherwise, EUS-GBD can be performed again but the gallbladder wall is thick and hard due to chronic inflammation and the procedure may be technically difficult.

25.6 Potential Pitfalls

Stent misdeployment is one of the pitfalls of EUS-GBD using a plastic stent, which leads to a serious sequel such as peritonitis. Since the double pigtail stent is inserted as straightened over the guidewire (and the inner sheath) and the endoscopic view is limited during stent insertion/deployment, the distal stent end can be mistakenly deployed inside the gallbladder or in the peritoneum. A double pigtail stent with fluoroscopy markers or with a retrieval system are useful but its availability is limited. Thus, endoscopists should understand the length of pigtail part before stent insertion. The insertion of the first pigtail is performed under EUS and fluoroscopy guidance. The puncture tract with a guidewire should be visualized on EUS to keep the alignment, and once the pigtail part is inserted enough in the gallbladder, the first pigtail part should be released in the gallbladder. Then, the remaining stent with the second part of the gallbladder should be deployed under endoscopy and fluoroscopy guidance. To achieve this, the echoendoscope should be gradually withdrawn as the stent is pushed out of the scope. The endoscopist should make sure the first pigtail is kept in the gallbladder on fluoroscopy. Once the second pigtail is fully out of the echoendoscope, the stent can be carefully deployed. Even if the stent end is in the duodenum, the stent can advance out of the duodenum when the guidewire is pulled out. We even experienced migration of a double pigtail stent at stent deployment as the pigtail curled up by guidewire removal [8].

In case of stent misdeployment, if the guidewire is still in place, then, another double pigtail stent placement can be tried with or without retrieval of a migrated stent [9]. If failed, then, after surgical consultation, percutaneous transhepatic gallbladder drainage can be an option. Additional percutaneous peritoneal drainage might be necessary if bile leakage is significant. It is important to place some kind of drainage once gallbladder is punctured and the tract is dilated.

References

1. Isayama H, Kawabe T, Nakai Y, Tsujino T, Sasahira N, Yamamoto N, et al. Cholecystitis after metallic stent placement in patients with malignant distal biliary obstruction. Clinical gastroenterology and hepatology: the official clinical practice journal of the American Gastroenterological Association. 2006;4(9):1148–53.
2. Nakai Y, Isayama H, Kawakubo K, Kogure H, Hamada T, Togawa O, et al. Metallic stent with high axial force as a risk factor for cholecystitis in distal malignant biliary obstruction. J Gastroenterol Hepatol. 2014;29(7):1557–62.
3. Teoh AYB. Outcomes and limitations in EUS-guided gallbladder drainage. Endoscopic ultrasound. 2019;8(Suppl 1):S40–s3.
4. Imai H, Kitano M, Omoto S, Kadosaka K, Kamata K, Miyata T, et al. EUS-guided gallbladder drainage for rescue treatment of malignant distal biliary obstruction after unsuccessful ERCP. Gastrointest Endosc. 2016;84(1):147–51.
5. Irani S, Ngamruengphong S, Teoh A, Will U, Nieto J, Abu Dayyeh BK, et al. Similar efficacies of endoscopic ultrasound gallbladder drainage with a lumen-apposing metal stent versus percutaneous transhepatic gallbladder drainage for acute cholecystitis. Clinical gastroenterology and hepatology: the official clinical practice journal of the American Gastroenterological Association. 2017;15(5):738–45.
6. Amano M, Ogura T, Onda S, Takagi W, Sano T, Okuda A, et al. Prospective clinical study of endoscopic ultrasound-guided biliary drainage using novel balloon catheter (with video). J Gastroenterol Hepatol. 2017;32(3):716–20.

7. Nakai Y, Kogure H, Koike K. Double-guidewire technique for endoscopic ultrasound-guided pancreatic duct drainage. Digestive endoscopy: official journal of the Japan Gastroenterological Endoscopy Society. 2019;31(Suppl 1):65–6.
8. Nakai Y, Isayama H, Umefune G, Mizuno S, Kogure H, Yamamoto N, et al. Percutaneous transhepatic cholangioscopy-assisted repositioning of misplaced endoscopic ultrasound-guided pancreatic duct stent. Endoscopy. 2016;48(Suppl 1):E129–30.
9. Nishiyama M, Ishii S, Fujisawa T, Saito H, Isayama H. Endoscopic removal of a migrated plastic stent from the peritoneal cavity after an EUS-guided gallbladder drainage procedure. VideoGIE: an official video journal of the American Society for Gastrointestinal Endoscopy. 2019;4(6):266–8.

26 Cholecystoscopy with Advanced Gallbladder Interventions

Shannon Melissa Chan
and Anthony Y.B. Teoh

26.1 Background

EUS-guided gallbladder drainage (EGBD) has increasingly been recognized as an alternative to percutaneous transhepatic gallbladder drainage for surgically high-risk patients with acute cholecystitis. With the development of EGBD with lumen apposing stent (LAMS), gallbladder access via the stent was made possible [1]. Through this access, advanced endoscopic evaluation and therapeutic interventions can be performed [2]. For diagnostic purposes, narrow-band imaging (NBI), biopsy, endoscopic ultrasound (EUS), and cholecystogram can be performed. For therapeutic purposes, stones can be cleared with different instruments and the LAMS can be removed. This is a relatively new procedure and the definite clinical indications and long-term efficacy have yet to be determined.

Supplementary Information The online version contains supplementary material available at [https://doi.org/10.1007/978-981-16-9340-3_26].

S. M. Chan · A. Y.B. Teoh (✉)
Department of Surgery, The Prince of Wales Hospital, The Chinese University of Hong Kong, Shatin, Hong Kong SAR, China
e-mail: shannonchan@surgery.cuhk.edu.hk; anthonyteoh@surgery.cuhk.edu.hk

26.2 Case History

An 80-year old lady with multiple co-morbidities was previously admitted four weeks ago for acute cholecystitis. EGBD has been performed with LAMS. She was scheduled to have a cholecystoscopy.

26.3 Procedural Plan

As EGBD is still a relatively new procedure, the long-term management plan of whether the gallstones and the LAMS should be removed is still controversial. The main concerns about keeping the LAMS long term are stent erosion causing bleeding and stent migration. On the other hand, the rate of recurrent cholecystitis after removing the LAMS has to be considered. In a cohort of 56 patients, two cases of stent migration at 170 and 303 days after stent placement occurred and there were 2 cases of recurrent cholecystitis [3]. On the other hand, in another cohort of 8 patients in which the stents were removed without stent replacement, there was no recurrence cholecystitis in a mean follow-up of 304 days [4]. In a recent review published in 2019, the authors suggested that for patients with an expected short-term survival, permanent stent placement may be suitable in order to avoid reintervention and recurrence of acute cholecystitis. In patients with longer expected survival, stent removal may be

A. Y.B. Teoh et al. (eds.), *Atlas of Interventional EUS*, https://doi.org/10.1007/978-981-16-9340-3_26

more suitable to reduce stent-related complications [5]. Therefore, before proceeding to cholecystoscopy, the patients expected time of survival, risk of further endoscopic procedures, and patients' wish have to be carefully considered.

The aim of the cholecystoscopy is mainly for gallstone and stent removal. We published the first case series on peroral cholecystoscopy. The overall stone clearance rate was 88% after an average of 1.25 sessions [2]. The procedure is performed with a standard forward-viewing endoscope, preferably equipped with a water-jet function under carbon dioxide insufflation. For diagnostic purposes, a narrow-band magnifying endoscopy with a short cap can be used. Endocytoscopy and confocal laser microscopy can also be performed. To detect the depth of involvement of any lesions, endoscopic ultrasound with miniprobe can be used. Biopsies can also be taken to confirm the endoscopic suspicion of malignancies. In the presence of gallstones, different instruments can be used to remove the stones. These instruments include rat-tooth or alligator forceps, snare, basket, Roth net, etc. For larger stones, mechanical basket lithotripsy or laser lithotripsy could be used. Multiple sessions may be needed. For gallbladder polyps, they can be removed with a cold biopsy or polypectomy. Cholecystogram and cholangiogram can be performed with fluoroscopic guidance.

After stone clearance was achieved and the stent removed, the insertion of a double pigtail catheter after removal of LAMS may be able to prevent recurrent cholecystitis or facilitate salvage of the fistulous tract when cholecystitis recur. However, given the low rates of recurrent cholecystitis, it is doubtful whether this is necessary.

26.4 Description of the Procedure (Video 26.1)

The procedure is performed with a forward-viewing endoscope with a water-jet function. Patient was in left lateral position. The endoscope entered the first part of duodenum where the LAMS was seen. The endoscope then entered the gallbladder and saw a 2 cm gallstone. There were also some gallbladder polyps. Narrow-band magnifying endoscopy was performed which showed an increase in vascularity but a regular capillary pattern on the polyps (Fig. 26.1). In view of the large size of the gallstone, the gallstone was fragmented with holmium laser lithotripsy (VersaPulse PowerSuite; UHS, Minneapolis, Minn, USA) (Fig. 26.2). The use of fluoroscopy aided the assessment of the depth of the laser lithotripsy (Fig. 26.3), which was repeated multiple times till the gallstones were small enough to be removed through the stent. Initially, snare (Olympus Medical, Tokyo, Japan) was used to retrieve the fragments, but the fragments were too soft and the gallstones were cut through. Subsequently, a Roth net (US Endoscopy, Mentor, Ohio, USA) was used to retrieve the fragments to the stomach (Fig. 26.4). After clearance of the gallstones, the stent was removed with alligator forceps. The gallbladder was re-entered to clear the residual stones. An 8.5-Fr 5 cm double pigtail catheter was inserted (Figs. 26.5 and 26.6).

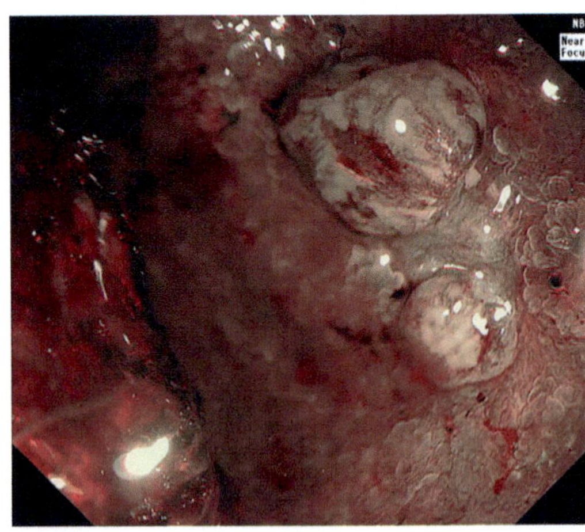

Fig. 26.1 Narrow-band magnifying imaging of the gallbladder polyps

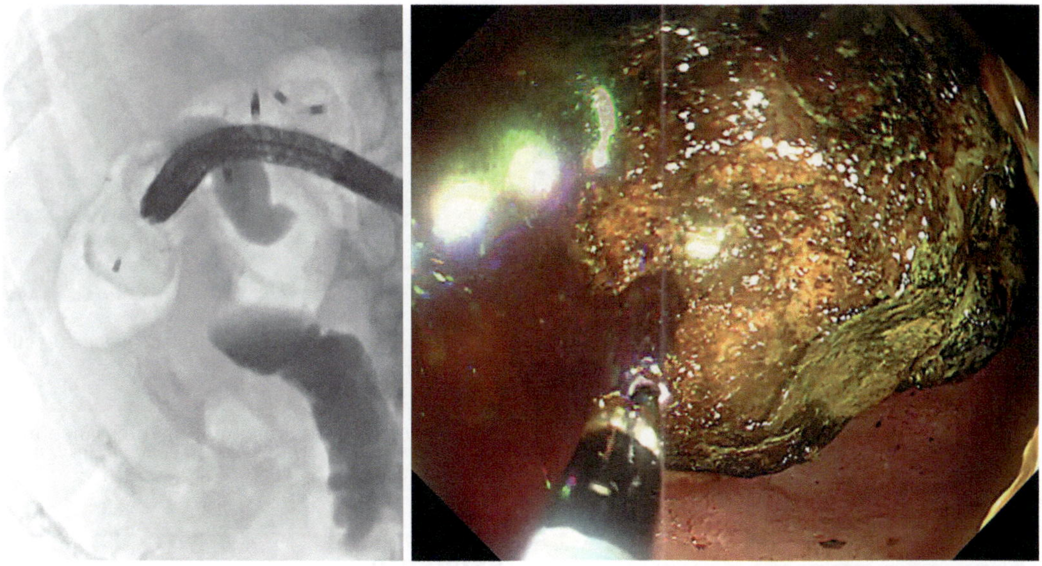

Fig. 26.2 The use of holmium laser lithotripsy

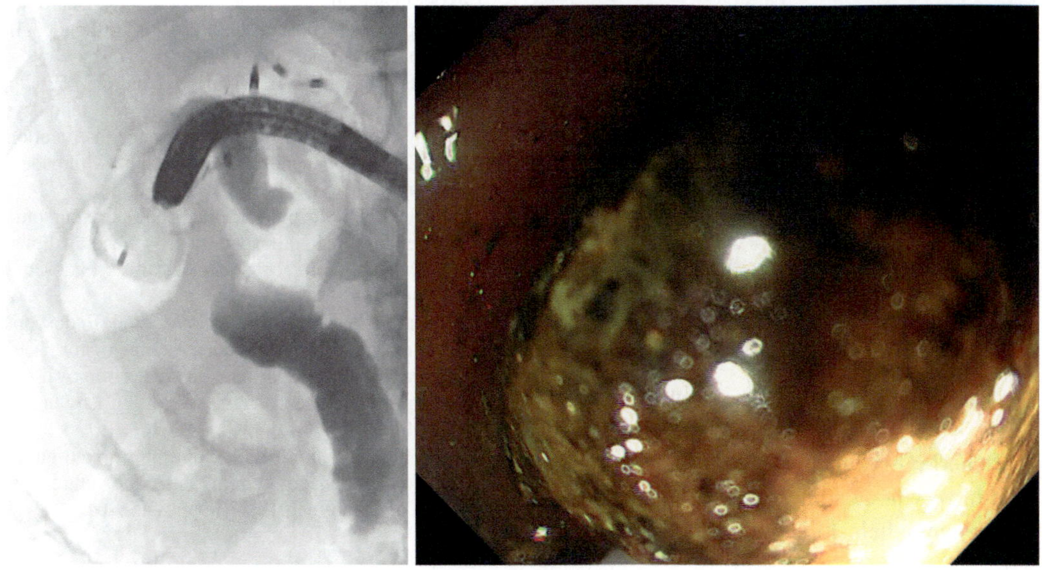

Fig. 26.3 The use of fluoroscopy to guide the depth of the laser lithotripsy

26.5 Post-procedural Management

Patient can be resumed on normal diet and discharged on the same day. Multiple sessions may be required for the complete removal of the gallstones.

26.6 Potential Pitfalls

This is a relatively safe procedure. However, it is important to bear in mind that the gallbladder has very thin walls. All manipulations must be done gently and with caution. It is in particular during laser lithotripsy where the dissipated

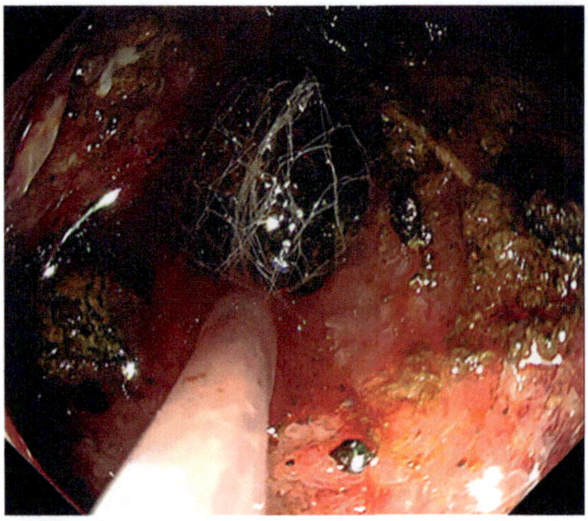

Fig. 26.4 The use of Roth net to remove the fragments

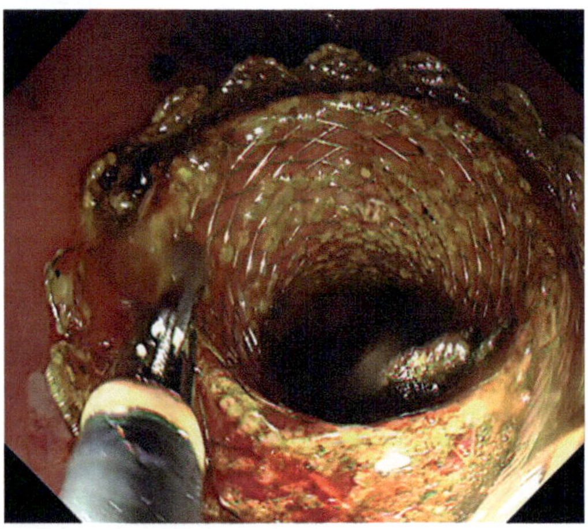

Fig. 26.5 The removal of LAMS with alligator forceps

heat energy may theoretically lead to perforation. In very large stones, the assistance of fluoroscopy may help to estimate the depth of the stone. Multiple sessions of stone clearance may be required.

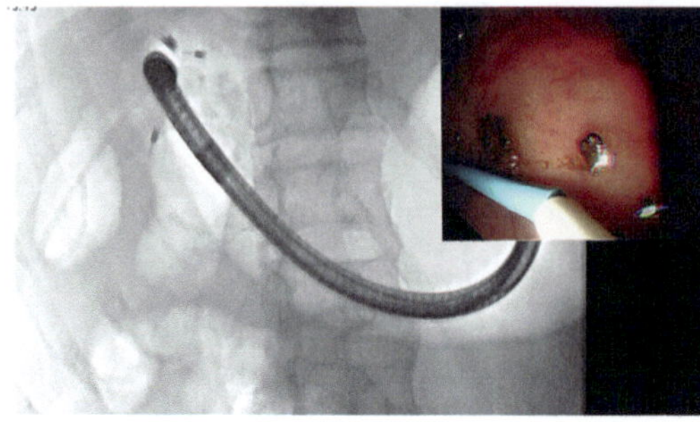

Fig. 26.6 The insertion of double pigtail to the gallbladder

References

1. Mori Y, Itoi T, Baron TH, et al. Tokyo guidelines 2018: management strategies for gallbladder drainage in patients with acute cholecystitis (with videos). J Hepatobiliary Pancreat Sci. 2018;25:87–95.
2. Chan SM, Teoh AYB, Yip HC, Wong VWY, Chiu PWY, Ng EKW. Feasibility of per-oral cholecystoscopy and advanced gallbladder interventions after EUS-guided gallbladder stenting (with video). Gastrointest Endosc. 2017;85:1225–32.
3. Choi JH, Lee SS, Choi JH, et al. Long-term outcomes after endoscopic ultrasonography-guided gallbladder drainage for acute cholecystitis. Endoscopy. 2014;46:656–61.
4. Kamata K, Takenaka M, Kitano M, et al. Endoscopic ultrasound-guided gallbladder drainage for acute cholecystitis: long-term outcomes after removal of a self-expandable metal stent. World J Gastroenterol. 2017;23:661–7.
5. Ogura T, Higuchi K. Endoscopic ultrasound-guided gallbladder drainage: current status and future prospects. Dig Endosc. 2019;31(Suppl 1):55–64.

Part VI

EUS-Guided Gastroenterostomy

27 EUS-Guided Gastroenterostomy: Balloon Technique

Saad Alrajhi and Yen-I Chen

27.1 Background

Endoscopic ultrasound-guided gastroenterostomy (EUS-GE) is a novel approach in the management of malignant gastric outlet obstruction that has gained attention with the advent of the lumen apposing metal stent (LAMS) [1]. EUS-GE allows for a luminal bypass of the tumor obstruction, which has been shown to decrease the risk for stent dysfunction and re-intervention when compared to traditional enteral stenting. In addition, the endoscopic approach avoids the morbidity of surgery and has been shown to be similar in safety as enteral stenting [2]. Various techniques have been described to perform EUS-GE including the direct technique and endoscopic ultrasonography-guided double-balloon-occluded gastrojejunostomy bypass (EPASS). The following describes the balloon-assisted gastroenteromy (BAGE) method, which is one of the first described techniques for EUS-GE.

Supplementary Information The online version contains supplementary material available at [https://doi.org/10.1007/978-981-16-9340-3_27].

S. Alrajhi
Division of Gastroenterology and Hepatology, McGill University Health Centre, McGill University, Montreal, QC, Canada
e-mail: saad.alrajhi@mail.mcgill.ca

Y.-I. Chen (✉)
Division of Gastroenterology and Hepatology, McGill University Health Centre, McGill University, Montreal, QC, Canada
e-mail: yen-i.chen@mcgill.ca

27.2 Case History

A 71-year-old male known for unresectable pancreatic cancer treated with multiple lines of chemotherapy presented to the emergency room with a one-week history of recurrent vomiting and epigastric discomfort. Computer tomography (CT) suggested gastric outlet obstruction with a transition point in the third–fourth portion of the duodenum due to the extension of the pancreatic body mass (Fig. 27.1). A diagnostic esophagogastroduodenoscopy was performed confirming the presence of external compression and obstruction at the third–fourth portion of the duodenum (D3–D4). A decision was taken with the patient and his family to proceed with EUS-GE. The choice of EUS-GE over enteral stenting was mostly due to the fact that the patient was quite robust despite the diagnosis of pancreatic cancer and likely had several months of high quality of life, which would really benefit from a procedure that would decrease the risk for stent dysfunction and re-intervention.

A. Y.B. Teoh et al. (eds.), *Atlas of Interventional EUS*, https://doi.org/10.1007/978-981-16-9340-3_27

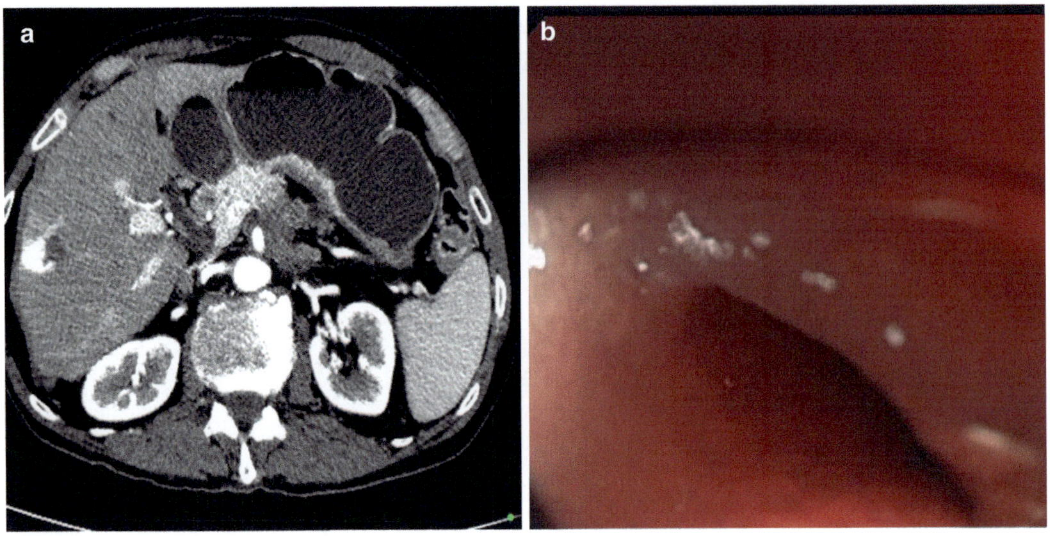

Fig. 27.1 (**a**) CT image showing pancreatic body mass leading to external compression and obstruction of D3–D4 confirmed on (**b**) endoscopy

27.3 Procedural Plan

Given its complexity, the procedure was planned for general anesthesia in the therapeutic endoscopy suite with both EUS and fluoroscopic availability. The BAGE technique was chosen over the water infusion technique due to the fact the obstruction was quite distal and outside the reach of a gastroscopy, which would make the infusion of fluid across the obstruction difficult. In addition, the BAGE technique has the potential to be more simply salvaged in case of stent misdeployment given that re-stenting is easily performed after having achieved wire capture and wire control at both ends. Lastly, the BAGE technique can be performed with a "cold" non-cautery-assisted LAMS, which is significantly less costly than a cautery-assisted LAMS. A 15 mm LAMS is generally used for EUS-GE. A 20 mm LAMS could be considered; however, clinical success has been shown to be excellent with the 15 mm LAMS and the use of 20 mm LAMS can be challenging given the greater distance needed for stent deployment in a relatively small space, which could lead to increased risk for misdeployment. In terms of anatomical considerations, we generally aim to target the jejunal loop at the ligament of Treitz given that it is usually the closest to the stomach. The ultimate goal was to perform EUS-GE using the BAGE technique with enteral stenting as the backup modality if needed.

- Enteroscope with overtube: needed for initial wire insertion across the obstruction with the overtube eventually serving as a facilitator for balloon catheter insertion.
- Therapeutic linear echoendoscope for LAMS insertion.
- Two 0.035 inch guidewire: one for balloon insertion and the other to be captured following transgastric puncture of the small bowel using EUS.
- 20 mm dilated balloon or ERCP basket
- Fine needle aspiration needle (19-gauge) for initial transgastric puncture and access to the small bowel.
- 4 mm dilating balloon to dilate the gastroenterotomy tract to facilitate stent insertion if "cold" LAMS is used
- "Cold" 15 mm LAMS (could also use "hot" LAMS but not required for BAGE).

27.4 Description of the Procedure

The procedure was performed with the patient in the supine position under general anesthesia. An enteroscope fitted with a single balloon overtube was first inserted in the patient's mouth and advanced to the level of the obstruction. An 0.035-inch stiff guidewire was then inserted across the obstruction using fluoroscopic guidance and advanced deep into the small bowel. The enteroscope was then removed via exchange over the wire while keeping the overtube in place. The primary role of the overtube is to facilitate instrument advancement across the greater curvature of the stomach, which tends to cause extensive looping. A 20 mm dilating balloon was then inserted over the wire through the overtube and advanced through the obstruction to the ligament of Treitz with fluoroscopic guidance. The balloon is then inflated serving as a target for the gastroenterostomy. Alternatively, an ERCP basket can be used instead of the balloon. The overtube was then removed and a therapeutic linear echoendsocope was inserted. The balloon or basket is then located via EUS and punctured through a transgastric approach. Once the needle is inside a second 0.035 wire is advanced through the needle and curled inside the balloon or through the basket. The collapsed balloon with the captured wire is then pulled back through the patient's mouth along with the wire, which allows the endoscopist to have control on both ends of the wire. Anecdotally, wire capture with the basket is much easier and prevents slippage and loss of the wire during withdrawal. By having access to both ends of the wire, optimal traction and wire tension can be provided. Given a "cold" LAMS was used in this case for economic reasons, a 4 mm dilating balloon was inserted through this wire to dilate the GE tract. This is then followed by advancement of the LAMS over the wire with deployment of the distal and proximal flange using sonographic and endoscopic guidance. Note that if a "hot" LAMS was used then dilation would not be needed. Due to potential stent migration, we do not routinely dilate the stent post-LAMS insertion [3]. An enterogram is then performed through the LAMS to confirm successful gastroenterostomy. The major advantage of the BAGE technique lies in the ability to easily remove a misdeployed LAMS over the wire and to insert a second LAMS using the same wire with minimal to no clinical consequence. This of course is not the case with the water infusion technique where the LAMS is inserted freehand with cautery assistance, which leads to a difficult to salvage perforation in case of stent misdeployment.

—Please discuss if any difficulties have been encountered.

No difficulties were encountered in this case. Generally, the most challenging part of the procedure is the advancement of the balloon through the greater curvature of the stomach. An overtube is essential in facilitating this process. In addition, as aforementioned, wire capture can sometimes be unreliable using the balloon and a basket may be preferred to prevent wire loss.

27.5 Post-procedural Management

The patient's diet was advanced to a low residue regiment after 48 hours of clear fluid. Caution should be taken in advancing the diet too quickly, which may lead to food impaction secondary to incomplete stent expansion. If a decision was taken to dilate the stent, then the diet can be advanced within 24 hours. No follow-up procedures are needed unless dictated by symptoms that suggest potential stent obstruction or migration. Given the palliative nature of the procedure, there is a limited role of long-term follow-up.

—Please also provide follow-up images.

No follow-up images available.

27.6 Potential Pitfalls

Although generally very safe and comparable to enteral stenting [2], the most feared pitfall of EUS-GE is the risk for perforation with stent misdeployment. The use of the BAGE technique nearly completely eliminates the risk for perforation given the ease of salvaging any stent misdepolyments. Wire capture using the BAGE approach; however, can be challenging and time-consuming. Indeed a comparative study assessing the BAGE and water infusion technique showed a significantly longer procedure time with the BAGE (89.9 minutes vs 35.7 minutes) [4]. Anecdotally, the use of a basket is much easier and faster than the balloon and may be preferred. Overall, the choice of the most appropriate technique largely depends on endoscopist's preference and expertise. However, for endoscopists who are only beginning to perform EUS-GE, the BAGE technique may be the preferred method given its more forgiving nature.

References

1. Chen YI, James TW, Agarwal A, et al. EUS-guided gastroenterostomy in management of benign gastric outlet obstruction. Endosc Int Open. 2018;6:E363–8.
2. Chen YI, Itoi T, Baron TH, et al. EUS-guided gastroenterostomy is comparable to enteral stenting with fewer re-interventions in malignant gastric outlet obstruction. Surg Endosc. 2017;31:2946–52.
3. Chen YI, Haito-Chavez Y, Bueno RP, et al. Displaced endoscopic ultrasound-guided gastroenterostomy stent rescued with natural orifice transluminal endoscopic surgery. Gastroenterology. 2017;153:15–6.
4. Chen YI, Kunda R, Storm AC, et al. EUS-guided gastroenterostomy: a multicenter study comparing the direct and balloon-assisted techniques. Gastrointest Endosc. 2018;87:1215–21.

28 EUS-guided Gastroenterostomy: The Direct Method

Jennifer T. Higa and Shayan S. Irani

28.1 Background

There is an evolving role for interventional endoscopy in the management of benign and malignant gastric outlet obstruction (GOO) with the creation of an EUS-guided gastroenterostomy (EUS-GE) using a lumen-apposing metal stent (LAMS). Multiple series have documented favorable outcomes for patients who undergo EUS-GE for the treatment of malignant and benign GOO as a non-operative alternative [1–4]. The direct puncture method is a favorable approach due to the shorter procedure time [5] and appears to be safe and effective when performed by experienced interventional endosonographers. Low reintervention rates (15.1%) were reported in one long-term cohort which was followed for a median of 196 days in malignant GOO and 319.5 days in benign GOO following direct EUS-GE [6]. We present a case of EUS-GE performed using a direct method for malignant GOO in a patient with metastatic disease who failed prior enteral stenting.

Supplementary Information The online version contains supplementary material available at [https://doi.org/10.1007/978-981-16-9340-3_28].

J. T. Higa (✉)
Division of Gastroenterology and Hepatology, Fox Chase Cancer Center, Philadelphia, PA, USA
e-mail: Jennifer.higa@fccc.edu

S. S. Irani
Division of Gastroenterology and Hepatology, Virginia Mason Medical Center, Seattle, WA, USA
e-mail: shayan.irani@virginiamason.org

28.2 Case History

The patient was a 65-year-old female with a history of metastatic pancreatic adenocarcinoma. She had undergone enteral stent placement for gastric outlet obstruction due to stenosis of the third portion of the duodenum (D3) by a large pancreas body mass. She re-presented a few weeks later with nausea and vomiting due to tissue ingrowth of the previously placed stent. A second enteral stent was placed; however, the distal flange was inadvertently placed through the distal interstices of the first stent (Fig. 28.1). Consequently, the second stent could not fully open and the patient's gastric outlet obstruction remained un-attenuated. A third procedure confirmed the malpositioned stent, and given her poor surgical candidacy, a decision was made to proceed with an EUS-guided gastroenterostomy to definitively treat her obstruction.

28.3 Procedural Plan

Several techniques have been used to perform EUS-GE; the well-published iterations include a balloon-assisted method and a direct method

A. Y.B. Teoh et al. (eds.), *Atlas of Interventional EUS*, https://doi.org/10.1007/978-981-16-9340-3_28

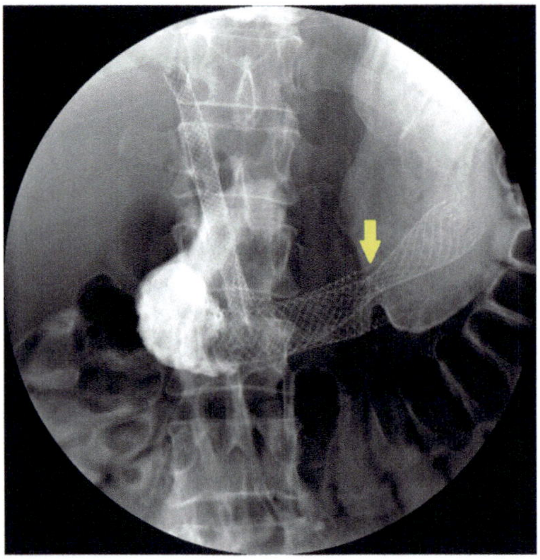

Fig. 28.1 Upper GI series without any contrast extravasation through the enteral stents due to placement of the second stent through the interstices of the first stent (arrow) leading to a gastric outlet obstruction

(antegrade) [3, 5]. The direct method requires an antegrade EUS approach with a free-hand puncture of the small bowel using a cautery-enhanced LAMS (Hot-Axios Boston Scientific Corp. Natick, MA, USA) without using a guidewire. First, the distal duodenum and jejunum are infused with a solution of saline and methylene blue +/− contrast material. Approximately 500 cc of fluid is needed to adequately distend the bowel. Saline is preferred by some to minimize the theoretical risk of iatrogenic hyponatremia, particularly if larger volumes of fluid are instilled. The infusion can be performed using a forward-viewing endoscope, by placing a nasobiliary catheter (7 French) beyond the obstruction into the downstream small bowel, or by instillation via the EUS scope itself. Enough fluid must be instilled to adequately distend the lumen to visualize a window for LAMS placement. Intervening tissue should be less than 10 mm between the stomach and the small bowel. Fluoroscopy provides confirmation of scope position, ideally within a dependent portion of the stomach to facilitate gastric emptying and PO tolerance. Glucagon (1 mg dosed intravenously) or other anti-spasmodic medication, can be administered prior to puncture to minimize small bowel peristalsis.

After the bowel is sufficiently distended with the solution, a 19-gauge "finder" needle is used to puncture the bowel and aspirate methylene blue-tinged fluid thereby confirming needle placement within the jejunum. This insures against unintentional colonic stent placement. The needle is then withdrawn and a cautery-enhanced LAMS is deployed under EUS-guidance. A rush of blue fluid from the anastomosed small bowel is the initial confirmation of adequate stent placement. Balloon dilation of the LAMS using a hydrostatic balloon dilator (e.g. 12–15 mm CRE balloon dilator, Boston Scientific, Natick, MA) expedites stent expansion which facilitates PO intake and provides the immediate benefit of adequate visualization of the downstream small bowel to confirm successful stent placement. Balloon dilation of the stent is neither standard practice nor strictly necessary, however, as there are some anecdotal reports of bleeding post-dilation.

28.4 Description of the Procedure (Video 28.1)

EUS-GE was successfully performed using the direct method in this case (VIDEO). Pre-procedure antibiotics were administered (typically an IV fluoroquinolone or cephalosporin). Exam was performed under general anesthesia to minimize the risk of aspiration. A single-channel therapeutic upper endoscope (GIF-HQ190, Olympus America, Center Valley, Pennsylvania, USA) was advanced to the obstructed distal flange of the enteral stent in the third portion of the duodenum. A guidewire was advanced under fluoroscopic guidance into the proximal jejunum and was exchanged for a nasobiliary drain catheter (7 French) with the distal end of the catheter coiled within the proximal jejunum (Fig. 28.2). Saline mixed with methylene blue plus contrast was infused into the small bowel to distend the lumen. A therapeutic linear echoendoscope (GF-UCT180, Olympus America, Center Valley,

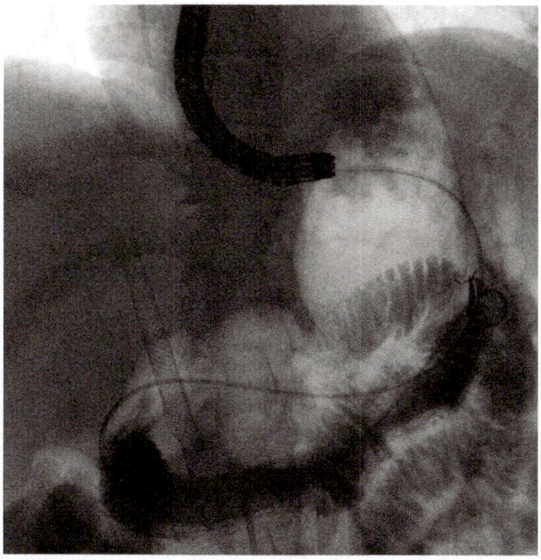

Fig. 28.2 Fluoroscopic image of a nasobiliary drain advanced into the proximal jejunum with endoscope removed

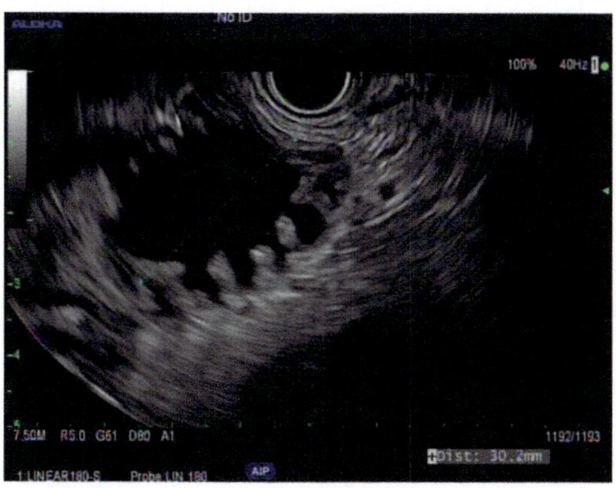

Fig. 28.3 EUS view of the targeted proximal jejunum (pre-puncture) with the lumen adequately distended with fluid and measuring >30 mm

Pennsylvania, USA) was used to identify a sufficiently distended loop of small bowel through the gastric body (Fig. 28.3). A 19 gauge "finder" needle was used to puncture the targeted small bowel with confirmatory aspiration of blue-tinged fluid. A cautery-enhanced 15 mm LAMS was then advanced directly into the jejunum (sans guidewire) and successfully deployed to create the gastroenterostomy (Fig. 28.4). The stent was dilated using a 15 mm CRE balloon dilator and

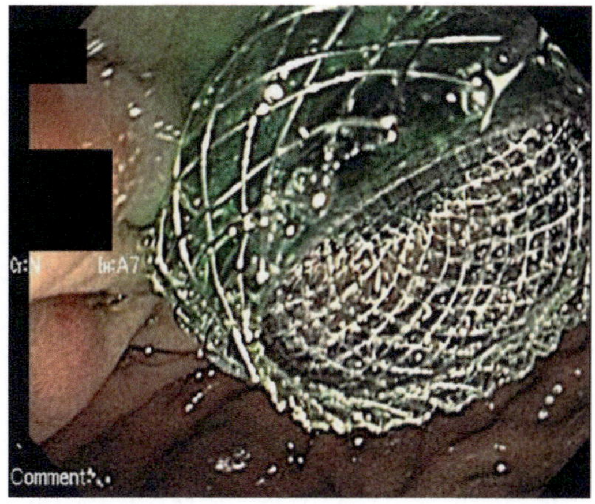

Fig. 28.4 Endoscopic view of the gastric flange following the deployment of the lumen-apposing metal stent (LAMS)

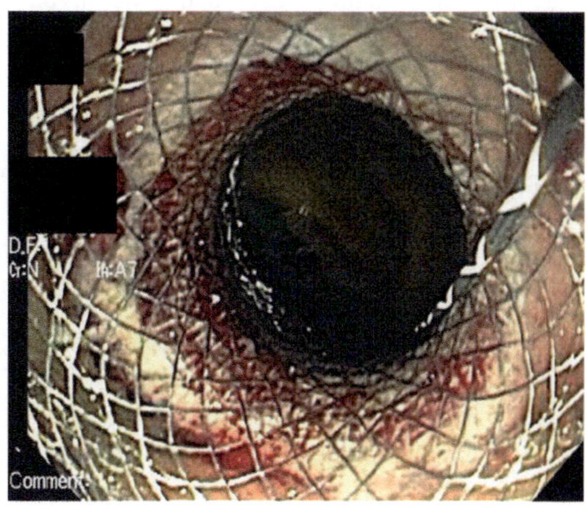

Fig. 28.5 Endoscopic view of the gastric flange post-balloon dilation with visualization of the newly anastomosed jejunum

the small bowel was visualized through the lumen of the stent for confirmation (Fig. 28.5).

28.5 Post-procedural Management

Patients are typically admitted for overnight observation. If the patient is doing well, then the diet is advanced as tolerated typically starting with a liquid diet immediately post-procedure followed by low residue diet on post-procedure day #1. This is followed by advancement to an unrestricted diet per the patient's tolerance. If there is any concern for stent migration, extraluminal leak, or stent occlusion, then an upper GI series can be obtained prior to advancing oral intake. Non-steroidal anti-inflammatory drugs (NSAIDs) are avoided for 2 weeks after stent placement. Stents are left indefinitely without indication for routine follow-up endoscopy.

28.6 Potential Pitfalls

The advantage of using the direct method for EUS-GE is faster deployment [5] due to the reduced number of steps compared to other published methods including: antegrade EUS-GE with rendezvous, retrograde EUS-GE *entero*gastrostomy, and balloon-occluded GE bypass (EPASS) [6, 7]. Another advantage of the direct method is the eliminated use of a guidewire during LAMS deployment that might potentially push the targeted small bowel away from the penetrating LAMS, which is the most commonly reported adverse event for EUS-GE [8].

Successfully performing the direct method requires a careful assessment of the length of intervening tissue between the stomach and the jejunum; ideally <10 mm. We offer a word of caution when performing this procedure in patients with large-volume ascites. This procedure should likewise be avoided in the presence of intervening tumor.

Methylene blue is useful at two key portions of the procedure; during the EUS-guided needle aspiration to confirm appropriate intended lumen for LAMS deployment, and immediately after successful LAMS insertion with a confirmatory rush of fluid from the newly anastomosed downstream bowel. If a large volume of methylene blue-tinged fluid is infused into the bowel and refluxes back into the gastric lumen, this can be mistaken as a sign of proper stent deployment. Aspirating blue contents from the targeted lumen also reduces the risk of inadvertent gastro-colonic stenting. Careful inspection after LAMS deployment is critical to assure proper stent placement; and balloon dilation facilitates adequate visualization of the downstream small bowel.

We leave these stents indefinitely and have observed rapid structuring of the GE anastomosis in cases of spontaneous stent migration. Lastly, this procedure is technically challenging even for experienced endosonographers and should be reserved for tertiary referral endoscopy centers.

References

1. Tyberg A, Kumta N, Karia K, Zerbo S, Sharaiha RZ, Kahaleh M. EUS-guided gastrojejunostomy after failed enteral stenting. Gastrointest Endosc. 2015;81(4):1011–2.
2. Khashab MA, Tieu AH, Azola A, Ngamruengphong S, El Zein MH, Kumbhari V. EUS-guided gastrojejunostomy for management of complete gastric outlet obstruction. Gastrointest Endosc. 2015;82(4):745.
3. Khashab MA, Kumbhari V, Grimm IS, Ngamruengphong S, Aguila G, El Zein M, et al. EUS-guided gastroenterostomy: the first U.S. clinical experience (with video). Gastrointest Endosc. 2015;82(5):932–8.
4. Tyberg A, Perez-Miranda M, Sanchez-Ocana R, Penas I, de la Serna C, Shah J, et al. Endoscopic ultrasound-guided gastrojejunostomy with a lumen-apposing metal stent: a multicenter, international experience. Endosc Int Open. 2016;4(3):E276–81.
5. Chen YI, Kunda R, Storm AC, Aridi HD, Thompson CC, Nieto J, et al. EUS-guided gastroenterostomy: a multicenter study comparing the direct and balloon-assisted techniques. Gastrointest Endosc. 2018;87(5):1215–21.
6. Kerdsirichairat T, Irani S, Yang J, Brewer Gutierrez OI, Moran R, Sanaei O, et al. Durability and long-term outcomes of direct EUS-guided gastroenterostomy using lumen-apposing metal stents for gastric outlet obstruction. Endosc Int Open. 2019;7(2):E144–E50.
7. Irani S, Itoi T, Baron TH, Khashab M. EUS-guided gastroenterostomy: techniques from east to west. VideoGIE. 2020;5(2):48–50.
8. Khashab MA. EUS-guided gastroenterostomy vs duodenal stenting for the palliation of malignant gastric outlet obstruction. Gastroenterol Hepatol (N Y). 2019;15(6):323–5.

EUS-Guided Balloon Occluded Gastrojejunostomy Bypass

29

Yukitoshi Matsunami and Takao Itoi

29.1 Background

Malignant gastric outlet obstruction (GOO) is often observed in patients with advanced pancreatobiliary and gastroduodenal cancers. In recent years, endoscopic ultrasonography-guided gastroenterostomy (EUS-GE) using a lumen-apposing metal stent (LAMS) has emerged as an alternative to conventional surgical gastroenterostomy and endoscopic enteral stenting for symptomatic GOO. EUS-GE using LAMS is a technique of interventional EUS, in which an anastomosis of the stomach and small intestine is created using LAMS, and enables a shortcut of the food pathway, similar to a surgical bypass. To date, there have been several reports of EUS-GE using LAMS [1–3]. Overall, the technical success rate of EUS-GE using LAMS is approximately 90%, and it has a lower rate of symptom recurrence than endoscopic enteral stenting [4]. We have previously developed a novel technique, which is a EUS-GE that uses LAMS and a special double-balloon enteric tube (EUS-guided double-balloon occluded gastroenterostomy bypass: EPASS) [5]. Herein, we describe a case of EPASS for symptomatic malignant GOO.

Supplementary Information The online version contains supplementary material available at [https://doi.org/10.1007/978-981-16-9340-3_29].

Y. Matsunami · T. Itoi (✉)
Department of Gastroenterology and Hepatology, Tokyo Medical University, Tokyo, Japan
e-mail: itoi@tokyo-med.ac.jp

29.2 Case History

A 68-year-old man who was diagnosed with gastric cancer of the antrum with multiple liver metastases 4 months before the procedure and had been received chemotherapy, was admitted for vomiting and anorexia. Physical examination showed upper quadrant tenderness. Computed tomography (CT) showed stricture in the antrum of the stomach with dilation of the oral side of the lesion with large amounts of food residue (Fig. 29.1a). The features were compatible with GOO owing to the tumor invasion, however, he had no indication of curative resection and was critically ill, with no tolerance for surgical GE. The patient did not opt for the endoscopic enteral stenting, owing to its high rate of symptom recurrence, and finally he was referred to our institution to undergo the EPASS.

29.3 Procedural Plan

CT showed that stricture was only located in the antrum of the stomach, and there were no obvious ascites. Blood examination showed no coagulopathy or thrombocytopenia, and he did not

A. Y.B. Teoh et al. (eds.), *Atlas of Interventional EUS*, https://doi.org/10.1007/978-981-16-9340-3_29

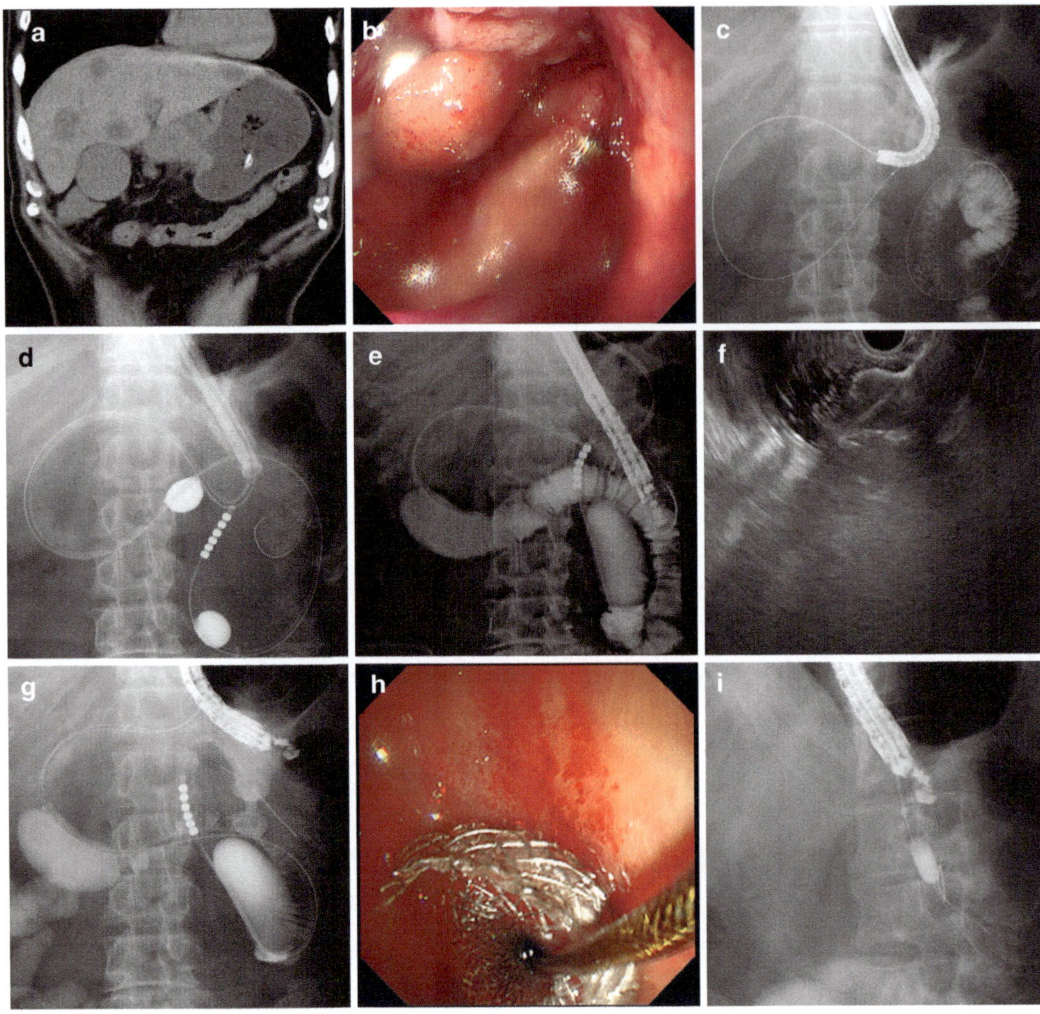

Fig. 29.1 Images of the EPASS procedure. (**a**) Coronal CT view of a patient with stomach cancer displaying a stricture in the antrum of the stomach. (**b**) Endoscopic view of the site of GOO in the antrum caused by stomach cancer. (**c**) A stiff guidewire is inserted as far as possible using an ERCP catheter through the stenotic site into the jejunum loop beyond the ligament of Treitz. (**d**) A double-balloon enteric tube is advanced into the appropriate area over the wire, and 2 balloons are inflated with saline and contrast medium to occlude the intestine. (**e**) A sufficient amount of normal saline with contrast material is introduced into the space between the 2 balloons to distend the small intestinal lumen. (**f**) An EUS image of the deployed distal flange in the jejunum. (**g**) A fluoroscopic view of stent deployment. (**h**) An endoscopic view of stent deployment. (**i**) The lumen of the deployed stent is dilated using a dilating balloon

take anti-thrombotic medicine. There were no contraindications and was considered to be an agreeable indication of EPASS. To date, several EUS-GE techniques have been reported from various institutions [3, 6, 7]. However, most of the previously reported EUS-GE techniques require a rapid infusion of a large volume of saline to dilate the jejunum sufficiently, as the injected saline immediately flows to the anal side, causing the targeted small intestine to shrink. Injection of a large amount of fluid may distend not only the targeted jejunum, but also the large bowel unintentionally, which may lead to mispuncture into the large bowel. On the other hand, regarding the EPASS, theory of double-balloon occluded gastroenterostomy is that filling saline into the limited area of the jejunum near the ligament of Treitz, which is anatomically the nearest site between the stomach and jejunum [8]. Inflated two balloons, which are attached to the special enteric tube, can occlude the small intestine, and enable limited water filling in the proper area. The space occluded by two balloons is easily dilated without shrinking, and the needle easily goes into the jejunum because the jejunal wall has tension. EPASS is divided into 2 procedures according to the type of LAMS, namely, a one-step procedure (the so-called freestyle technique), which uses the Hot-AXIOS system (Boston Scientific, Natick MA, USA), which is LAMS including an electrocautery tip, and a two-step procedure (the so-called standard technique), which uses the AXIOS™ stent [6, 9]. Hot-AXIOS system has made it possible to place the stent in place without needle puncture and guidewire placement. When the flanges are fully opened, the anchor flanges have a diameter of 24 mm, which is almost double that of the saddle section (15 mm). The stent anchors are designed to distribute pressure evenly over the luminal wall and to securely anchor the stent to prevent migration. Owing to its simplicity and safety of the procedure, one-step procedure is preferable. The patient was to be offered a one-step EPASS.

29.4 Description of the Procedure

Firstly, a standard upper gastrointestinal (GI) endoscope was advanced into the front of the stenosis area (Fig. 29.1b) (Video 29.1). A stiff guidewire was inserted using an ERCP catheter through the stenotic site into the duodenum or jejunum loop beyond the ligament of Treitz, as far as possible (Fig. 29.1c). After removing the upper GI endoscope, leaving the guidewire in place, the special double-balloon enteric tube was advanced over the wire to the proper area. Next, two balloons were inflated with saline and a contrast medium to occlude the intestine (Fig. 29.1d). After inserting the linear EUS endoscope, the saline and contrast medium was injected through the enteric tube and directly delivered into the lumen, which was occluded by the 2 inflated balloons. Generally, a total of 150 mL of fluid is sufficient to dilate the small intestine. The dilated intestine was detected by EUS and fluoroscopy (Fig. 29.1e). The Hot-AXIOS system was used to directly puncture the dilated intestine using the cautery tip and to deploy the distal anchor flange under EUS guidance (Fig. 29.1f). Then, the stent was pulled back to the stomach side to connect the stomach wall and jejunum wall, and to deploy the proximal flange (Fig. 29.1g, h). Additionally, the lumen of the deployed stent was dilated using a 12-mm dilating balloon (Fig. 29.1i).

29.5 Post-Procedural Management

Periprocedural intravenous antibiotics are continued for 3 to 5 days. A liquid diet is begun 1 or 2 days after the procedure with confirmation of the absence of a fever and abdominal pain. Then, the diet is advanced as tolerated by the patient, to a low-residue or full diet. The status of food intake is evaluated using the gastric outlet obstruction scoring system (GOOSS) [10]. Patients are discharged after an improvement of at least 2 points from their baseline GOOSS is achieved.

29.6 Potential Pitfalls

CT images are useful for determining the stricture site before the procedure. Owing to that anastomosis is created in the body of the stomach and beyond the fourth portion of the duodenum, if the tumor has invaded the body of the stomach or beyond the fourth portion of the duodenum, EPASS may not be technically possible. The patients with multiple GI tract strictures and complete GOO in whom guidewire advancement is impossible may not be suitable for this procedure. Regarding the presence of ascites, a small amount of ascites may be acceptable; however, patients with an uncontrollable excessive amount of ascites should avoid this procedure. Patients with the condition of coagulopathy and/or thrombocytopenia should be treated their general condition before the procedure. The rate of adverse events (AEs) of EUS-GE, including EPASS was reported to be approximately 10%, which includes misdeployment of the stent, bleeding, pneumoperitoneum, peritonitis, abdominal pain, and gastrocolonic fistula [4]. The rate of serious AEs was reported to be 5.6% [11]. Misdeployment of the stent, which is a common AE, may be caused by the difficulty in accurately puncturing the small intestine, as well as owing to the long procedure time. As the stomach and jejunum are anatomically not adjacent, it leads to the small intestine being pushed away from the stomach. It is noted that misdeployment of a stent may be fatal in end-stage cancer patients with a poor general condition. Avoiding such situations, enough dilation of small intestine and minimalizing the procedure time is mandatory. Additionally, to confirm the correct stent deployment to the targeted jejunum, injection of saline with indigo carmine through the special enteric tube into the small intestine, and checking the backflow of indigo carmine through the stent to the stomach is recommended. It should be also noted that previously published data of EUS-GE, including EPASS, are mostly retrospective, and the procedures were performed by experts in high-volume tertiary referral centers. Therefore, at present, it should be performed only by highly skilled experts of interventional EUS under a multidisciplinary setting.

References

1. Itoi T, Itokawa F, Uraoka T, et al. Novel EUS-guided gastroenterostomy technique using a new double-balloon enteric tube and lumen-apposing metal stent (with videos). Gastrointest Endosc. 2013;78:934–9.
2. Khashab MA, Kumbhari V, Grimm IS, et al. EUS-guided gastroenterostomy: the first U.S. clinical experience (with video). Gastrointest Endosc. 2015;82:932–8.
3. Tyberg A, Perez-Miranda M, Sanchez-Ocana R, et al. Endoscopic ultrasound-guided gastrojejunostomy with a lumen-apposing metal stent: a multicenter, international experience. Endosc Int Open. 2016;4:E276–81.
4. Iqbal U, Khara HS, Hu Y, et al. EUS-guided gastroenterostomy for the management of gastric outlet obstruction: a systematic review and meta-analysis. Endosc ultrasound. 2020;9(1):16–23.
5. Itoi T, Tsuchiya T, Tonozuka R, et al. Novel EUS-guided double balloon-occluded gastrojejunostomy bypass. Gastrointest Endosc. 2016;83:461–2.
6. Itoi T, Ishii K, Ikeuchi N, et al. Prospective evaluation of endoscopic ultrasonography-guided double-balloon-occluded gastrojejunostomy bypass (EPASS) for malignant gastric outlet obstruction. Gut. 2016;65:193–5.
7. Khashab MA, Bukhari M, Baron TH, et al. International multicenter comparative trial of endoscopic ultrasonography-guided gastroenterostomy versus surgical gastrojejunostomy for the treatment of malignant gastric outlet obstruction. Endosc Int Open. 2017;5:E275–81.
8. Itoi T, Tsuchiya T, Matsunami Y, et al. EUS-guided gastrojejunostomy: double-balloon occlusion theory with experimental study (with video). J Hepatobiliary Pancreat Sci. 2020;27:791–2.
9. Itoi T, Baron TH, Khashab MA, et al. Technical review of endoscopic ultrasonography-guided gastroenterostomy in 2017. Digestive Endosc. 2017;29: 495–502.
10. Adler DG, Baron TH. Endoscopic palliation of malignant gastric outlet obstruction using self-expanding metal stents: experience in 36 pa- tients. Am J Gastroenterol. 2002;97:72–8.
11. McCarty TR, Garg R, Thompson CC, et al. Efficacy and safety of EUS-guided gastroenterostomy for benign and malignant gastric outlet obstruction: a systematic review and meta-analysis. Endosc Int Open. 2019;07:E1474–82.

30 One-Stage EUS-Guided Gastrogastrostomy and ERCP in Roux-n-Y Gastric Bypass Anatomy

Rahman Nakshabendi and Todd H. Baron

30.1 Background

EUS-guided gastrogastrostomy using lumen-apposing metal stents (LAMS) is gaining popularity for allowing access to the papilla to perform ERCP as an alternative to device-assisted ERCP (DA-ERCP) (e.g., enteroscopy-assisted) and laparoscopic-assisted ERCP (LA-ERCP) for patients with Roux-en-Y gastric bypass (RYGB) anatomy. The procedure was first described by Kahaleh's group with the acronym EDGE (EUS-directed transgastric ERCP) [1]. The procedure has been shown to be associated with high technical success and low adverse event rates [2]. In one study EDGE was shown to have similar technical success and adverse events compared to LA-ERCP, with significantly shorter procedure times and hospital stay and without significant weight gain. In a decision model comparing EDGE to DA-ERCP and LA-ERCP in post-RYGB anatomy, EDGE was the most cost-effective modality in post-RYGB anatomy for treatment of pancreaticobiliary diseases [3]. The gastrogastrostomy can be used for other interventions and is referred to as EUS-directed transgastric intervention (EDGI) [4], which can allow for other interventions such as passage of an echoendoscope to the duodenum for evaluation of the pancreatic head and subsequent fine needle aspiration and biopsy.

30.2 Case History

A 48-year-old female with remote cholecystectomy and Roux-en-Y gastric bypass performed six months prior presented with clinically mild acute gallstone pancreatitis; serum lipase was >40,000 U/L, and AST/ALT were 1419 and 1091 IU/L, respectively. Abdominal CT showed changes of acute pancreatitis with peripancreatic fluid and stranding but no pancreatic necrosis was seen. The common bile duct was dilated in caliber without visible stones. Forty-eight hours later EDGE was undertaken.

30.3 Procedural Plan

EDGE can be performed via a gastrogastric or jejunogastric [5] approach, the latter entry point is usually just beyond the gastrojejunal anastomosis.

Supplementary Information The online version contains supplementary material available at [https://doi.org/10.1007/978-981-16-9340-3_30].

R. Nakshabendi · T. H. Baron (✉)
Division of Gastroenterology & Hepatology, University of North Carolina, Chapel Hill, NC, USA
e-mail: todd_baron@med.unc.edu

A. Y.B. Teoh et al. (eds.), *Atlas of Interventional EUS*, https://doi.org/10.1007/978-981-16-9340-3_30

We perform EDGE using a cautery-enhanced lumen apposing metallic stent (LAMS) because it greatly simplifies the procedure and reduces procedural time and need for device exchange.

If the indication for ERCP is elective, we prefer to perform it after a duration of 10 or more days following LAMS placement to allow the tract to mature in the event of stent dislodgement, which may occur when ERCP is performed at the same session as EDGE.

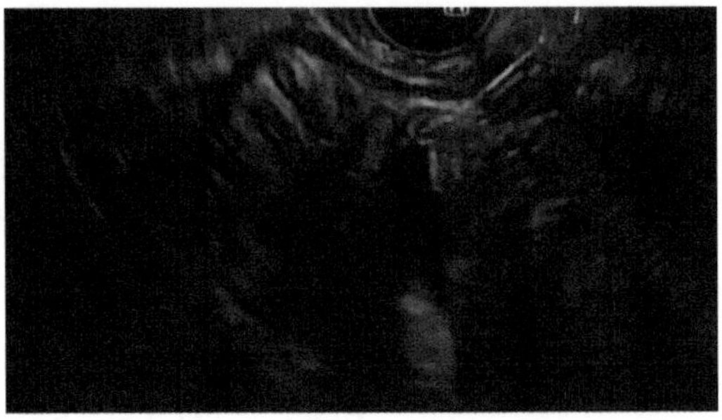

Fig. 30.2 19 G FNA needle used to inject contrast to confirm position and to distend the lumen

30.4 Description of the Procedure

General anesthesia was administered. No antibiotics were given. The procedure was performed with the patient in the supine position and CO_2 insufflation. The anastomosis was performed with a cautery-enhanced lumen apposing metal stent (LAMS) via the gastrogastrostomy approach using a standard, oblique-viewing linear echoendoscope. The excluded stomach was identified echosonographically and is often seen as the Starfish Sign [6]. An area without intervening blood vessels was located (Fig. 30.1) (Video 30.1). The excluded stomach was punctured with a standard 19-gauge FNA needle (Fig. 30.2, Video 30.1). Water-soluble contrast was injected under fluoroscopic guidance to confirm entry into the excluded stomach (Video 30.1). The needle was then attached to a standard endoscopic water irrigation pump and approximately 500 cc of sterile saline was instilled into the excluded stomach to distend the lumen and create an easy target for "freehand" LAMS deployment. The FNA needle was removed and the 20 mm × 10 mm LAMS cautery-enhanced delivery system was passed into the excluded stomach using pure cutting current (Fig. 30.3). The distal flange was opened under EUS guidance (Fig. 30.4). Rather than pull the stent back against the inner wall of the excluded stomach, it was left more distally. The endoscope was withdrawn with the stent delivery system until the black marker was seen endoscopically on the catheter and then opened and deployed (Fig. 30.5) (Video 30.1). We do not routinely dilate the stent after deployment unless a one-stage EDGE is performed, as in this case; the stent lumen was balloon dilated to 20 mm (Fig. 30.6, Video 30.1). The echoendoscope was removed and a standard duodenoscope was inserted and passed through the LAMS to the papilla. ERCP, sphincterotomy, and stone extrac-

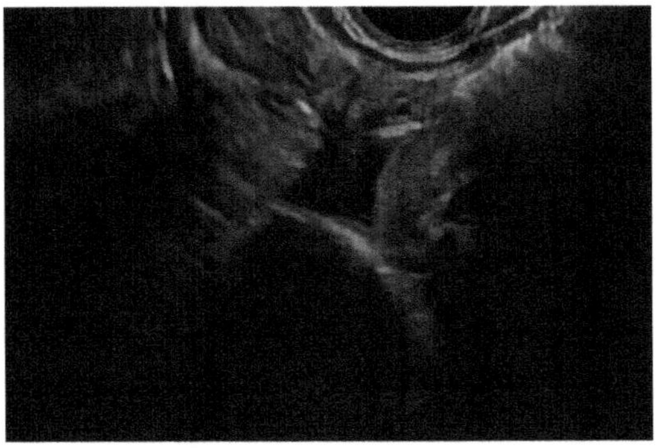

Fig. 30.3 Inner flange of the LAMS deployed in the excluded stomach

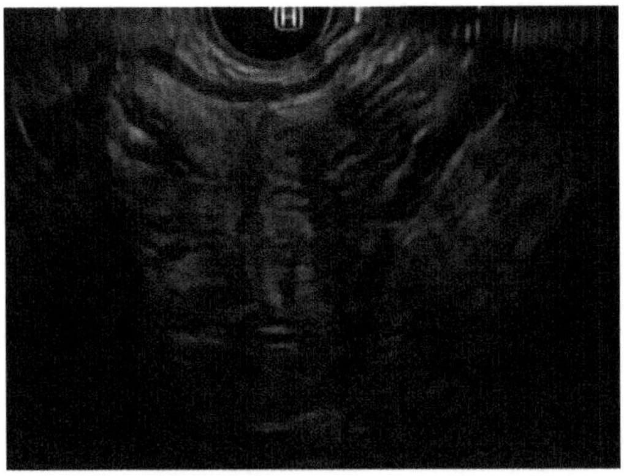

Fig. 30.1 Echosonographic appearance of the excluded stomach

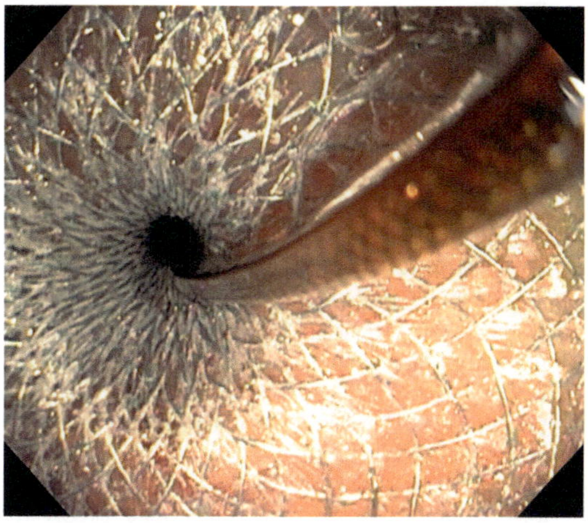

Fig. 30.4 Endoscopic view immediately after deployment of LAMS within the gastric pouch

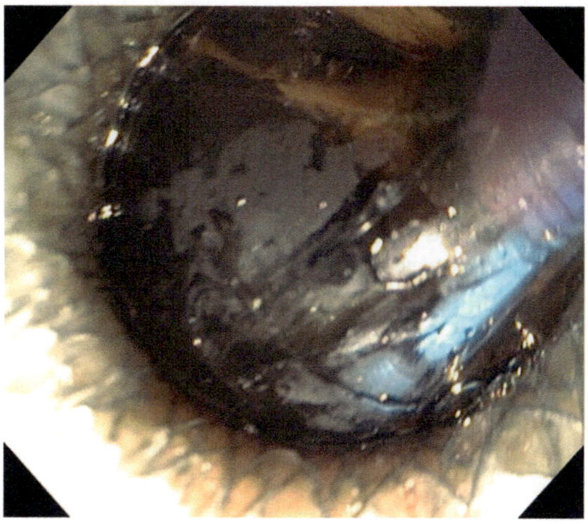

Fig. 30.5 Endoscopic view of LAMS during balloon dilation

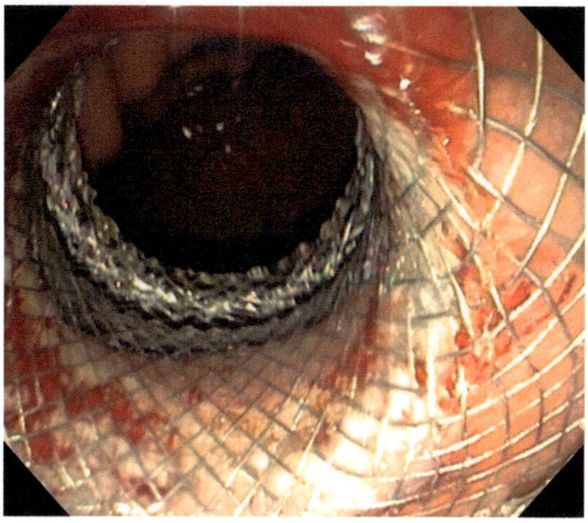

Fig. 30.6 Endoscopic view after balloon dilation

tion were performed (Video 30.1). As the duodenoscope was withdrawn across the LAMS, the stone extraction balloon and guidewire used for the ERCP were advanced so that they remained in the duodenum while inspecting for LAMS dislodgement. If it had, the catheter would have been exchanged leaving the wire in place and a 6-cm long, fully covered TTS esophageal stent would then be passed through the LAMS to salvage the procedure and prevent leakage.

30.5 Post-Procedural Management

A diet was resumed the same day. The patient was discharged home later the same day as her pancreatitis was already clinically resolving. There were no adverse events and she underwent elective outpatient upper endoscopy 6 weeks later to remove the LAMS using a standard forward-viewing endoscope. The LAMS was removed using alligator/rat-toothed forceps. The fistula tract was cauterized with argon plasma coagulation to promote closure (Fig. 30.7).

30.6 Potential Pitfalls

The potential adverse events after EDGE include misdeployment of the stent, migration / dislodgement, perforation, and bleeding. In the case of stent misdeployment, management

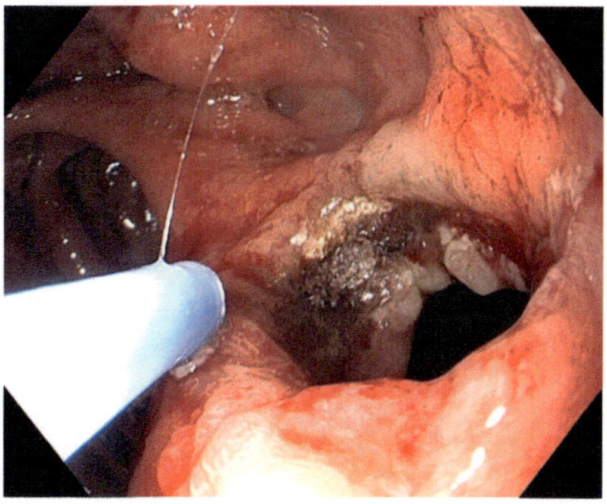

Fig. 30.7 Argon plasma coagulation of the gastrogastric fistula

depends on whether a guidewire had been passed. If a guidewire is still in place, a 20-mm diameter covered TTS esophageal stent is passed through the LAMS and /or tract to bridge the two lumens. If there is no wire access, a therapeutic upper endoscope is used to identify the site and pass a wire from the pouch or jejunum into the excluded stomach to regain access and allow a bridging stent to be placed. Percutaneous drainage or surgery may be required to manage this adverse event. For patients undergoing same session ERCP, stent dislodgement can be prevented by endoscopically suturing the LAMS in place and dilating the LAMS lumen to its maximal 20 mm diameter prior to passage of a duodenoscope. Weight regain may occur if the fistula does not close after LAMS removal, which occurs in up to 10% of patients [7]. Primary fistula closure at the time of LAMS removal via suturing or over-the-scope clip devices, or other novel tacking systems can be used. Similarly, delayed closure may be achieved with over-the-scope clip application or endoscopic suturing. It is important to follow patients closely for weight regain as a sign of persistent fistula. Alternatively, an upper endoscopy or upper GI barium series can be obtained, and should be obtained to document successful endoscopic closure, when performed.

References

1. Internal EUS-directed transgastric ERCP (EDGE): game over Kedia P, Sharaiha RZ, Kumta NA, Kahaleh M. Gastroenterology. 2014 Sep;147(3):566-568.
2. Forster E, Elmunzer BJ. Endoscopic Retrograde Cholangiopancreatography in Patients With Roux-en-Y Gastric Bypass. Am J Gastroenterol. 2020 Feb;115(2):155–7.
3. James HJ, James TW, Wheeler SB, Spencer JC, Baron TH. Cost-effectiveness of endoscopic ultrasound-directed transgastric ERCP compared with device-assisted and laparoscopic-assisted ERCP in patients with Roux-en-Y anatomy. Endoscopy. 2019 Nov;51(11):1051–8.
4. The EDGI new take on EDGE: EUS-directed transgastric intervention (EDGI), other than ERCP, for Roux-en-Y gastric bypass anatomy: a multicenter study. Krafft MR, Hsueh W, James TW, Runge TM, Baron TH, Khashab MA, Irani SS, Nasr JYEndosc Int Open 2019 Oct;7(10):E1231–E1240.
5. Tyberg A, Nieto J, Salgado S, Weaver K, Kedia P, Sharaiha RZ, Gaidhane M, Kahaleh M. Endoscopic Ultrasound (EUS)-Directed Transgastric Endoscopic Retrograde Cholangiopancreatography or EUS: Mid-Term Analysis of an Emerging Procedure. Clin Endosc. 2017 Mar;50(2):185–90.
6. Siddiki H, Baron TH. The sand dollar sign: a reliable EUS image to identify the excluded stomach during EUS-guided gastrogastrostomy. Gastrointest Endosc. 2018 Aug;88(2):398–9.
7. James TW, Baron TH. Endoscopic Ultrasound-Directed Transgastric ERCP (EDGE): a Single-Center US Experience with Follow-up Data on Fistula Closure. Obes Surg. 2019 Feb;29(2):451–6.

31 Afferent Limb Obstruction

Rastislav Kunda

31.1 Background

Afferent limb obstruction, also frequently called afferent loop syndrome, is a rare complication that can occur after surgical procedures involving anastomosis of the stomach, esophagus, and also other segments of upper gastrointestinal tract to the jejunum. The afferent loop is the duodenojejunal loop proximal to the gastrojejunal (or other) anastomosis and syndrome is the result of partial or complete mechanical obstruction of the afferent limb or at its anastomosis. It is typically described following Billroth II gastrojejunostomy, Roux-en-Y gastrojejunostomy, and cephalic duodenopancreatectomy, regardless of the type of reconstruction used [1].

The afferent limb transfers bile, pancreatic, and proximal intestinal secretions distally toward the anastomosis (gastrojejunostomy in Billroth II/Whipple procedures and jejunojejunostomy in Roux-en-Y reconstructions). The efferent loop receives and transfers the ingested food and liquids. Afferent limb obstruction is defined by a distal obstruction causing distension of the afferent limb secondary to the accumulation of bile, pancreatic fluid, and proximal small bowel secretions [2].

The incidence of significant afferent limb obstruction after these procedures is low (0.3% to 1.0%) and is similar for both open and laparoscopic surgeries [3–5]. The etiologies of afferent limb obstruction include postoperative adhesions/kinking, internal herniation, volvulus and intussusception of the afferent loop, ulceration in the anastomosis and its scarring, local recurrence of cancer, peritoneal carcinomatosis, radiation enteritis, and others.

Although both acute and chronic forms of afferent loop syndrome have been described, chronic partial obstruction is the more common clinical manifestation. The classic presentation of chronic afferent loop syndrome is postprandial abdominal pain relieved by bilious vomiting, but the latter may be lacking if Roux-en-Y postsurgical anatomy is present. Secretions accumulate in the afferent limb and thereby give bowel distention which is painful and when severe can lead to perforation, leakage of the bowel content, and peritonitis. Less frequently jaundice, cholangitis, or pancreatitis may be part of the clinical presentation, especially in cases of more severe obstruction [6–8].

Treatment options have evolved in recent years from surgical revision and percutaneous

Supplementary Information The online version contains supplementary material available at [https://doi.org/10.1007/978-981-16-9340-3_31].

R. Kunda (✉)
Department of Surgery, Department of Advanced Interventional Endoscopy and Department of Gastroenterology-Hepatology, Universitair Ziekenhuis Brussel, Vrije Universiteit Brussel, Brussels, Belgium
e-mail: rkunda@uzbrussel.be

A. Y.B. Teoh et al. (eds.), *Atlas of Interventional EUS*, https://doi.org/10.1007/978-981-16-9340-3_31

drainage to full endoscopic management [9]. Endoscopic treatment is not always feasible but therapeutic possibilities using endoscopic ultrasound are increasing thanks to new devices [10]. Endoscopic ultrasound-guided gastrojejunostomy or gastroenterostomy have been used in the treatment of benign or malignant gastric outlet obstruction but can also be used in the treatment of afferent limb obstruction and afferent loop syndrome [11, 12]. When compared with surgical gastroenteroanastomosis, EUS-guided gastroenterostomy shows significantly fewer adverse events [13]. When performing EUS-guided gastroenterostomy, we try to access the jejunum or duodenum endosonographically, from the stomach or jejunum, while using a lumen apposing metal stent.

31.2 Case History

A 55-year-old female patient presented with abdominal pain, vomiting, and high fever to the emergency department. She had a history of pancreatic adenocarcinoma (T3N1M0) and had undergone a pancreatoduodenectomy 18 months ago, followed by adjuvant chemotherapy. She had reduced oral intake in the last two weeks as it aggravated her symptoms. This resulted in significant weight loss and dehydration. Blood pressure at admission was 97/63 mm Hg, heart rate 112 per minute, respiratory rate of 20 per minute, and body temperature of 38.9 C. Physical examination revealed painful palpation of the upper abdomen and scleral icterus. Complete blood count showed white blood cells of 21,000/mm^3, hemoglobin of 8.3 g/dL and platelet of 115.000/mm^3. Blood chemistry tests were total bilirubin 4.6 mg/dL, direct bilirubin 3.9 mg/dL AST/ALT 54/69 IU/L, alkaline phosphatase 270 IU/L, and glutamyl transpeptidase 644 IU/L. Laboratory tests suggested sepsis secondary to obstructive jaundice and ascending cholangitis. Abdominal CT scan after intravenous rehydration confirmed dilatation of the biliary tree and remarkable distention of the afferent limb due to regional pancreatic cancer recurrence. Patient was diagnosed with afferent loop syndrome and empiric antibiotics were started. EUS-guided gastrojejunostomy to drain the afferent limb was indicated and offered to patient.

31.3 Procedural Plan

Conventionally, treatment options include percutaneous biliary drainage or surgical bypass. By standard endoscopy, access to the afferent limb, for balloon dilatation or stenting, may be technically challenging because of long enteric loop, tight angulations, multiple strictures, or totally obstructing malignant lesion. Transanastomotic stenting may also compromise flow through and occlude efferent part of the anastomosis.

EUS-guided anastomosis in cases of afferent limb obstruction is typically performed from the stomach, but it can be done also from the efferent limb of jejunum. Patients with recurrent malignancies have a rather dubious prognosis and limited life expectancy. Therefore, positioning of the anastomosis may not be as crucial. Transjejunal approach may be considered in some benign cases. But there is no clear clinical evidence supporting the benefit of either approach. Both strategies work well in terms of symptom relief. However, both approaches may be also considered in terms of potential further endoscopic access into the enteric lumen of the afferent limb and eventual need for endoscopic interventions on bile ducts or pancreatic duct.

We prefer to use electrocautery enhanced LAMS, which facilitates to create "kissing" tension-free anastomosis in between two lumens/organs. It allows performance of freestyle technique, where the use of guidewire or EUS-needle is not required or needed. Distended afferent limb typically presents as an good target for this technique, due to enhanced ultrasound coupling by accumulated fluid contents in it. We typically prefer 10 mm in diameter LAMS in majority of cases and 15 mm in diameter LAMS, only in those cases where further interventions through the stent may be warranted. Smaller or larger diameters of LAMS are available; however, they would be either too small to drain afferent limb or too large when essentially only fluid content needs to be drained.

31.4 Description of the Procedure

EUS-guided gastrojejunostomy was performed with the electrocautery-enhanced lumen-apposing metal stent (LAMS). The distended afferent loop following previous pancreatic surgery, was identified. As it is typically filled with a large volume of fluid content, it does not require additional measures to enhance its ultrasound coupling and visualization. The freestyle technique is used and the loop is punctured directly by the tip of electrocautery-enhanced LAMS introducer. The first flange of LAMS is opened in the lumen of jejunum. The delivery system is then pulled back and the second flange is then deployed in the endoscope channel and then fully deployed by pushing it out of the channel. EUS-guided anastomosis in between afferent limb and stomach is thus created.

We do not routinely dilate the stent after the procedure as the LAMS usually fully expands within 24 hours. The afferent limb typically contains only fluids and even incomplete stent expansion is sufficient for their evacuation and drainage.

31.5 Post-Procedural Management

Patient may resume oral intake almost immediately, right after recovery from conscious sedation or general anesthesia. It is recommended to start with the fluid diet within first 24 hours. Typically, symptoms of pain, fullness, nausea, and vomiting resolve within 24 hours. In case of jaundice and/or cholangitis, resolution of these symptoms may take a longer time. Created EUS-guided gastroenteric anastomosis facilitates endoscopic access through this anastomosis, if needed, as it serves now not only to drain the afferent limb but also as the access point for the bile and pancreatic ducts, respectively. Other options in cases of severe cholangitis include percutaneous transhepatic biliary drainage and EUS-guided hepaticogastrostomy.

31.6 Potential Pitfalls

Potential adverse events related to EUS guided management of afferent limb obstruction may include misdeployment of the stent, its migration, perforation, and bleeding. In a few cases, especially in recurrent malignancies, additional obstruction(s) may be present or develop later, both on afferent and on efferent limbs, resulting in incomplete resolution of symptoms (Figs. 31.1, 31.2, 31.3, 31.4, and 31.5).

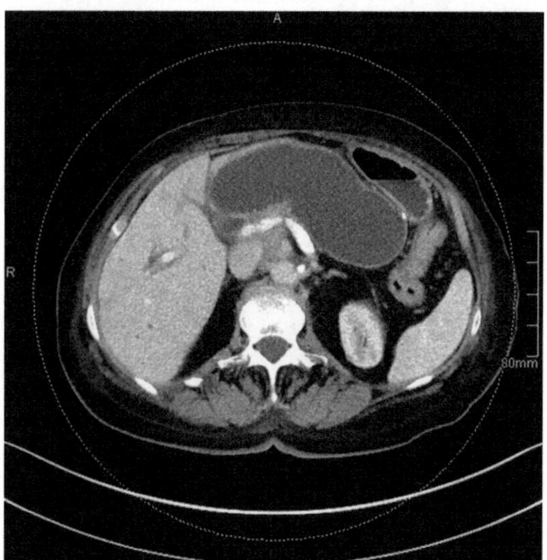

Fig. 31.1 Computer tomography demonstrating afferent limb obstruction—axial plane

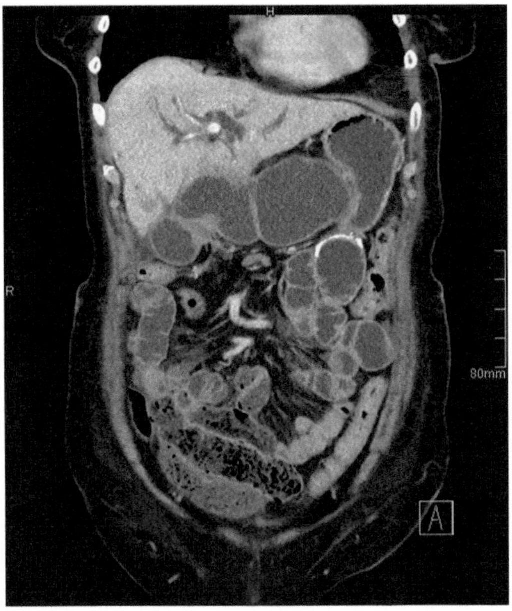

Fig. 31.2 Computer tomography demonstrating afferent limb obstruction with bile duct dilation—coronal plane

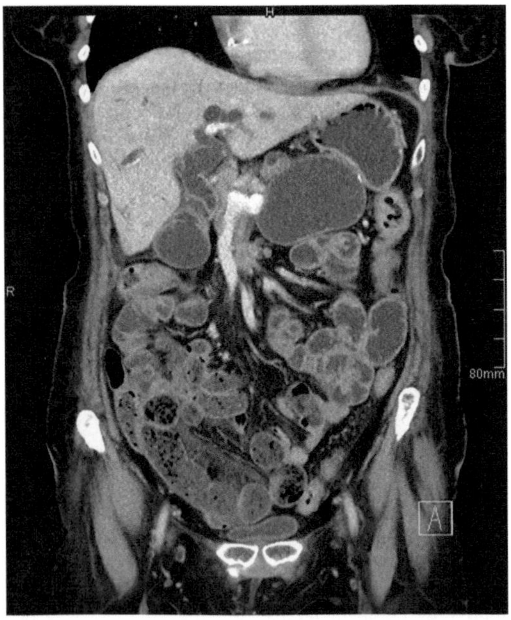

Fig. 31.3 Computer tomography demonstrating afferent limb obstruction—coronal plane

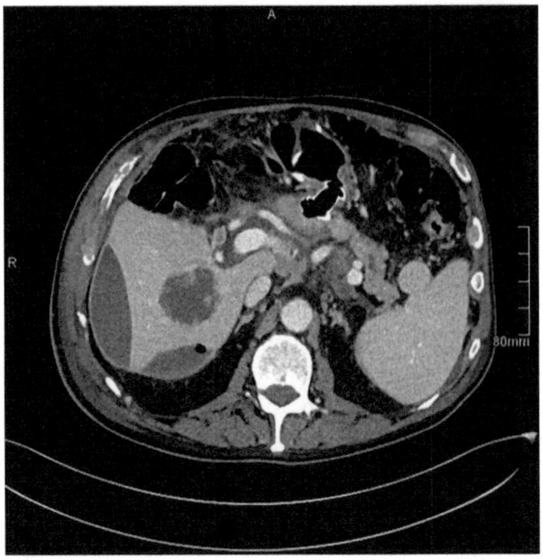

Fig. 31.4 Computer tomography showing resolution of afferent limb obstruction by LAMS—axial plane

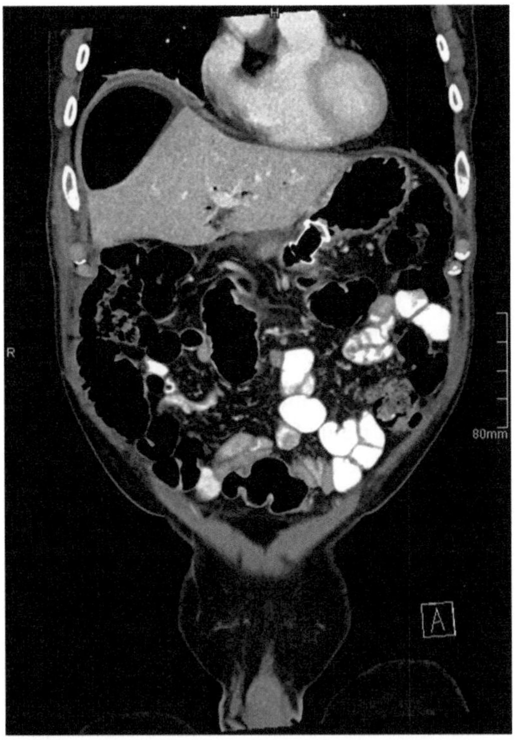

Fig. 31.5 Computer tomography showing resolution of afferent limb obstruction by LAMS—coronal plane

References

1. Nageswaran H, Belgaumkar A, Kumar R, et al. Acute afferent loop syndrome in the early postoperative period following pancreaticoduodenectomy. Ann R Coll Surg Engl. 2015;97(5):349–53.
2. Kawamoto Y, Ome Y, Kouda Y, Saga K, Park T, Kawamoto K. Pancreaticoduodenectomy following gastrectomy reconstructed with Billroth II or roux-en-Y method: case series and literature review. Int J Surg Case Rep. 2017;35:106–9.
3. Cao Y, Kong X, Yang D, Li S. Endoscopic nasogastric tube insertion for treatment of benign afferent loop obstruction after radical gastrectomy for gastric cancer: a 16-year retrospective single-center study. Medicine (Baltimore). 2019;98(28):e16475.
4. Kim DJ, Lee JH, Kim W. Afferent loop obstruction following laparoscopic distal gastrectomy with Billroth-II gastrojejunostomy. J Korean Surg Soc. 2013;84(5):281–6.
5. Aoki M, Saka M, Morita S, Fukagawa T, Katai H. Afferent loop obstruction after distal gastrectomy with Roux-en-Y reconstruction. World J Surg. 2010;34(10):2389–92.
6. Uriu Y, Kuriyama A, Ueno A, Ikegami T. Afferent loop syndrome of 10 years' onset after gastrectomy. Asian J Surg. 2019;42(10):935–7.
7. Katagiri H, Tahara K, Yoshikawa K, Lefor AK, Kubota T, Mizokami K. Afferent loop syndrome after Roux-en-Y Total gastrectomy caused by volvulus of the roux-limb. Case Rep Surg. 2016;2016:4930354.
8. Blouhos K, Boulas KA, Tsalis K, Hatzigeorgiadis A. Management of afferent loop obstruction: reoperation or endoscopic and percutaneous interventions? World J Gastrointest Surg. 2015;7(9):190–5.
9. Ratone JP, Caillol F, Bories E, Pesenti C, Godat S, Giovannini M. Hepatogastrostomy by EUS for malignant afferent loop obstruction after duodenopancreatectomy. Endosc Ultrasound. 2015;4(3):250–2.
10. Rimbas M, Larghi A, Costamagna G. Endoscopic ultrasound-guided gastroenterostomy: are we ready for prime time? Endosc Ultrasound. 2017;6(4):235–40.
11. Khashab MA, Bukhari M, Baron TH, et al. International multicenter comparative trial of endoscopic ultrasonography-guided gastroenterostomy versus surgical gastrojejunostomy for the treatment of malignant gastric outlet obstruction. Endosc Int Open. 2017;5(4):E275–81.
12. Brewer Gutierrez OI, Irani SS, Ngamruengphong S, et al. Endoscopic ultrasound-guided entero-enterostomy for the treatment of afferent loop syndrome: a multicenter experience. Endoscopy. 2018;50(9):891–5.
13. Carbajo AY, Kahaleh M, Tyberg A. Clinical review of EUS-guided gastroenterostomy (EUS-GE). J Clin Gastroenterol. 2020;54(1):1–7.

32 EUS Gastric Access for Therapeutic Endoscopy for Management of a Walled Off Necrosis with a LAM Stent in Gastric Bypass Anatomy

Javier Tejedor-Tejada, Ameya Deshmukh, Ahmed Mohammed Elmeligui, and Jose Nieto

32.1 Background

Gastric bypass is a common surgical procedure to induce weight loss in patients with severe obesity [1]. Gastric Access Temporary for Endoscopy (GATE) is a new and emerging endoscopic procedure. It is an alternative to device-assisted enteroscopy or surgery in patients with gastric bypass [2]. During the GATE procedure, a lumen apposing metal stent (LAM) is inserted from the gastric remnant into the excluded stomach for access to allow for various biliary/pancreatic endoscopy procedures, including transmural drainage of a pancreatic pseudocyst [3]. Another name for GATE described in other studies is endoscopic ultrasound-directed transgastric ERCP (EDGE) [4].

Supplementary Information The online version contains supplementary material available at [https://doi.org/10.1007/978-981-16-9340-3_32].

J. Tejedor-Tejada
Department of Gastroenterology, Hepatology and Endoscopy, Hospital Universitario Rio Hortega, Valladolid, Spain

A. Deshmukh
Department of Internal Medicine, Saint Louis University – School of Medicine, St. Louis, MO, USA
e-mail: ameya.deshmukh@health.slu.edu

32.2 Case History

A 60-year-old female presented with nausea, vomiting, and epigastric pain. She had a history of gastric bypass surgery and multiple comorbidities, admitted with the diagnosis of acute biliary pancreatitis. A control CT scan held after 10 days identified a walled off necrosis (WON) occupying more than 50% of the pancreatic parenchyma and retroperitoneal free liquid. Endoscopic drainage was chosen as this patient met the criteria including a fully walled off necrosis, the fluid collection was adjoined to the stomach/duodenum and the fluid collection was greater than or equal to 6 cm in size.

A. Mohammed Elmeligui
Division of Gastroenterology, Hepatology and Endoscopy, Kasr Alainy School of Medicine, Cairo, Egypt
e-mail: Ahmed.elmeligui@kasralainy.edu.eg

J. Nieto (✉)
Division of Gastroenterology, Hepatology and Endoscopy, Baptist Medical Center Jacksonville, Jacksonville, FL, USA

A. Y.B. Teoh et al. (eds.), *Atlas of Interventional EUS*, https://doi.org/10.1007/978-981-16-9340-3_32

32.3 Procedural Plan

The procedure can be performed in a single or two sessions. Single session are preferred for urgent cases. In both situations, the first is to create a gastric anastomosis to the excluded stomach. Then, ERCP, EUS, or therapeutic endoscopy through the LAMS can be performed in the excluded gastrointestinal tract.

First, an anastomosis is created from the gastric pouch to the excluded stomach using LAMS. A balloon dilatation catheter is used to dilate the LAMS and the stent is anchored with Overstitch endoscopic suture (Apollo Endosurgery, Texas, USA). The echoendoscope (EUS) is then inserted into the excluded stomach. An additional LAMS is then placed from the excluded stomach to the WON for EUS-guided drainage and subsequent endoscopic necrosectomy. Two sessions of endoscopic necrosectomy were required (Video 32.1).

32.4 Description of the Procedure

A curvilinear echoendoscope (GF-UCT180, Olympus, America, Center Valley, PA) was forwarded into the gastric pouch to visualize the excluded stomach on EUS (Fig. 32.1). Color Doppler imaging was used to verify the absence of significant vascular structures obstructing the needle's path before insertion. A 19-gauge FNA needle was used to create a gastric-gastric access. Contrast or water (> 200 cc) was instilled into the cavity to fill the remnant stomach and to optimize the target size (Fig. 32.2). Then, under fluoroscopic, endosonographic, and endoscopic guidance, one 20 mm × 10 mm LAMS (AXIOS, Boston Scientific, Marlborough, MA) was deployed with cautery enhancement across the tract (Fig. 32.3). Finally, an 18-mm balloon dilatation catheter (CRE Pro Wire-guided, Boston Scientific, Marlborough, MA) was used to dilate the LAMS lumen (Fig. 32.4). Overstitch sutures were then applied to the LAMS to prevent stent dislodgment.

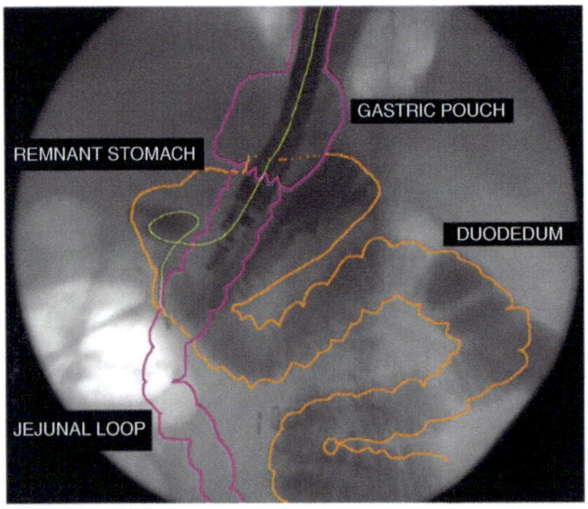

Fig. 32.1 Gastric bypass anatomy. Visualization of possible access site for GATE

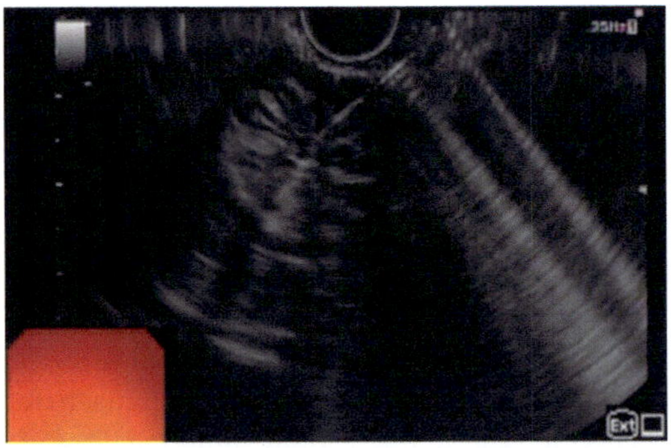

Fig. 32.2 Needle puncturing from gastric pouch into the remnant stomach

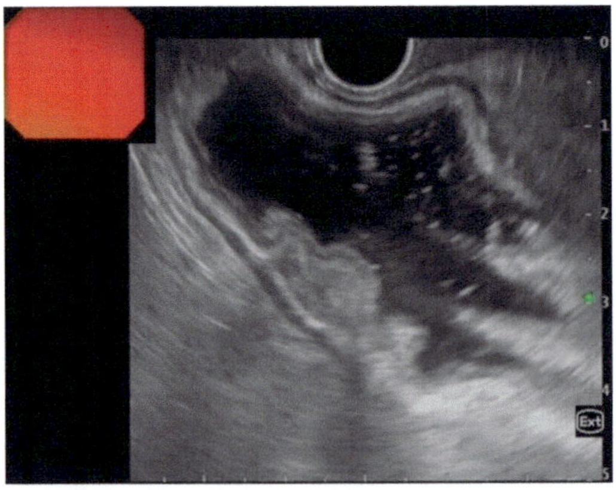

Fig. 32.3 Water injected to confirm target and to increase target size

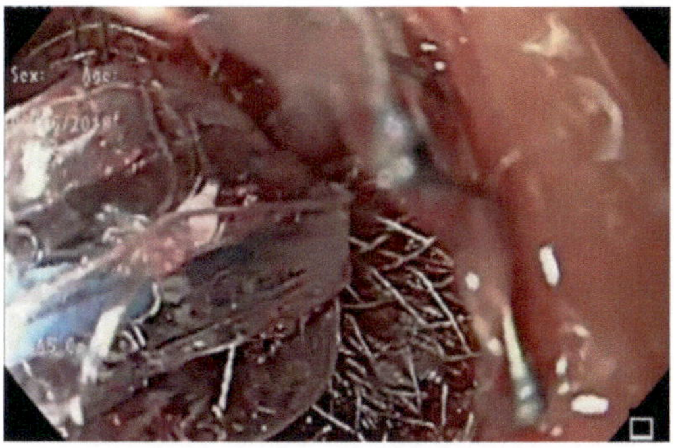

Fig. 32.4 Balloon dilate the LAMS lumen up to 20 mm in diameter

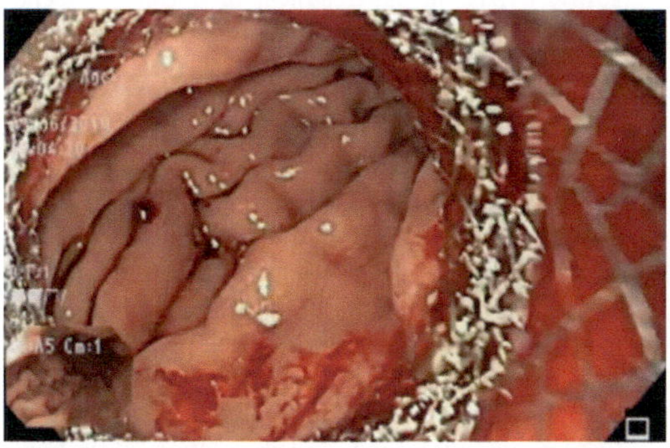

Fig. 32.5 Endoscopic images of deployed and dilated LAMS

Transgastric endoscopic ultrasound-guided drainage of WON was then completed utilizing one 15 mm × 10 mm LAMS. The stent was deployed using cautery, directly into the WON followed by deployment of the distal flange and then the proximal flange (Figs. 32.5 and 32.6). Necrosectomy was performed with a gastroscope using a snare. One additional session of endoscopic necrosectomy was performed three weeks later for complete removal of the necrotic material. Both LAMS were removed during the follow-up session. The gastric pouch to exclude stomach anastomosis was then closed using the overstitch to prevent persistent opening of the fistula (Figs. 32.7 and 32.8).

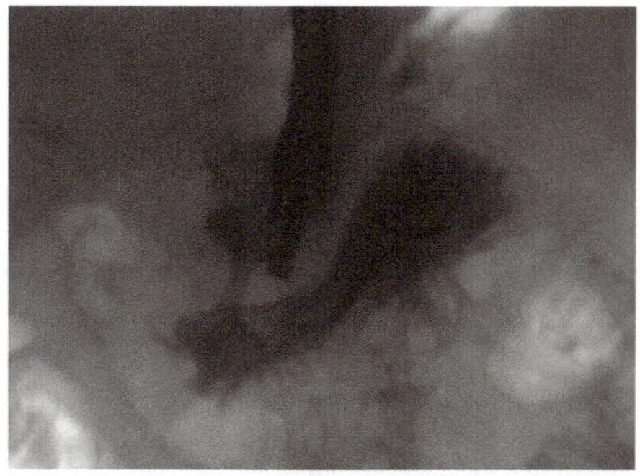

Fig. 32.6 Fluoroscopic image of the GATE

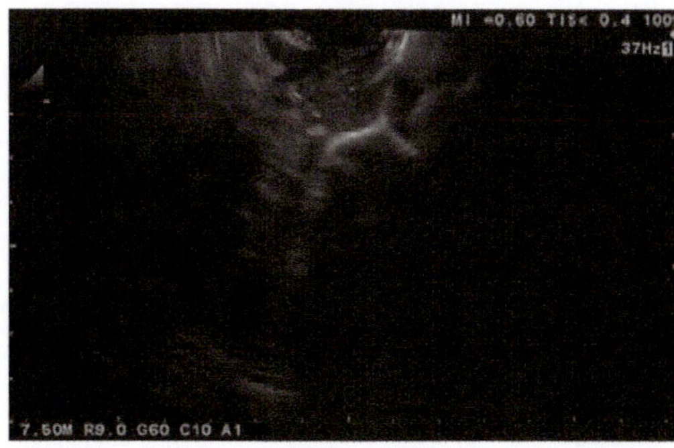

Fig. 32.7 The stent delivery system is inserted directly into the pseudocyst using cautery followed by expansion of the distal flange and subsequent

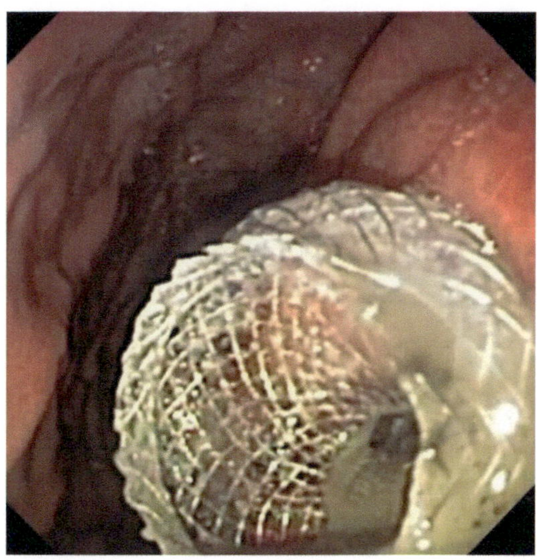

Fig. 32.8 Expansion of the proximal flange of the LAMS under endoscopic control

32.5 Post-Procedural Management

The patients were monitored for approximately 30 minutes to one hour after the GATE procedure. Analgesics were given as needed. Patients who developed pain are observed for longer periods of time. Additionally, fluoroquinolone or other broad-spectrum antibiotics are given for seven days. A clear liquid diet is encouraged for the first 24 hours and advanced slowly to small low-fat meals. There are no activity restrictions. Patients are recommended to have follow-up clinic visits at two- and four weeks post-procedure for evaluation of any adverse events.

32.6 Potential Pitfalls

GATE remains a highly technically challenging endoscopic procedure and is only to be performed by highly experienced advanced endoscopists with experience in interventional EUS. The complications for this procedure include bleeding at the access site, risk of incomplete fistula closure, reversal of the metabolic effect of the bariatric surgery, and the risk of LAMS dislodgement during the procedure [1]. In one study, two out of six patients were found to have LAMS dislodgment during ERCP with successful repositioning. One patient out of twelve was found to have a persistent transgastric fistula after LAMS removal requiring closure using endoscopic suturing. All patients had clinical success [4].

References

1. Morales-Maza J, Rodriguez-Quintero JH, Sanchez-Morales GE, Sanchez Garcia-Ramos E, Romero-Velez G, Aguilar-Frasco JL, et al. Laparoscopic roux-en-Y gastric bypass in the treatment of obesity: evidence based update through randomized clinical trials and meta-analyses. G Chir. 2020;41(1):5–17.
2. Kedia P, Tyberg A, Kumta NA, Gaidhane M, Karia K, Sharaiha RZ, et al. EUS-directed transgastric ERCP for roux-en-Y gastric bypass anatomy: a minimally invasive approach. Gastrointest Endosc. 2015;82(3):560–5.
3. Wang TJ, Thompson CC, Ryou M. Gastric access temporary for endoscopy (GATE): a proposed algorithm for EUS-directed transgastric ERCP in gastric bypass patients. Surg Endosc. 2019;33(6):2024–33.
4. Ngamruengphong S, Nieto J, Kunda R, et al. Endoscopic ultrasound-guided creation of a transgastric fistula for the management of hepatobiliary disease in patients with roux-en-Y gastric bypass. Endoscopy. 2017;49(6):549–52. https://doi.org/10.1055/s-0043-105072.

Part VII

EUS-Guided Pancreatic Cyst Ablation

EUS-Guided Pancreatic Cyst Ablation with Alcohol

33

Dongwook Oh and Dong-Wan Seo

33.1 Background

Pancreatic cystic lesions represent a wide spectrum of biologic behavior, ranging from benign to malignant [1]. With widespread use of cross-sectional imaging studies, the number of incidental pancreatic cystic lesions has increased. Management of pancreatic cyst is challenging, particularly when a lesion is located in the pancreas head, because surgical resection of pancreatic cysts is associated with a substantial morbidity of 20–40% and a mortality rate of 2% [2, 3].

Endoscopic ultrasound-guided pancreatic cyst ablation (EUS-PCA) with ethanol and/or other ablative agents has been investigated in clinical trials. EUS-PCA can be performed safely, with fewer adverse events and avoids the risks associated with surgical treatment [1, 4, 5]. EUS-PCA may be an effective, alternative treatment option, particularly for patients with high surgical risk.

D. Oh · D.-W. Seo (✉)
Department of Gastroenterology, University of Ulsan College of Medicine, Asan Medical Center, Seoul, Korea
e-mail: dwseoamc@amc.seoul.kr

33.2 Case History

A 47-year-old woman was referred for a 5-cm-sized pancreatic cyst detected on transabdominal ultrasonography during a health maintenance examination. She was regularly followed up over 4 years for a cystic lesion at the body of the pancreas (Fig. 33.1). The patient had no history of pancreatitis or specific symptoms related to the cystic lesion. The cystic lesion measured 4.6 × 2.6 cm on EUS. It was a unilocular cyst without septation (Fig. 33.2). Computed tomography (CT) did not reveal parenchymal change in the pancreas, which is suggestive of pancreatitis. No communication between the cyst and the pancreatic duct was evident in endoscopic retrograde pancreatography (ERP). As the clinical diagnosis was based on all available clinical data and imaging studies, including CT, ERP, and EUS findings, mucinous cystic neoplasm was suspected. Surgical resection of the cystic lesion was considered due to malignant potential, but the patient declined. Therefore, EUS-PCA was performed as an alternative treatment (Fig. 33.2).

On serial CT scan at 3 and 9 months after ablation, cyst has decreased and complete ablation was achieved. On the last CT scan (9 years after ablation), cyst was not identified (Fig. 33.3).

A. Y.B. Teoh et al. (eds.), *Atlas of Interventional EUS*, https://doi.org/10.1007/978-981-16-9340-3_33

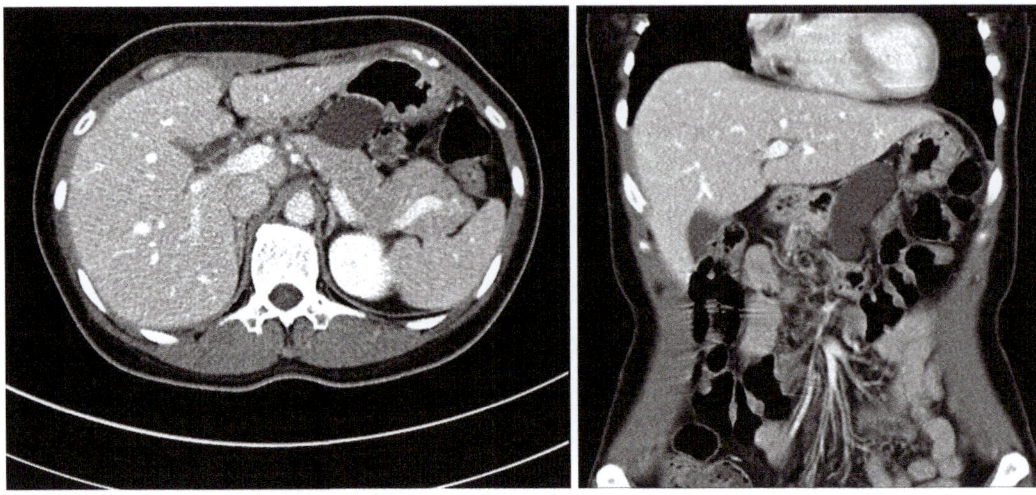

Fig. 33.1 Initial CT scan. A 5-cm-sized cyst located at the body of pancreas

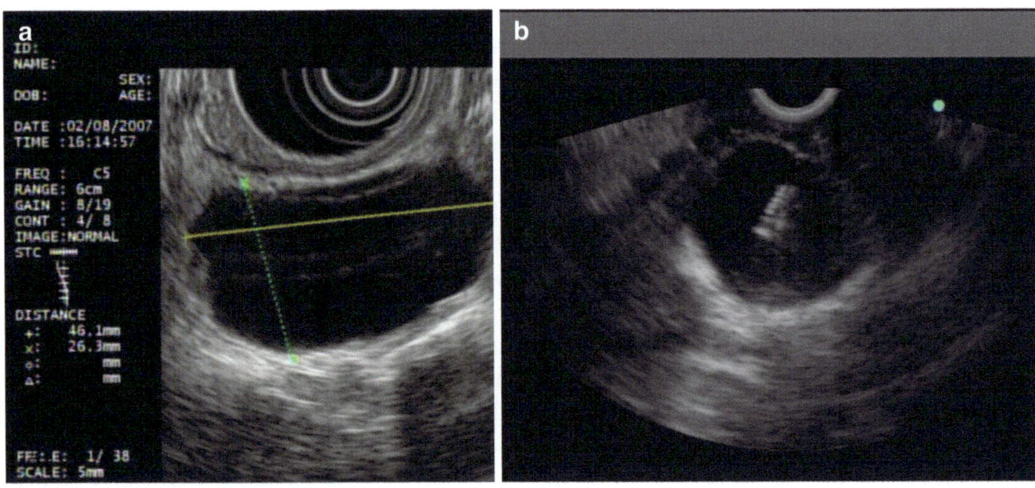

Fig. 33.2 Endoscopic ultrasound image. (**a**) EUS shows a unilocular cyst. (**b**) EUS-guided pancreatic cyst ablation

33.3 Procedural Plan

Before EUS-guided ablation, careful EUS examination is mandatory to determine the anatomical and morphologic features of lesions. For effective and safe ablation, the suitable location for the procedure (stable scope position) and the cyst characteristics (size, septation, wall thickness, mural nodule, communication with the pancreatic duct) should be evaluated [6]. In patients with mucinous cysts (branch duct intraduct papillary mucinous cystic neoplasm [BD-IPMN] or mucinous cystic neoplasm [MCN]), contrast-enhanced EUS (CE-EUS) may help avoid the overdiagnosis of presence of mural nodules [7]. EUS-guided FNA is performed for cyst evacuation. A 22-gauge needle is usually used in most cases. Currently, most reports describing EUS-PCA have used a 22-gauge needle [1, 4, 5, 8–11]. A 19-gauge needle can be used if the mucin takes too much time to aspirate; however, it has a risk of leakage. If a 22-gauge needle is used, suction is applied with a 20-mL or larger syringe. A 25-gauge needle is not appropriate for aspiration and injection.

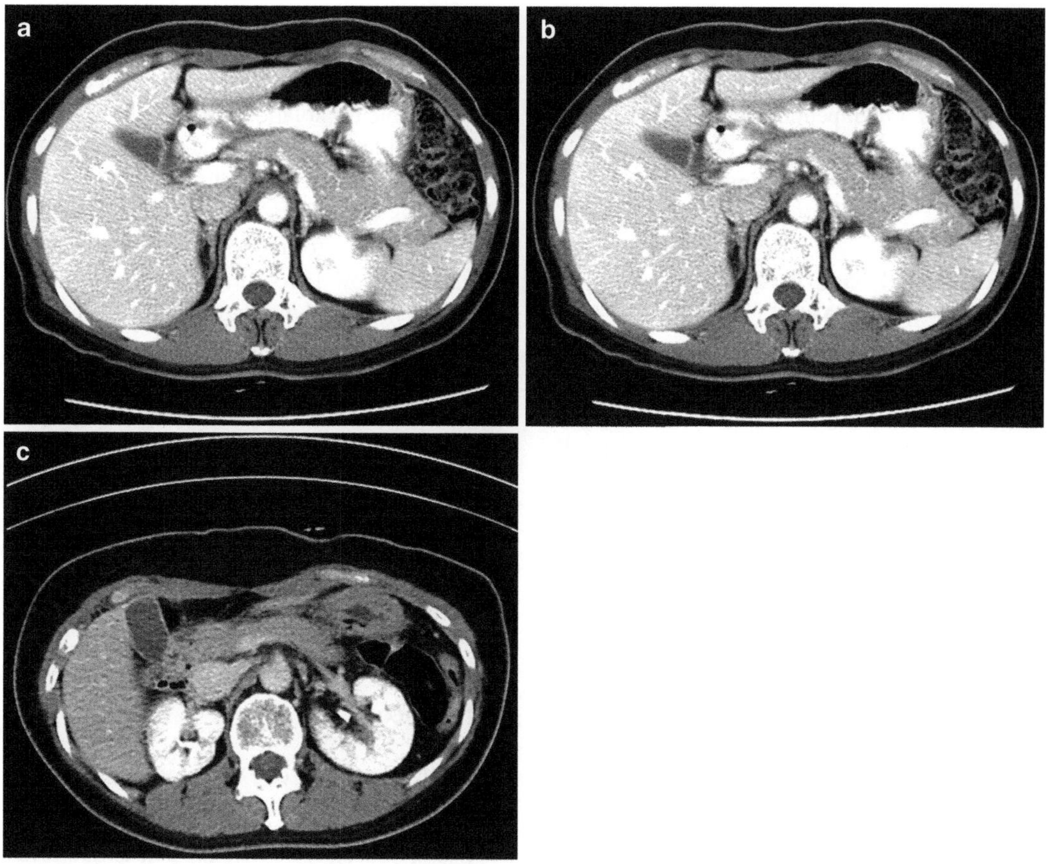

Fig. 33.3 (**a**) A follow-up CT after 3 months shows cyst had decreased. (**b**) A follow-up CT after 9 months shows complete ablation. (**c**) A last CT after 9 years shows no residual cyst

33.4 Description of the Procedure

After identification of the cystic lesion, a 22-gauge needle is inserted into the cyst under EUS guidance. After successful puncture of the cyst, a syringe is attached to the proximal end of the needle and the maximum possible volume of cyst fluid is aspirated. The amount of aspirated fluid should be recorded, and the fluid should be sent for further examination (e.g., amylase and carcinoembryonic antigen examination). To ensure that the cyst is not completely collapsed, the needle remains within the cyst before injection of the ethanol. Then, 99% ethanol is injected into the cyst in a volume equal to that of the originally aspirated fluid, followed by reaspiration of injected ethanol immediately. Then, 99% ethanol can be injected into the cyst again, followed by reaspiration. This repeated injection and reaspiration of ethanol is called lavage. Generally, ethanol lavage can be repeated 3–4 times. In cases of large cyst, repeated injection and reaspiration takes too much time and technically challenging. Ethanol retention therapy can be an alternative option. After aspiration of cystic fluid, 99% ethanol can be injected into the cyst. Then the needle and echoendoscope can be removed. To get even contact of ethanol and cyst wall, the patient position can be changed from supine, left lateral decubitus, prone, and right lateral decubitus. At each position, 5 minutes are given for the action of ethanol. After 20–40 minutes of retention time, injected ethanol can be reaspirated. If necessary, paclitaxel injection can be added after full aspiration of injected ethanol and left in the cyst. Paclitaxel is a therapeutic drug that can be used for pancreatic cancer. It can evade septal walls and causing apoptosis of lining tumor cells.

33.5 Post-Procedural Management

All patients should be closely monitored for possible adverse events including abdominal pain, bleeding, pancreatitis, and infection in the 24 hours after treatment. A simple abdominal radiograph and blood tests are checked for adverse events on the next day. Diet can be resumed 24 hours after procedure. Other studies can be performed depending on the clinical signs and symptoms. The first follow-up computed tomography (CT) scan was performed 3 months after EUS-PCA. Further follow-up CTs were performed at 6-month intervals until cyst resolution and yearly thereafter. For long-term follow-up for evaluation of treatment response, contrast-enhanced CT may be the mainstay for imaging of treated patients.

33.6 Potential Pitfalls

Although EUS-PCA may not be yet the definitive treatment of all pancreatic cysts, it can be used as a useful bridge until the presence of clinical stigmata that requires definite surgical resection. To maximize the therapeutic efficacy, careful patient selection is required. Endosonographers should consider following factors for the ideal candidate for EUS-PCA [1]: morphology: unilocular or oligolocular [2], size: 2–5 cm [3], no communication between main pancreatic duct and pancreatic cyst on imaging studies including, magnetic resonance pancreatography or ERP [4], cysts that increases in size during the follow-up, and [5] patients who refuse surgery or who have high surgical risk [8]. The ideal cyst size for ablation is based on two competing factors; the malignant risk and the success rate [12]. Large cyst (>3 to 4 cm in diameter) may have an increased malignant potential. On the other hand, in terms of feasibility and safety, cyst less than 2 cm in diameter is not suitable for ablation. MCN is the ideal indication for ablative treatment because it has malignant potential and is often a unilocular cyst. BD-IPMNs seems to be unilocular cyst, however, they often have a tortuous septated configuration or have a narrow 1- to 2-mm duct that forms the side branch throughout the cyst. These morphologic characteristics make treatment of some BD-IPMNs difficult if not impossible because the injected ablative agent may not safely come in contact with the entire cyst [13]. In addition, the presence of septations within the cyst is not good indication of ablation because of the presence of often hundreds of small cysts that do not permit uniform application or retention of the ablative liquid agent [5, 13].

References

1. Oh HC, Seo DW, Lee TY, et al. New treatment for cystic tumors of the pancreas: EUS-guided ethanol lavage with paclitaxel injection. Gastrointest Endosc. 2008;67:636–42. https://doi.org/10.1016/j.gie.2007.09.038.
2. Brugge WR, Lauwers GY, Sahani D, et al. Cystic neoplasms of the pancreas. N Engl J Med. 2004;351:1218–26. https://doi.org/10.1056/NEJMra031623.
3. Allen PJ, D'Angelica M, Gonen M, et al. A selective approach to the resection of cystic lesions of the pancreas: results from 539 consecutive patients. Ann Surg. 2006;244:572–82. https://doi.org/10.1097/01.sla.0000237652.84466.54.
4. Oh HC, Seo DW, Song TJ, et al. Endoscopic ultrasonography-guided ethanol lavage with paclitaxel injection treats patients with pancreatic cysts. Gastroenterology. 2011;140:172–9. https://doi.org/10.1053/j.gastro.2010.10.001.
5. Oh HC, Seo DW, Kim SC, et al. Septated cystic tumors of the pancreas: is it possible to treat them by endoscopic ultrasonography-guided intervention? Scand J Gastroenterol. 2009;44:242–7. https://doi.org/10.1080/00365520802495537.
6. Cho MK, Choi JH, Seo DW. Endoscopic ultrasound-guided ablation therapy for pancreatic cysts. Endosc Ultrasound. 2015;4:293–8. https://doi.org/10.4103/2303-9027.170414.
7. Fujita M, Itoi T, Ikeuchi N, et al. Effectiveness of contrast-enhanced endoscopic ultrasound for detecting mural nodules in intraductal papillary mucinous neoplasm of the pancreas and for making therapeutic

decisions. Endosc Ultrasound. 2016;5:377–83. https://doi.org/10.4103/2303-9027.190927.
8. Choi JH, Seo DW, Song TJ, et al. Long-term outcomes after endoscopic ultrasound-guided ablation of pancreatic cysts. Endoscopy. 2017;49:866–73. https://doi.org/10.1055/s-0043-110030.
9. Oh HC, Seo DW. Endoscopic ultrasonography-guided pancreatic cyst ablation (with video). J Hepatobiliary Pancreat Sci. 2015;22:16–9. https://doi.org/10.1002/jhbp.179.
10. Caillol F, Poincloux L, Bories E, et al. Ethanol lavage of 14 mucinous cysts of the pancreas: a retrospective study in two tertiary centers. Endosc Ultrasound. 2012;1:48–52. https://doi.org/10.7178/eus.01.008.
11. DiMaio CJ, DeWitt JM, Brugge WR. Ablation of pancreatic cystic lesions: the use of multiple endoscopic ultrasound-guided ethanol lavage sessions. Pancreas. 2011;40:664–8. https://doi.org/10.1097/MPA.0b013e3182128d06.
12. Oh HC, Brugge WR. EUS-guided pancreatic cyst ablation: a critical review (with video). Gastrointest Endosc. 2013;77:526–33. https://doi.org/10.1016/j.gie.2012.10.033.
13. DeWitt J. Endoscopic ultrasound-guided pancreatic cyst ablation. Gastrointest Endosc Clin N Am. 2012;22(291–302):ix–x. https://doi.org/10.1016/j.giec.2012.04.001.

34 EUS-Guided Pancreatic Cyst Ablation with Alcohol and Paclitaxel

John DeWitt

34.1 Background

Pancreatic cysts are classified as: (1) those complicating acute or chronic pancreatitis (acute fluid collections and pseudocysts) or (2) pancreatic cystic neoplasms (PCNs) lined by epithelium. The former possess no epithelial lining and therefore no malignant potential. Epithelium from PCNs may have either negligible malignant potential (serous cysts [SCNs]) or represent either premalignant (intraductal papillary mucinous neoplasms [IPMNs] or mucinous cystic neoplasms [MCNs]) or malignant tumors [1]. These lesions present either incidentally on imaging studies [2, 3] or during evaluation of symptoms such as abdominal pain, weight loss, or jaundice. Traditionally, surgery has been advocated to remove premalignant cysts >3 cm in diameter, those associated with high-risk imaging stigmata or the presence of related symptoms such as weight loss or jaundice [4]. However, pancreatic resection is associated with frequent morbidity and rare mortality. Pancreatic cyst ablation (PCA) has been evaluated as a possible alternative to surgery or clinical observation for selected benign PCNs [5–8]. Published studies show that ablation with ethanol and paclitaxel or alternatively an alcohol-free regimen of gemcitabine and paclitaxel produces imaged-defined cyst ablation in 50–65% of patients with durable results in >90% of those treated.

34.2 Case History

A 53-year-old female presented with vague lower abdominal discomfort. Physical examination and laboratory studies were all normal. CT scan performed on February 16, 2014, demonstrated a 3-cm cyst at the body–tail junction of the pancreas. The remaining pancreas was normal. She denied upper abdominal pain, weight loss, jaundice, or a history of pancreatitis.

EUS at outside hospital in March 2014 showed a 3-cm cyst at the body–tail junction with internal septations, but no nodules. EUS-FNA disclosed no atypical epithelial cells and a cyst fluid CEA of 1089 ng/mL. The clinical diagnosis was a mucinous cystic neoplasm. Repeat CT at outside hospital in July 2014 demonstrated the cyst to be unchanged. The patient was offered surgical resection, observation with repeat imaging in one year, or endoscopic cyst ablation. She elected to undergo ablation.

Supplementary Information The online version contains supplementary material available at [https://doi.org/10.1007/978-981-16-9340-3_34].

J. DeWitt (✉)
Division of Gastroenterology & Hepatology, Indiana University Health Medical Center, Indianapolis, IN, USA
e-mail: jodewitt@iu.edu

A. Y.B. Teoh et al. (eds.), *Atlas of Interventional EUS*, https://doi.org/10.1007/978-981-16-9340-3_34

34.3 Procedural Plan

Pancreatic cyst ablation can generally be performed in 10–15 minutes and therefore with conscious sedation alone. If excessive movement such as coughing, retching, or excessive respiratory movement is felt to be likely, general anesthesia with paralysis should be considered. The lavage agent (i.e., ethanol or saline) and chemotherapy (i.e., paclitaxel or paclitaxel + gemcitabine) should be prepared prior to the procedure. Antibiotics are recommended to decrease the risk of post-procedure infection.

Saline and ethanol are non-viscous solutions that pass easily through a 22-gauge or 19-gauge needle. However, paclitaxel at the full concentration of 6 mg/mL as supplied in the United States, is viscous and requires dilution to 3 mg/mL or less to permit instillation by either needle. A 22-gauge FNA needle is utilized for a cyst measuring 2–3 cm in diameter while reserving 19-gauge needles for cysts >3 cm in diameter or previously known to have highly viscous cyst fluid. Infusing the chemotherapy agent(s) typically requires high pressure, therefore a syringe strapped to a high-pressure gun or infusion device is usually used.

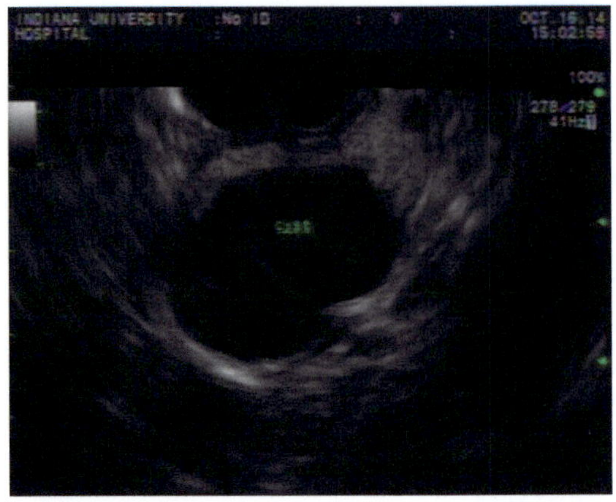

Fig. 34.1 Baseline EUS imaging of a 3.2 × 2.1 cm cyst at the junction of the pancreatic body and tail with a single septation

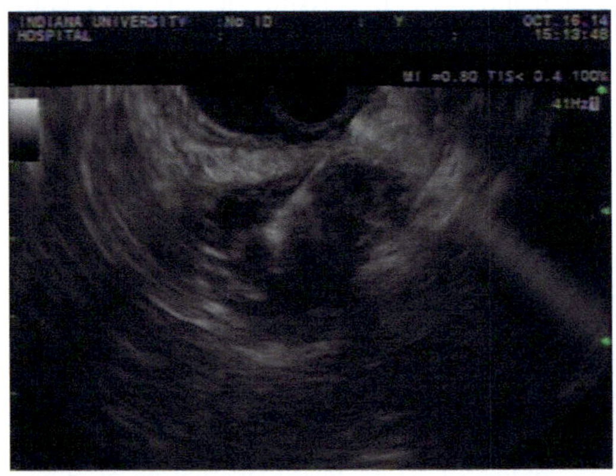

Fig. 34.2 EUS-guided lavage with ethanol

34.4 Description of the Procedure

Pancreatic cyst ablation was performed in October 2014 using a linear echoendoscope. Repeat measurement of the cyst prior to treatment was 3.2 × 2.1 cm in maximal diameter (Fig. 34.1). A 19-gauge needle was used to puncture the cyst and 5 mLs of moderately viscous fluid was retrieved. Then, 5 mLs of 98% ethanol was instilled as the lavage agent. Over 5 minutes, the cyst fluid/ethanol combination was aspirated, injected, and re-aspirated (Fig. 34.2). The cyst contents were then completely evacuated and 5 mL of dilute paclitaxel (3 mg/mL) was injected into the cyst (with the assistance of a high-pressure gun) and left in place (Fig. 34.3).

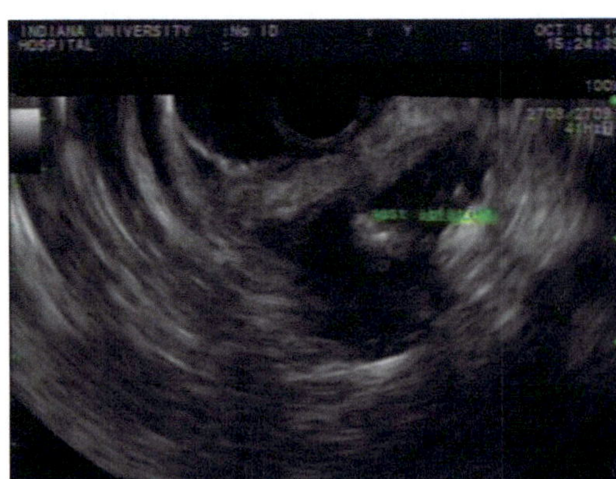

Fig. 34.3 Endosonographic image of the cyst immediately after paclitaxel injection and needle withdrawal

34.5 Post-Procedural Management

The patient developed abdominal pain following the procedure and was admitted for 36 hours with post-ablation pancreatitis. She was discharged, tolerated a soft diet for 3 days and subsequently resumed a regular diet without abdominal pain. Repeat CT scan 2 months after ablation showed the cyst had decreased in size to 17 mm × 10 mm (Fig. 34.4). CT scan 8 months after ablation showed the cyst measured 2 × 2 mm thus signifying a complete radiologic response (defined as <5% of the original cyst volume) (Fig. 34.4).

34.6 Potential Pitfalls

Pancreatic cyst ablation is a fairly easy procedure and theoretically anyone experienced in EUS-FNA should be able to perform this procedure after some mentoring and observation of an expert. However, acceptance of PCA by patients and surgeons as an alternative to surgery may require some education by endoscopists. Furthermore, oncologists, medical institutions, and institutional review boards must be involved with discussions and management of these patients to permit use of chemotherapy to treat these lesions.

After initial puncture, it is critical that the EUS-FNA needle is visualized during the entire procedure to ensure that the lavage agent and chemotherapy stay within the cyst cavity. This is best accomplished by leaving an anechoic (black) rim around the FNA needle during the entire procedure. If there is any uncertainty about whether the needle remains in the cyst, instillation of saline to enlarge the cyst may be considered.

Adverse events associated with pancreatic cyst ablation include abdominal pain in up to 15%, pancreatitis in 2–10%, and rarely peritonitis or venous thrombosis [8]. It has been presumed that these adverse events are nearly always related to use of ethanol. A recent randomized trial showed that alcohol-free chemotherapy ablation achieves image-defined ablation rates

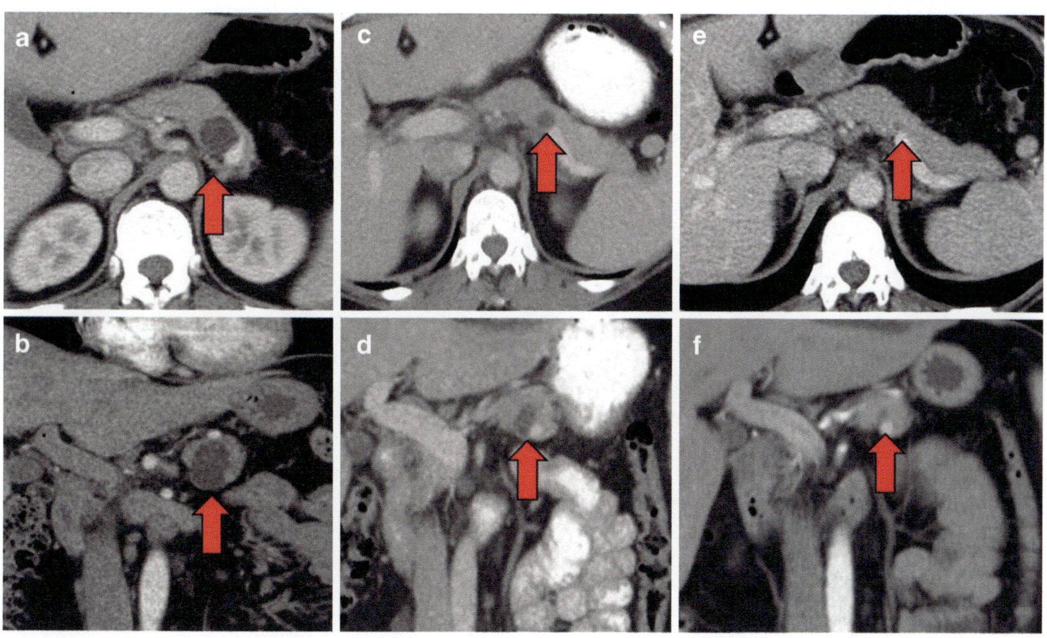

Fig. 34.4 Cross-sectional imaging of the pancreatic cyst before and after ablation. (**a, b**) Baseline axial and coronal CT showing a 3-cm cyst (red arrow) at the junction of the pancreatic body and tail. (**c, d**) Axial and coronal CT scan 2 months after ablation. The cyst (red arrow) decreased in size to 17 mm × 10 mm. (**e, f**) Axial and coronal CT scan 8 months after ablation demonstrating a residual 2 × 2 mm cyst (red arrow) consistent with complete ablation (<5% original the cyst volume)

similar to one that contains alcohol. Furthermore, elimination of alcohol from chemoablation decreases adverse events to 1–2%. For this reason, ablation with an initial saline (non-ethanol) lavage followed injection of a gemcitabine-paclitaxel admixture should be considered [9].

Follow-up imaging for all patients regardless of the degree of ablation is mandatory. Although current data suggests that nearly two-thirds of patients achieve radiologic resolution (<5% original cyst volume) following ablation, some patients have either a modest or a minimal response by follow-up imaging. This may represent incomplete epithelial ablation which is best followed with cross-sectional imaging annually or semi-annually to ensure that cyst regrowth does not occur. If regrowth occurs, repeat ablation or surgery may be offered.

References

1. Al-Haddad M, Schmidt MC, Sandrasegaran K, et al. Diagnosis and treatment of cystic pancreatic tumors. Clin Gastroenterol Hepatol. 2011;9:635–48.
2. Lee KS, Sekhar A, Rofsky NM, et al. Prevalence of incidental pancreatic cysts in the adult population on MR imaging. Am J Gastroenterol. 2010;105:2079–84.
3. de Jong K, Nio CY, Hermans JJ, et al. High prevalence of pancreatic cysts detected by screening magnetic resonance imaging examinations. Clin Gastroenterol Hepatol. 2010;8:806–11.
4. Tanaka M, Fernández-del Castillo C, Adsay V, et al. International consensus guidelines 2012 for the management of IPMN and MCN of the pancreas. Pancreatology. 2012;12:183–97.
5. DeWitt J, McGreevy K, Schmidt CM, et al. Endoscopic ultrasound-guided ethanol versus saline lavage for pancreatic cysts: a randomized double blinded study. Gastrointest Endosc. 2009;70:710–23.
6. DeWitt JM, Al-Haddad M, Sherman S, et al. Alterations in cyst fluid genetics following endoscopic ultrasound-guided pancreatic cyst ablation with ethanol and paclitaxel. Endoscopy. 2014;46:457–64.
7. Choi JH, Seo DW, Song TJ, et al. Long-term outcomes after endoscopic ultrasound-guided ablation of pancreatic cysts. Endoscopy. 2017;49:866–73.
8. Moyer MT, Sharzehi S, Mathew A, et al. The safety and efficacy of an alcohol-free pancreatic cyst ablation protocol. Gastroenterology. 2017;153:1295–303.
9. Moyer MT, Maranki JL, DeWitt JM. EUS-guided pancreatic cyst ablation: a clinical and technical review. Curr Gastroenterol Rep. 2019;21:19.

35 Alcohol-Free EUS-Guided Pancreatic Cyst Chemoablation

Leonard T. Walsh and Matthew T. Moyer

35.1 Background

EUS-guided pancreatic cyst chemoablation has emerged as an innovative and minimally invasive approach for the treatment of neoplastic pancreatic cysts. To date, ten published studies using randomized design have investigated the efficacy and safety of EUS-guided pancreatic cyst ablation using ethanol lavage or ethanol lavage followed by the infusion of paclitaxel [1–3]. Recently, a randomized prospective trial demonstrated that alcohol is not required for effective pancreatic cyst ablation when a chemoablation cocktail of paclitaxel and gemcitabine is used, and that when alcohol is removed from the ablation process, serious and minor adverse event rates which approximate that of EUS-FNA are achieved [4]. Alcohol-free pancreatic cyst ablation thus offers an effective treatment option for appropriately selected mucinous cyst tumors with a very attractive safety profile to a patient population otherwise facing the alternatives or a major pancreatic surgery [2, 4–7]. Additionally, a recent prospective long-term follow-up trial has shown that pancreatic cyst chemoablation has a durable treatment effect for patients who achieved complete EUS-guided pancreatic cyst ablation, with 98.3% remaining in remission at six-year follow up [8, 9].

35.2 Case History

A healthy 82-year-old female without significant medical history was incidentally found to have a 3.5 × 1.6 cm pancreatic cyst consistent with a mucinous type pancreatic cyst with one worrisome feature per 2017 Fukuoka consensus guidelines [10]. She underwent annual surveillance by MRI-MRCP for 3 years, however, due to an increase in size of the tumor, she was referred for EUS-guided chemoablation. MRI-MRCP of the abdomen (Fig. 35.1a, b) at time of referral showed a 3.6 × 3.2 cm cystic tumor in the uncinate process of the pancreas without main duct dilation, surrounding lymphadenopathy, or stigmata of malignancy. After a clinical evaluation and multidisciplinary review, she was offered and enthusiastically agreed to undergo alcohol-free, EUS-guided, and pancreatic cyst chemoablation. At 12 month follow-up, there was no residual

Supplementary Information The online version contains supplementary material available at [https://doi.org/10.1007/978-981-16-9340-3_35].

L. T. Walsh (✉)
Division of Gastroenterology and Hepatology, Guthrie Robert Packer Hospital, Sayre, PA, USA
e-mail: leonard.walsh@guthrie.org

M. T. Moyer
Division of Gastroenterology and Hepatology, Penn State Health Milton S. Hershey Medical Center, Hershey, PA, USA
e-mail: mmoyer@pennstatehealth.psu.edu

A. Y.B. Teoh et al. (eds.), *Atlas of Interventional EUS*, https://doi.org/10.1007/978-981-16-9340-3_35

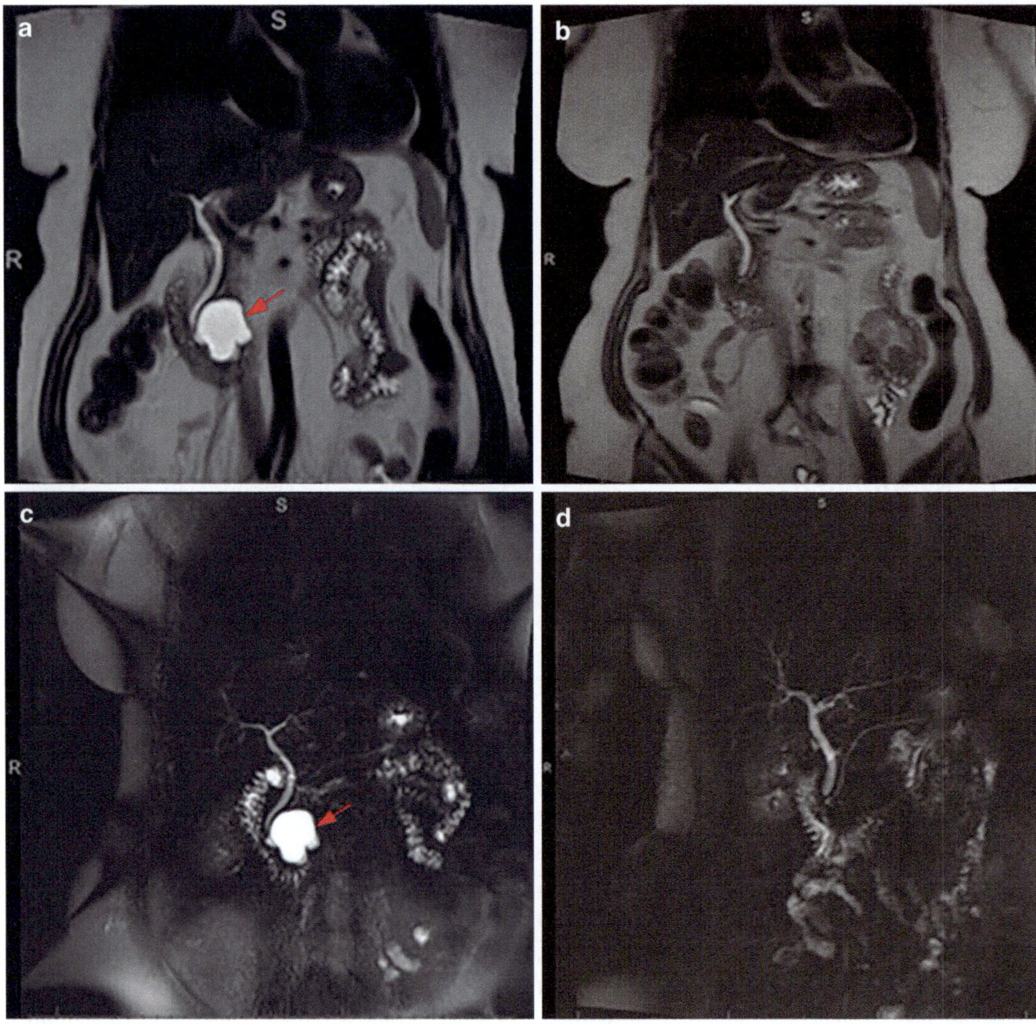

Fig. 35.1 T2 MRI (**a**) and MRCP (**b**) showing a 3.5 × 1.6 cm mucinous cystic neoplasm in the head of the pancreas prior to EUS-guided chemoablation. At three year follow up after alcohol-free EUS-guided pancreatic cyst chemoablation, T2 MRI (**c**) and MRCP (**d**) showed no evidence of residual cyst

cyst identified on high-resolution imaging, consistent with a complete ablation, and MRI-MRCP at 3 year follow-up (Fig. 35.1c, d) showed a sustained response with no residual cyst.

35.3 Procedural Plan

It is our recommendation that patients being considered for EUS-guided cyst ablation should undergo a full evaluation in a clinic setting where their clinical, radiographic, and endoscopic situation can be reviewed, and all options and areas of uncertainty discussed with the patient. Only cysts with a possibility for progression to malignancy with characteristics consistent with a mucinous-type cyst as per ASGE guidelines [11] and measuring between 2 and 6 cm should typically be considered candidates for ablation.

Contraindications for ablation include pregnancy, less than 3–5 year life expectancy, inability to safely undergo a 30–60 min procedure with monitored anesthesia, overt signs of malignancy, and benign cysts with little or no malignant potential. Relative contraindications for ablation include cysts with the following high-risk features: main pancreatic duct dilation >5 mm, epithelial type mural nodules, pathologically thick walls or septations, signs of common bile duct obstruction, solid mass component within or associated with a cyst, pathologic lymphadenopathy associated with the cyst, pancreatic duct stricture associated with tail atrophy, septated cysts with >4–5 discrete individual compartments, and/or irreversible coagulopathy, neutropenia, or severe thrombocytopenia.

35.4 Description of the Procedure

Patient preparation for pancreatic cyst ablation is similar to standard EUS-FNA. After a full endosonographic evaluation, the FNA needle is introduced into the center of the cyst (Fig. 35.2a) and the entire cyst contents are aspirated leaving only a rim of fluid around the needle tip to avoid possibly damaging the cyst wall or possibly injecting chemotherapy into the surrounding parenchyma (Fig. 35.2b). It is our practice to use a 22-gauge FNA needle for cysts measuring 2–3 cm in diameter, and a 19-gauge needle for cysts over 3 cm or previously known to have a highly viscous fluid. As soon as the aspiration is complete, the chemoablation cocktail, 3 mg/mL paclitaxel and 19 mg/mL gemcitabine (created by mixing 6 mg/mL paclitaxel with 38 mg/mL gemcitabine in a 1:1 ratio), is immediately infused under EUS guidance, replacing no more agent than is required to refill the cyst to its original volume and dimensions (Fig. 35.2c). Since Paclitaxel is highly viscous, infusion of the chemotherapy agent requires moderately high pressure to be done in a timely fashion, and an infusion apparatus such as a syringe strapped to a high-pressure gun or infusion device is often used (Fig. 35.3). Antibiotics are recommended as per ASGE guidelines [11] on pancreatic cyst management, and it has been our approach to observe these patients for one hour postoperatively.

35.5 Post-Procedural Management

The approach utilizes two to three alcohol-free, chemoablation treatments at three-month intervals. Residual cysts at the second or third endoscopies measuring >15 mm are retreated if otherwise appropriate. When a cyst is too small at ablation # 2 for re-treatment, ablation # 3 is cancelled. Treatments are followed by a clinic evaluation and follow-up cross-sectional imaging at 6 and 12 months to measure response and assess for complications. Treatment response is defined using the standardized metrics [3, 9] as complete (≥95% reduction of cyst volume ($V = 4/3\pi r^3$)), partial (94–75% reduction), or non-response (<75% reduction) at follow up. Patients then re-enter a surveillance program using the new size measurements as per guidelines on this subject [10, 12].

35.6 Potential Pitfalls

If EUS-guided cyst ablation is to be effective, it is our recommendation to avoid treating cysts with stigmata of malignancy which would be more appropriately treated by surgical resection and to avoid treating cysts with technical barriers to complete ablation (such as main duct dilation or multi-septated morphology). It is also important to note that ablation is technically challenging (and typically unnecessary) in most low-risk cysts ≤1.5 cm which would be more appropriate for routine surveillance as per guidelines [2, 3, 12].

Complete ablation of an appropriate mucinous cyst will not completely eliminate a patient's overall risk of developing pancreatic adenocarcinoma as up to a 2–4% residual chance of developing cancer elsewhere in the pancreas remains, which is true even after surgical resection of a mucinous tumor [13, 14]. For this reason, even in cases of complete ablation results, patients should remain in a surveillance program as per consensus guidelines as long as the patient's age and comorbidities make further surveillance reasonable [10, 15].

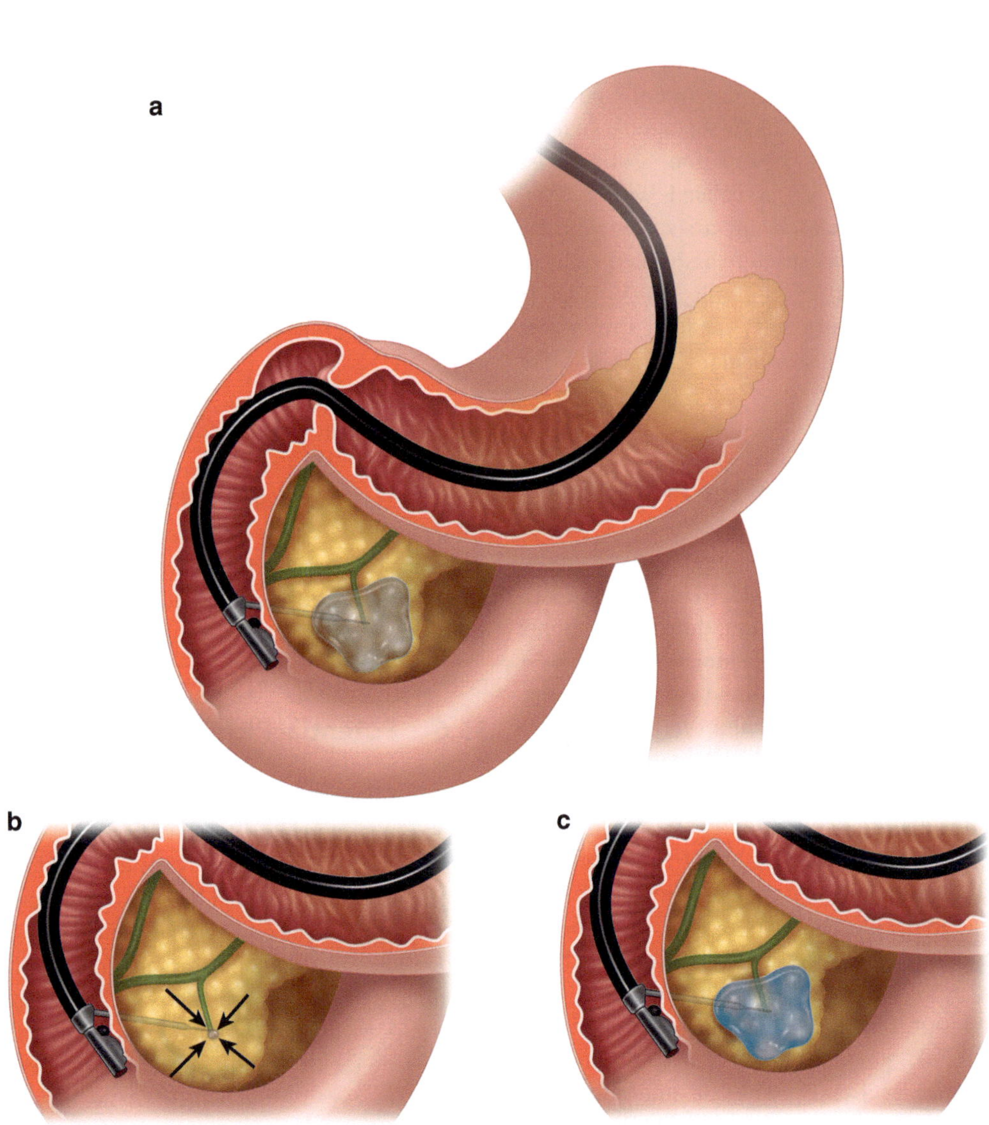

Fig. 35.2 The alcohol-free EUS-guided cyst ablation process: the FNA needle is introduced into the center of the cystic lesion (**a**). This is followed by near-complete aspiration of the mucinous fluid from all compartments, leaving a small amount of fluid around the needle tip to assure that the walls of the cyst are not damaged (**b**). The cyst is then immediately refilled with the chemoablation agent, infusing the same volume as was originally aspirated, reconstituting the cyst to its original dimensions and volume (**c**)

The most common serious adverse event related to EUS-guided pancreatic cyst ablation is post-procedure pancreatitis, however, this risk is largely mitigated with the removal of alcohol lavage from the ablation process. We also recommend that EUS-guided pancreatic cyst ablation be performed at high volume centers, by interventional endoscopists practicing in a multidisciplinary environment. Finally, we recommend that the procedure be performed by a dedicated endoscopy team to improve efficiency and prevent mistakes, and the procedure be part of an ongoing quality assurance process to assess and improve outcomes.

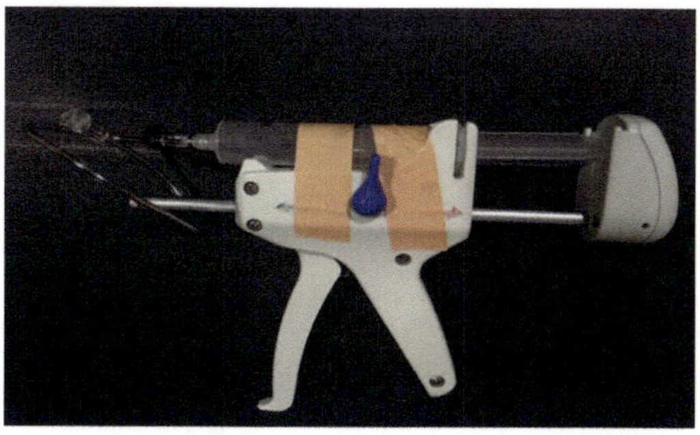

Fig. 35.3 A high-pressure gun, syringe, and short connector tubing assembly which can be used to quickly infuse viscous ablation agents into a cyst after the mucinous fluid is aspirated

This minimally invasive, emerging technique significantly expands treatment options for appropriately selected patients; however, areas of uncertainty and controversy exist as is typical in most novel and innovative procedures. Additional studies are needed to further develop the technique and to determine which patients are most appropriately offered this emerging treatment option based on efficacy, safety, patient satisfaction, and cost.

References

1. Canakis A, Law R, Baron T. An updated review on ablative treatment of pancreatic cystic lesions. Gastrointest Endosc. 2020;91(3):520–6.
2. Moyer MT, Maranki JL, DeWitt JM. EUS-guided pancreatic cyst ablation: a clinical and technical review. Curr Gastroenterol Rep. 2019;22(5):19.
3. Teoh AY, Seo DW, Brugge WR, Dewitt J, Kongkam P, Linghu E, et al. Position statement on EUS-guided ablation of pancreatic cystic neoplasms from an international expert panel. Endosc Int Open. 2019;7(9):1064–77.
4. Moyer MT, Sharzehi S, Mathew A, Levenick JM, Headlee BD, Blandford JT, et al. The safety and efficacy of an alcohol-free pancreatic cyst ablation protocol. Gastroenterology. 2017;153:1295–303.
5. Oh HC, Brugge WR. EUS-guided pancreatic cyst ablation: a critical review (with video). Gastrointest Endosc. 2013;77:526–33.
6. Cho MK, Choi JH, Seo DW. Endoscopic ultrasound-guided ablation therapy for pancreatic cysts. Endosc Ultrasound. 2015;4:293–8.
7. Walsh LT, Hartz K, Lester C, Groff A, Mathew A, Birkholz JH, et al. EUS-guided pancreatic cyst chemoablation as a minimally-invasive alternative to pancreaticoduodenectomy and distal pancreatectomy for the management of appropriately selected mucinous pancreatic cysts: a single center experience. Gastroenterology. 2020;158(6).
8. Choi JH, Seo DW, Song TJ, Park DH, Lee SS, Lee SK, et al. Long term outcomes after endoscopic ultrasound-guided ablation of pancreatic cysts. Endoscopy. 2017;49:866–73.
9. Lester C, Walsh LT, Hartz K, Mathew A, Levenick JM, Headlee BD, et al. The durability of endoscopic ultrasound-guided ablation of pancreatic cysts: a long term follow up of the Charm prospective, randomized, controlled clinical trial. Gastroenterology. 2020;158(6).
10. Tanaka M, Castillo CF, Kamisawa T, Jang JY, Levy P, Ohtsuka T, et al. Revisions of international consensus Fukuoka guidelines for the management of IPMN of the pancreas. Pancreatology. 2017;17(5):738–53.
11. ASGE Standards of Practice Committee. The role of endoscopy in the diagnosis and treatment of cystic pancreatic neoplasms. Gastrointest Endosc. 2016;84:1–9.
12. Basar O, Brugge WR. Pancreatic cyst guidelines: which one to live by? Gastrointest Endosc. 2017;85(5):1032–5.
13. Maguchi H, Tanno S, Mizuno N, Hanada K, Kobayashi G, Hatori T, et al. Natural history of branch duct intraductal papillary mucinous neoplasms of the pancreas: a multicenter study in Japan. Pancreas. 2011;40:364–70.
14. Tanno S, Nakano Y, Koizumi K, Sugiyama Y, Nakamura K, Sasajima J, et al. Pancreatic ductal adenocarcinomas in long-term follow-up patients with branch duct intraductal papillary mucinous neoplasms. Pancreas. 2010;39:36–40.
15. Elta GH, Enestvedt BK, Sauer BG, Marie LA. ACG clinical guideline: diagnosis and management of pancreatic cysts. Am J Gastroenterol. 2018;113:464–79.

Part VIII

EUS-Guided Tumor Ablations

36 EUS-Guided Radiofrequency Ablation of Pancreatic Cyst

Marc Barthet

Abbreviations

CEH EUS	contrast-enhanced harmonic EUS
EUS	endoscopic ultrasonography
IPMN	intraductal papillary mucinous neoplasm
MRI	magnetic resonance imaging
PCN	pancreatic cystic neoplasm
RF	radiofrequency
RFA	radiofrequency ablation

36.1 Background

PCNs are frequent pancreatic lesions mainly discovered fortuitously [1–4]. Most of these PCN are benign and only a few of them would undergo malignant change, including intraductal papillary mucinous neoplasm (IPMN) and mucinous cystadenoma (MCA). Branch duct IPMN could develop malignancy in about 5 to 10% of the patients, requiring imaging follow-up [1–3]. PCN presenting with worrisome features (presence of mural nodules greater than 5 mm and cyst size> 3 cm), are at increased risk for malignancy [2–4]. An interesting alternative to surgery could be ablation with endoscopic radiofrequency (RF) [5–8].

Supplementary Information The online version contains supplementary material available at [https://doi.org/10.1007/978-981-16-9340-3_36].

M. Barthet (✉)
Department of Gastroenterology, Aix Marseille Université, Hôpital Nord, Marseille, France
e-mail: marc.barthet@ap-hm.fr

36.2 Case History

A 56 years old man presented with repeated attacks of mild acute pancreatitis. MRI showed non-dilated main pancreatic duct (MPD) but a cystic lesion located in the neck of the pancreas, measuring 30 mm with mural nodules of up to 5 mm. The pancreatic gland was not infiltrated and no suspicious area surrounding the cystic lesion could be demonstrated. A slight communication between the cystic lesion and the MPD was shown.

A diagnosis of side-branched IPMN with worrisome features was made and pancreaticoduodenectomy was advised. The patient refused surgery and was referred for consideration of EUS-guided RFA.

36.3 Procedural Plan

ERCP with pancreatic sphincterotomy and short-term stenting was first performed to decrease the risk of pancreatitis and followed by EUS-guided RFA for treating the PCN.

A. Y.B. Teoh et al. (eds.), *Atlas of Interventional EUS*, https://doi.org/10.1007/978-981-16-9340-3_36

Pancreatic sphincterotomy has been shown to be effective in about 80% of the cases for reducing the risk of pancreatitis in symptomatic side-branched IPMN (SB-IPMN) with recurrent pancreatitis without evolution towards malignancy [9]. This was the background of the first step of endoscopic management. EUS-guided RFA has also been shown to be effective in ablating SB-IPMN in at least two-third of the cases and resulting in 100% for the disappearance of mural nodules [10].

36.4 Description of the Procedure

ERCP was first done to perform a large pancreatic sphincterotomy and insertion of a 7 Fr 7 cm plastic stent for 6 months. One week later, EUS-guided RFA was performed. The patient received prophylactic rectal diclofenac and antibiotics (amoxicillin and clavulanic acid) 30 mins before the procedure. Multiple 3 mm to 5 mm mural nodules were demonstrated inside the SB-IPMN. CEH EUS was performed that showed intense enhancement of the mural nodules.

EUS-RFA was performed with a 19G RFA needle (Starmed, Taewong, Korea) with double setting availability, applying a 50 W current in Continuance Mode until impedance reaching 100 Ohms (white bubbles appearance will be seen around the needle) and not overpassing 500 Ohms. RFA was stopped either when the operator saw white bubbles on US images coming alongside the needle and outside the targeted lesions or when the impedance exceeded 100 Ohms. Before applying RFA, suction of the main part of the fluid content was done to avoid excessive and uncontrolled RF application. Three shots were applied to treat as much as possible the mural nodules and the epithelium lining the SB-IPMN (Video 36.1).

36.5 Post-procedural Management

Patient was fasted the day after operation and was then allowed regular diet. The post-operative course was uneventful except mild pain which was treated successfully with tramadol and paracetamol for 5 days.

6 months later, the patient did not experience any more attacks of acute pancreatitis. EUS showed absence of mural nodules, no suspicious lesions and no dilatation of the MPD. The pancreatic stent was retrieved (Video 36.2).

36.6 Potential Pitfalls

3 studies about EUS-guided RFA of PCN have been published, two of them being prospective including 6 to 17 patients [10–12]. Furthermore, the follow-up time was limited to one year (10–13 months). Hence, the long-term results are still unknown and the clinicians should be wary of risk of recurrences or malignant change [10–12].

Our team have published the long-term results of EUS-guided RFA for PCN. Significant response (disappearance or size decreasing >50%) was showed in 69.8% at one year versus 66.6% at the end of the follow-up. Patients who had RFA Failures (no change in size or decrease <50%) remained stable and occurred in one third of the patients. The median size of the cyst in patients in RFA failure group was greater [(35 mm (25–76)) than those with complete ablation 18 mm (11–37)) or size decrease >50% (12 mm (9–32)). Mural nodules were found in 12 out of the 17 patients and all disappeared RFA. Even in patients with failure, three patients previously had a mural nodule which disappeared completely. As for EUS-guided RFA, the initial protocol study scheduled a one-shot treatment within the cystic lesions. After the end of this study, we applied now two to three shots for filling the lumen of the cyst with white bubbles. We never overpass three shots since we had a biliary leakage in the patient with IPMN located in the head of the pancreas undergoing 7 shots in a second RFA session. The biliary leakage was treated after one-year biliary stenting without any stenosis (Fig. 36.1).

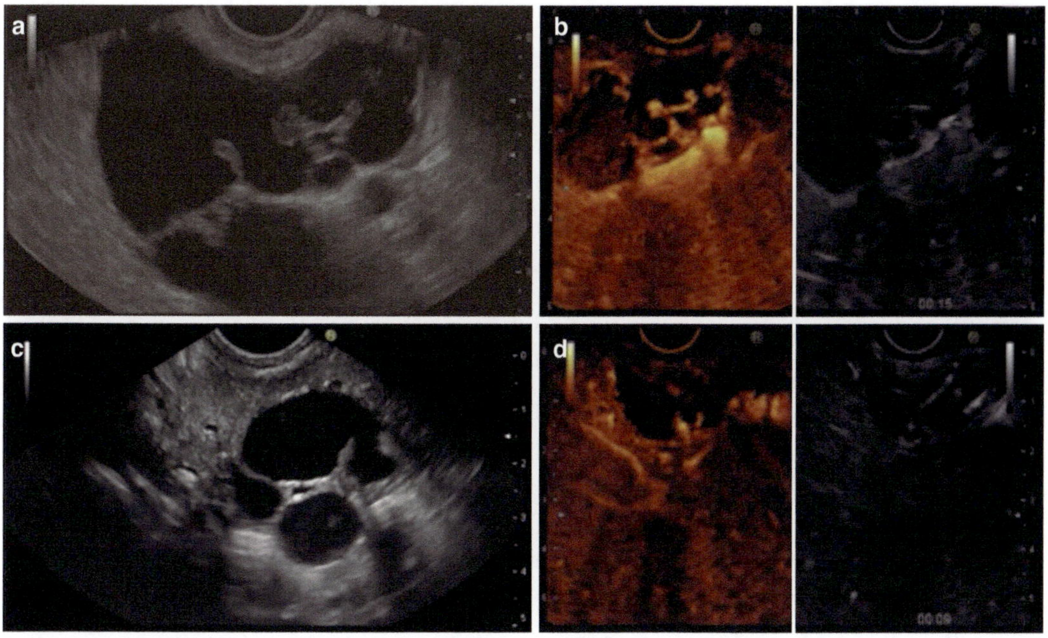

Fig. 36.1 EUS-guided RFA for IPMN with mural nodules. (**a**) EUS view showing a large IPMN with mural nodules located in the body of the pancreas; (**b**) CEH EUS showing enhancement of the mural nodules; (**c**) Follow-up at 6 months after EUS-RFA showing no disappearance of the cystic lesion but complete disappearance of mural nodules; (**d**) Follow-up at 6 months with CEH EUS showing no enhancement of mural nodule

References

1. Farrell JJ. Prevalence, diagnosis and management of pancreatic cystic neoplasms: current status and future directions. Gut Liver. 2015;9:571–89.
2. Tanaka M, Fernández-Del Castillo C, Kamisawa T, et al. Revisions of international consensus Fukuoka guidelines for the management of IPMN of the pancreas. Pancreatol Off J Int Assoc Pancreatol IAP Al. 2017;17:738–53.
3. Brugge WR, Lewandrowski K, Lee-Lewandrowski E, et al. Diagnosis of pancreatic cystic neoplasms: a report of the cooperative pancreatic cyst study. Gastroenterology. 2004;126:1330–6.
4. Okabayashi T, Kobayashi M, Nishimori I, et al. Clinicopathological features and medical management of intraductal papillary mucinous neoplasms. J Gastroenterol Hepatol. 2006;21:462–7.
5. Lakhtakia S, Seo D-W. Endoscopic ultrasonography-guided tumor ablation. Dig Endosc Off J Jpn Gastroenterol Endosc Soc. 2017;29:486–94.
6. Zacharoulis D, Lazoura O, Rountas C, et al. Experimental animal study of a novel radiofrequency endovascular occlusion device. Am J Surg. 2011;202:103–9.
7. Sethi A, Ellrichmann M, Dhar S, et al. Endoscopic ultrasound-guided lymph node ablation with a novel radiofrequency ablation probe: feasibility study in an acute porcine model. Endoscopy. 2014;46:411–5.
8. Kim HJ, Seo D-W, Hassanuddin A, et al. EUS-guided radiofrequency ablation of the porcine pancreas. Gastrointest Endosc. 2012;76:1039–43.
9. Gonzalez JM, Lorenzo D, Ratone JP, et al. Pancreatic sphincterotomy improves symptoms due to branch duct IPMN without worrisome features: a multicenter study. Endosc Int Open. 2019;9:E1130–4.
10. Barthet M, Giovannini M, Lesavre N, et al. Endoscopic ultrasound guided radiofrequency ablation for pancreatic neuroendocrine tumors and pancreatic cystic neoplasms: a prospective multicenter study. Endoscopy. 2019;51:836–42.
11. Pai M, Habib N, Senturk H, et al. Endoscopic ultrasound guided radiofrequency ablation, for pancreatic cystic neoplasms and neuroendocrine tumors. World J Gastrointest Surg. 2015;7:52–9.
12. Canakis A, Law R, Baron T. An updated review on ablative treatment of pancreatic cystic lesions. Gastrointest Endosc. 2020;91:520–6.

EUS-Guided Radiofrequency Ablation of Pancreatic Ductal Adenocarcinoma

37

Pradermchai Kongkam

37.1 Background

In the past 5 years, novel needle electrodes have been adapted to be connected to a radio frequency (RF) generator and inserted through the Endoscopic Ultrasonography (EUS) directly into the pancreas. As a result, an endosonographer began performing EUS-guided radio frequency ablation (EUS-RFA) in pancreatic adenocarcinoma (PDAC) [1].

37.2 Case History

A 51-year-old male patient presented with abdominal pain and weight loss for 2 kilograms over 2 months. His pain score was 8 out of 10. His ECOG score was 1 and Karnofsky scale was 90. There was no fever or jaundice. Past medical history was unremarkable. No heavy alcoholic drinking. No significant smoking history. Upper abdominal endoscopy revealed unremarkable examination. Computer tomography of the upper abdomen demonstrated a 4.7 × 6.9 × 4.2 cm enhancing soft tissue mass involving pancreatic body and tail with encased celiac trunk and splenic artery and obliterated superior mesenteric vein and splenic vein with evidence of collateral vessels from portal vein and isolated gastric varices at fundus (Fig. 37.1). The rest of the pancreas appears unremarkable. A 3.1 × 2.9 × 2.9 cm hypovascular mass suspected of liver metastases was identified at segment 8 of the liver. Multiple sub-centimeter

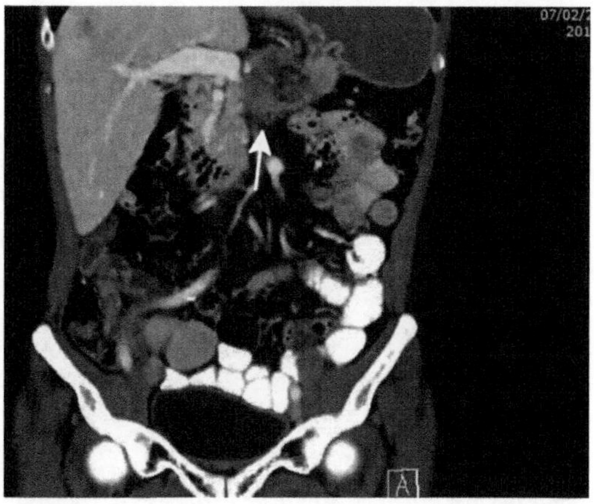

Fig. 37.1 Computer tomography of the upper abdomen demonstrated a 4.7 × 6.9 × 4.2 cm enhancing soft tissue mass involving pancreatic body and tail with encased celiac trunk and splenic artery and obliterated superior mesenteric vein and splenic vein with evidence of collateral vessels from portal vein and isolated gastric varices at fundus

Supplementary Information The online version contains supplementary material available at [https://doi.org/10.1007/978-981-16-9340-3_37].

P. Kongkam (✉)
Gastrointestinal Endoscopy Excellence Center and Division of Gastroenterology, Department of Medicine, Faculty of Medicine, Chulalongkorn University and King Chulalongkorn Memorial Hospital, Thai Red Cross Society, Bangkok, Thailand

Pancreas Research Unit, Department of Medicine, Faculty of Medicine, Chulalongkorn University, Bangkok, Thailand

A. Y.B. Teoh et al. (eds.), *Atlas of Interventional EUS*, https://doi.org/10.1007/978-981-16-9340-3_37

intra-abdominal lymph nodes (LNs) measuring up to 0.9 cm in diameter were present. Blood tests showed Hemoglobin 12.5 g/dL, WBC 4880 cell/HPF, neutrophil 58%, platelet 332,000 ul, INR 1.03, creatinine 0.74 mg/dL, total bilirubin 0.18 mg/dL, direct bilirubin 0.15 mg/dL, amylase 36 U/L, lipase 20 U/L, IgG4 119 mg/dL, CA 19-9 >1000 U/mL, and AFP 2.94 U/L.

37.3 Procedural Plan

Endoscopic ultrasound was performed to make a diagnosis. A large ill-defined hypoechoic mass measuring 1.7 × 2.8 cm in diameter was seen at the body and tail of the pancreas (Fig. 37.2). Trans-gastric EUS-guided fine needle biopsy (EUS-FNB) was performed. Pathological results showed moderately differentiated adenocarcinoma. The final diagnosis was then confirmed as unresectable pancreatic adenocarcinoma (Fig. 37.3).

After a lengthy discussion with the patient and family, we decided to perform endoscopic ultrasound-guided radio frequency ablation (EUS-RFA) plus systemic chemotherapy for his treatment.

37.4 Description of the Procedure

The echoendoscope was inserted into the gastrointestinal tract. Then, the echoendoscope was used to examine the pancreas to determine the location of the mass that needs to be ablated by radio frequency and evaluated if there are any interposing blood vessels. If there is none, the endosonographer will proceed to the next step.

The medical assistant turns on the needle electrode and installs the cooling system that is attached to the needle electrode cable to the RF

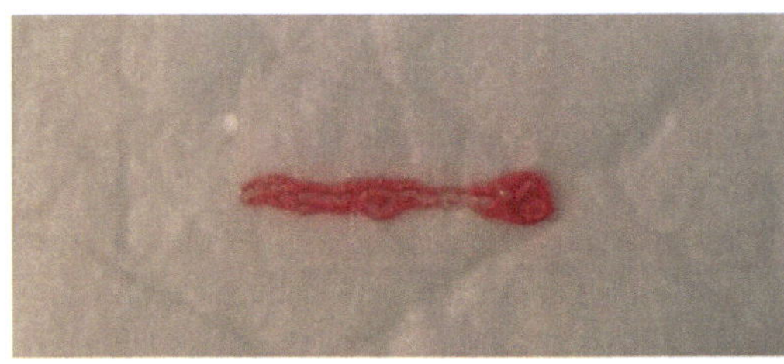

Fig. 37.3 Tissue was obtained from endoscopic ultrasound-guided fine-needle biopsy with a 20-G Procore needle. Final pathology showed moderately differentiated adenocarcinoma

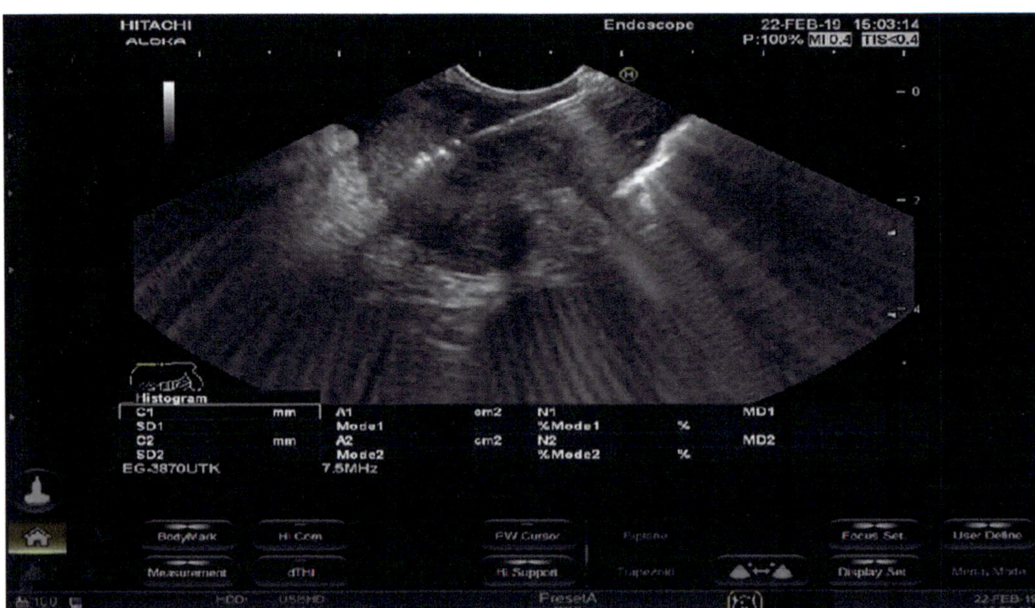

Fig. 37.2 Endoscopic ultrasound was performed. A large ill-defined hypoechoic mass measuring 1.7 × 2.8 cm in diameter was seen at the body and tail of the pancreas. Trans-gastric EUS-guided fine needle biopsy (EUS-FNB) was performed

generator. In our center, the King Chulalongkorn Memorial Hospital, the author and the team use the continuous mode, setting the maximum resistance at 50 watts (Fig. 37.4).

The endosonographer who performs the procedure inserts the needle electrode through the echoendoscope and pins it into the lesion according to the standard technique of EUS-guided needle electrode biopsy. When the needle is in the right position, the endosonographer then controls the start and stop of the radio frequency. In most cases, endosonographer defines the scope of the tumor using EUS images. The tumor is typically hypoechoic solid lesions. Sometimes, other technologies may be employed as well, for example, elastography technology, which can measure the hardness and softness of the target lesion. It is well known that consistency of pancreatic adenocarcinoma is hard. Therefore, using elastography technology, the cancer area will appear blue, specifying harder lesions. The softer ones are seen in green and red, respectively (Fig. 37.5).

At our center, the King Chulalongkorn Memorial Hospital, the endosonographer will ablate the lesion until it appears in white color, resulting from the heat. The endosonographer and medical team who perform the procedure will notice that the white image (Fig. 37.6) covers the desired area and is at least 5 millimeters away from the bile ducts, pancreatic duct, and blood vessels to avoid complications.

After the endosonographer ablates the desired area until a white image is seen, the endosonog-

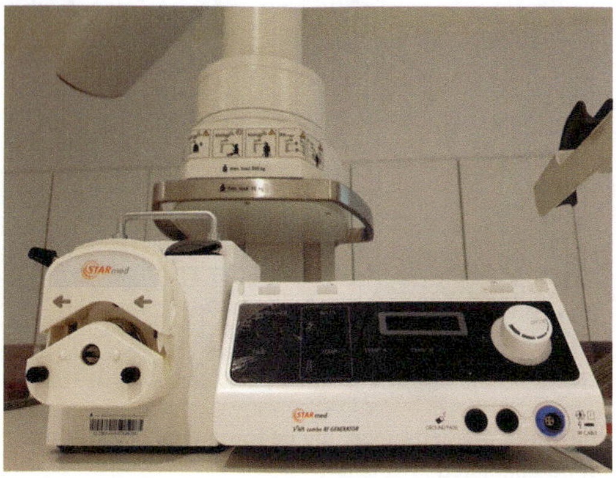

Fig. 37.4 Radio frequency generator was connected with the needle electrode and the cooling system was installed. In our center, at the King Chulalongkorn Memorial Hospital, the author and the team use the continuous mode, setting the maximum resistance at 50 watts

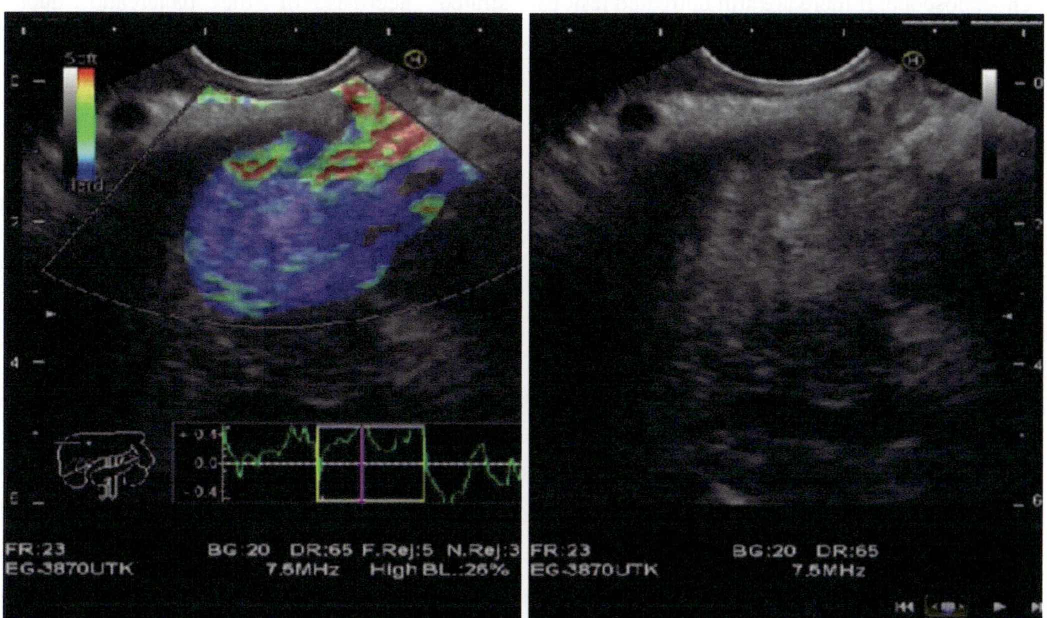

Fig. 37.5 Elastography technology, which can measure the hardness and softness of the target lesion is well known that consistency of pancreatic adenocarcinoma is hard. Therefore, using elastography technology, the cancer area will appear blue, specifying harder lesions. The softer ones are seen in green and red, respectively

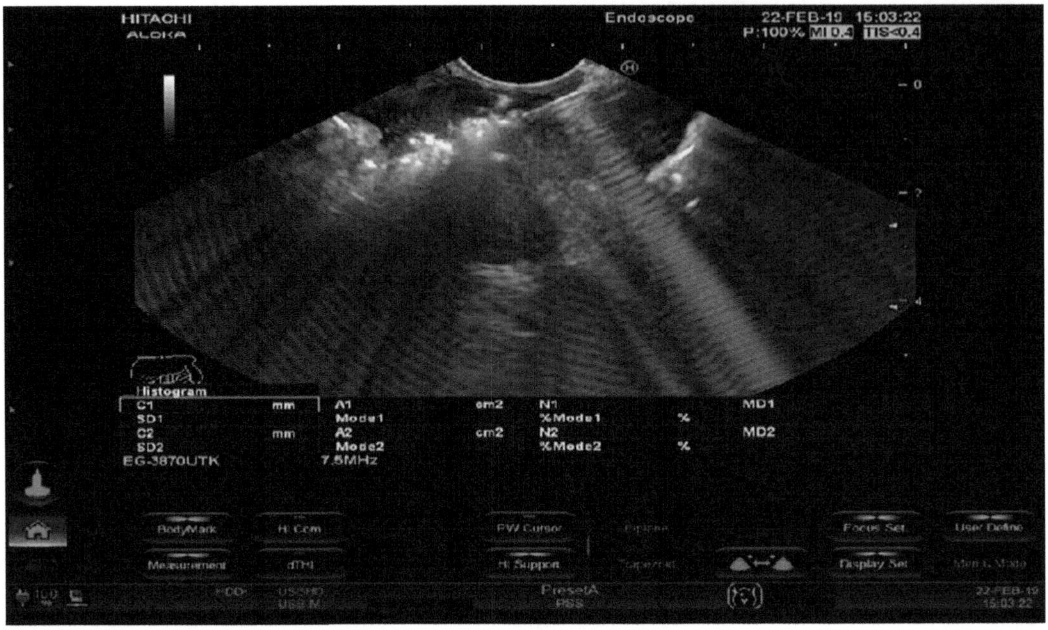

Fig. 37.6 The endosonographer ablates the desired area until a white image is seen, the endosonographer will move the needle electrode to the next area and repeat the actions until no unablated area is left

rapher will move the needle electrode to the next area and repeat the actions until no unablated area is left. The endosonographer then removes the needle and examines the lesion using an echoendoscope. If there are still untreated lesions left, the doctor will puncture the area, using the same methods until no unablated area is left or cannot continue so due to interposing blood vessels.

37.5 Post-Procedural Management

In our center, The EUS-RFA is repetitively performed every 2–4 weeks to the lesion until no more viable tissue to be operated. The procedure was performed concomitantly with systemic chemotherapy. In this current case, totally, within 6 months, the procedures were performed 6 times. No Intra- and post-procedural complications occurred after all procedures. At month 6, pain score had decreased to 1 without pain-controlled medication and the ECOG score was 1. No delayed scheduled chemotherapy as a result of EUS-RFA. After 6 times of EUS-RFA, computed tomography of the abdomen demonstrated necrosis of the pancreatic ductal adenocarcinoma.

In 2–4 weeks, the endosonographer makes an appointment for the patient to repeat EUS-RFA. If unablated lesions are detected and the endosonographer is able to ablate the cancer cells with needle electrodes without limitation, the endosonographer will repeat the treatment.

37.6 Potential Pitfalls

At the time of manuscript writing, there have been two studies using the same machine with the current case, both have reported adverse outcomes as follows. The first study by Song et al., published in 2016, examined 4 patients with pancreatic cancer and 2 patients with cancer spreading to the pancreas. This study reported complications in 2 patients with mild back pain after the procedure [1]. The second study, published in 2018, used EUS-guided RFA in 9 patients with pancreatic tumor, 8 of which had pancreatic adenocarcinoma and the other had kidney cancer which spread to the pancreas. There were 3 patients with slight abdominal pain after the procedure. In the remaining patients, no complications occurred at all, even after average 6-month follow-up [2].

References

1. Song TJ, Seo DW, Lakhtakia S, Reddy N, Oh DW, Park DH, et al. Initial experience of EUS-guided radiofrequency ablation of unresectable pancreatic cancer. Gastrointest Endosc. 2016 Feb;83(2):440–3.
2. Crinò SF, D'Onofrio M, Bernardoni L, Frulloni L, Iannelli M, Malleo G, et al. EUS-guided radiofrequency ablation (EUS-RFA) of solid pancreatic neoplasm using an 18-gauge needle electrode: feasibility, safety, and technical success. J Gastrointestin Liver Dis. 2018 Mar;27(1):67–72.

38 EUS-Guided Radiofrequency Ablation of Functional Pancreatic Neoplasms

Gianenrico Rizzatti and Alberto Larghi

38.1 Background

The mainstay treatment of both functional (F-PanNENs) and nonfunctional (NF-PanNENs) pancreatic neuroendocrine neoplasm is surgery, which however is associated with significant short- and long-term adverse events (AEs) [1]. Consequently, the possibility of performing locoregional treatments, such as EUS-guided ethanol and radiofrequency ablation, have been strongly advocated. EUS-guided radiofrequency ablation (EUS-RFA) of PanNENs has been mostly described in case reports, with only three case series available [2] [3] [4], for a total of 25 F-PanNENs patients (30 lesions) and 44 NF-PanNENs patients (51 lesions) treated so far [5]. For F-PanNENs, mostly insulinomas, available data demonstrated complete regression of the clinical syndrome in all but one case (96%), with only one patient who developed fever treated conservatively. For NF-PanNETs complete ablation, which is the treatment goal, was reached in 82.4% of the cases with a 2% rate of AEs. However, especially for NF-PanNETs, data fully assessing the safety of the procedure and the selection of patients who might benefit the most from this treatment are still limited [6].

Supplementary Information The online version contains supplementary material available at [https://doi.org/10.1007/978-981-16-9340-3_38].

G. Rizzatti · A. Larghi (✉)
Digestive Endoscopy Unit, Fondazione Policlinico Universitario A. Gemelli IRCCS—Università Cattolica del Sacro Cuore, Rome, Italy

CERTT, Center for Endoscopic Research Therapeutics and Training, Università Cattolica del Sacro Cuore, Rome, Italy
e-mail: alberto.larghi@policlinicogemelli.it

38.2 Case History

A 59-year-old male with a history of hypoglycemic episodes was found to have a lesion in the pancreatic body. After clinical confirmation of a diagnosis of insulinoma, he underwent distal pancreatectomy at an outside hospital. Unfortunately, hypoglycemic episodes recurred after surgery and subsequent MRI demonstrated presence of a second lesion (13 mm) in the pancreatic head/uncinate process, which was confirmed to be an insulinoma at diagnostic work-up. Pancreaticoduodenectomy was offered to the patient who refused a second surgical procedure. He was referred to us to perform EUS-RFA.

38.3 Procedural Plan

EUS-RFA is performed using a specifically developed 19-gauge needle electrode (140-cm long), a radiofrequency generator with 30–50 W delivery, and an inner cooling system that

A. Y.B. Teoh et al. (eds.), *Atlas of Interventional EUS*, https://doi.org/10.1007/978-981-16-9340-3_38

circulates chilled saline solution during the RFA procedure in order to dissipate the heating generated during the ablation. Energy is delivered by the exposed tip of needle electrode, which is available in 5–20 mm length. The 5 and 10 mm exposed tip electrode can produce, with one application, a maximum ablation area of about 15 and 25 mm, respectively, depending on wattage and application time. In addition to providing radiofrequency current, the generator allows control of physical power and impedance parameters. The patient herein described is part of an ongoing multicenter study (NCT03834701) for which we had a kick-off meeting to standardize the RFA procedure. In particular, it was decided to use the 5-mm tip for lesions with a diameter $\leq$ 10 mm and 10 or 15 mm tip for larger lesions, to utilize 50 W of power and to perform no more than three ablations for each session to avoid adverse events (AEs). Before ablation, we perform contrast-enhanced EUS (CH-EUS) to be able to compare pre-treatment contrast with CH-EUS performed in repeated procedure in case of failure. Prior to the procedure, indomethacin or diclofenac 100 mg suppository for acute pancreatitis prophylaxis and antibiotics to prevent infection were administered as suggested by Barthet and colleagues [3].

38.4 Description of the Procedure

EUS-RFA was performed via the transduodenal approach with a therapeutic linear echoendoscope. The insulinoma was located in the head/uncinated process close to the papilla and CH-EUS demonstrated the typical homogeneous hyperenhancing pattern in the arterial phase with rapid wash-out in the venous phase (Figs. 38.1 and 38.2). A window between the lesion and the papilla was found and the insulinoma was punctured directly with the 19-gauge needle electrode with a 10-mm exposed tip (Video 38.1). Once inside the target, the RF generator was activated until reaching the impedance limit. During the procedure, a slowly increasing hyperechoic zone can be visualized around (Fig. 38.3). The procedure was repeated a second time by reinserting the needle in the untreated portion of the lesion in order to obtain the largest possible ablation of the tumor.

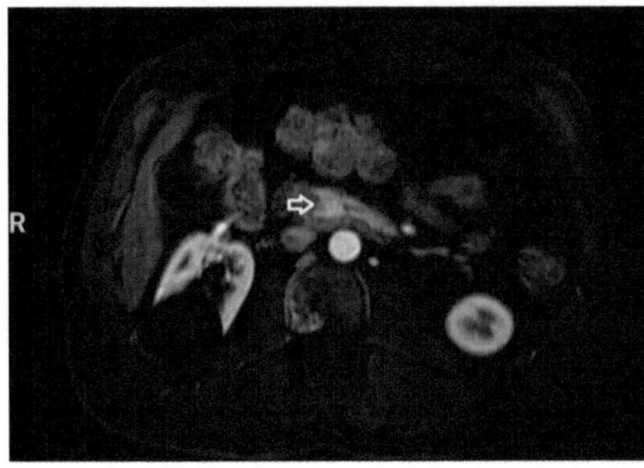

Fig. 38.1 Magnetic Resonance demonstrating hypervascular lesion of the uncinate process

38.5 Post-Procedural Management

The patient was hospitalized for the procedure and kept fast with continuous infusion of glucose 5% overnight. After the procedure, the patient was monitored for 24 h. The glycemia was normal by the subsequent morning and he was discharged home. We do not routinely perform control blood tests. Liquid intake was resumed after 12 h, and if well-tolerated food intake is resumed as well. For patients with F-PanNENs, follow up imaging is not routinely performed and treatment response is based on syndromic symptoms disappearance. Patients are given instructions to regularly monitor glycemic values and drugs to control symptomatic hypoglycemia are progressively reduced accordingly. For patients with NF-PanNENs a CH-EUS is scheduled at 1 month after the first treatment to evaluate for residual tissue to be ablated. In such cases, repeat EUS-RFA procedures are performed until all lesion is ablated. Follow-up CT or MRI is performed at 12 months to evaluate the overall treatment effectiveness.

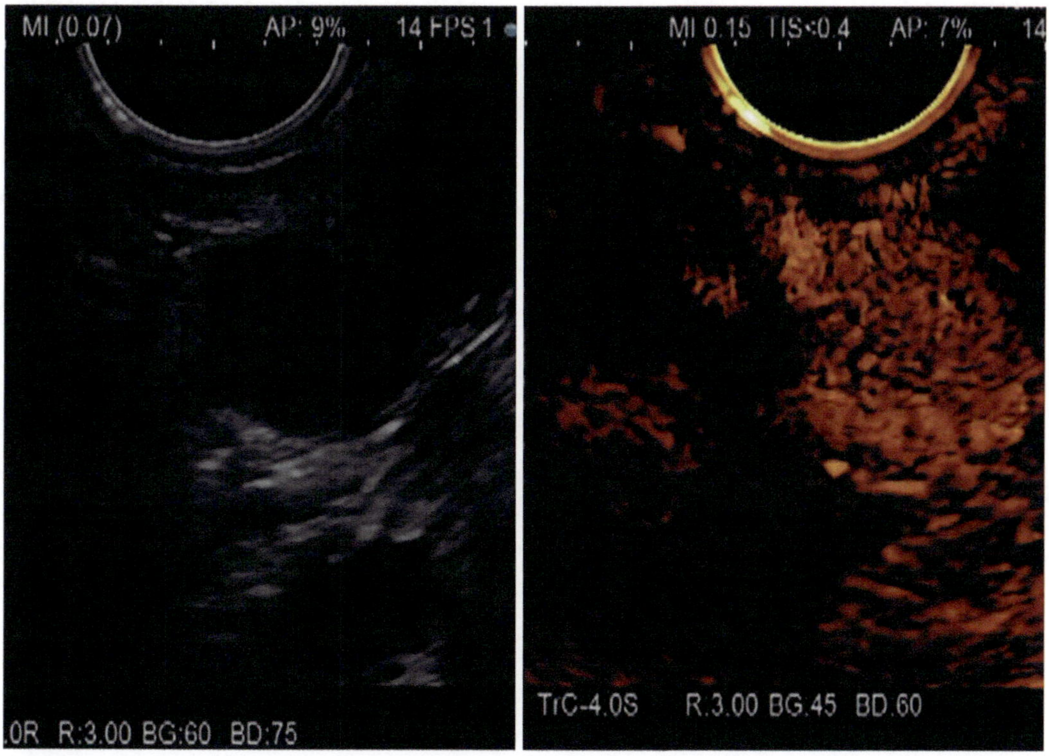

Fig. 38.2 Contrast-enhanced EUS demonstrating the typical homogeneous hyperenhancing pattern of the lesion

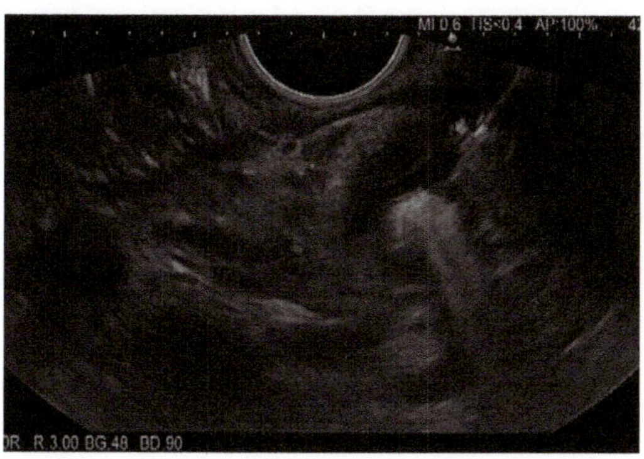

Fig. 38.3 Hyperechoic area in the ablation site at EUS

38.6 Potential Pitfalls

The most commonly reported AEs after EUS-RFA include abdominal pain and acute pancreatitis. Prophylaxis with indomethacin or diclofenac 100 mg suppository administered before the procedure has been empirically and successfully implemented by Barthet et al. [3]. To avoid the occurrence of main pancreatic duct (MPD) stenosis secondary to treatment of lesions too close to the MPD, it is advisable to treat only PanNENs with a distance of at least 2 mm from the MPD. Once the ablation is terminated, as documented by increasing the impedance, it is important to leave the needle for a few seconds inside the lesion before retracting it to avoid burning of the wall GI tract transversed by the ablation catheter.

References

1. Jilesen AP, van Eijck CH, in't Hof KH, van Dieren S, Gouma DJ, van Dijkum EJ. Postoperative complications, in-hospital mortality and 5-year survival after surgical resection for patients with a pancreatic neuroendocrine tumor: a systematic review. World J Surg 2016 Mar;40(3):729–748. Pubmed Central PMCID: 4746219.
2. Choi JH, Seo DW, Song TJ, Park DH, Lee SS, Lee SK, et al. Endoscopic ultrasound-guided radiofrequency

ablation for management of benign solid pancreatic tumors. Endoscopy 2018 Nov;50(11):1099–1104. PubMed PMID: 29727904.
3. Barthet M, Giovannini M, Lesavre N, Boustiere C, Napoleon B, Koch S, et al. Endoscopic ultrasound-guided radiofrequency ablation for pancreatic neuro-endocrine tumors and pancreatic cystic neoplasms: a prospective multicenter study. Endoscopy 2019 Sep;51(9):836–842. PubMed PMID: 30669161.
4. Oleinikov K, Dancour A, Epshtein J, Benson A, Mazeh H, Tal I, et al. Endoscopic ultrasound-guided radio-frequency ablation: a new therapeutic approach for pancreatic neuroendocrine tumors. J Clin Endocrinol Metab 2019 Jul 1;104(7):2637–2647. PubMed PMID: 31102458.
5. Rimbas M, Horumba M, Rizzatti G, Crino SF, Gasbarrini A, Costamagna G, et al. Interventional endoscopic ultrasound for pancreatic neuroendocrine neoplasms. Dig Endosc JGES 2020 Jan 29. PubMed PMID: 31995848.
6. Larghi A, Rizzatti G, Rimbas M, Crino SF, Gasbarrini A, Costamagna G. EUS-guided radiofrequency ablation as an alternative to surgery for pancreatic neuro-endocrine neoplasms: who should we treat? Endosc Ultrasound 2019 Jul–Aug;8(4):220–226. Pubmed Central PMCID: 6714479.

EUS-Guided Radiofrequency Ablation of a Functional Adrenal Tumor

39

Dongwook Oh and Dong-Wan Seo

39.1 Background

Radiofrequency ablation (RFA) uses a high-frequency alternating current, which generates heat energy that induces coagulative necrosis in the target lesion [1]. RFA has been applied percutaneously and intraoperatively for treating various tumors of the liver, kidney, and thyroid [2]. However, percutaneous RFA could not be used in cases of lesions with interposition of organs and/or vessels. Endoscopic ultrasound-guided RFA (EUS-RFA) provides real-time imaging of the target lesion, thus, RFA may be able to ablate the target lesion safely. Recently, several studies have shown that EUS-RFA is technically feasible, safe, and relatively effective for the management of various pancreatic tumors, including unresectable pancreatic cancer and benign solid pancreatic tumors [2–4].

39.2 Case History

A 62-year-old man was admitted for the evaluation of symptoms of Cushing's disease. His complaints were fatigue, weight gain of 5 kg in 2 months with gradual rounding of his face over the past 6 months. Overnight, 1 mg dexamethasone failed to suppress the morning level of cortisol, and the 24-hour urine cortisol level was elevated to 97 μg/day (normal range 0–50). Contrast-enhanced computed tomography (CT) showed a 2-cm left adrenal mass (Fig. 39.1) and the patient was diagnosed with Cushing's syndrome due to left adrenal adenoma. He refused surgery, thus EUS-RFA was performed.

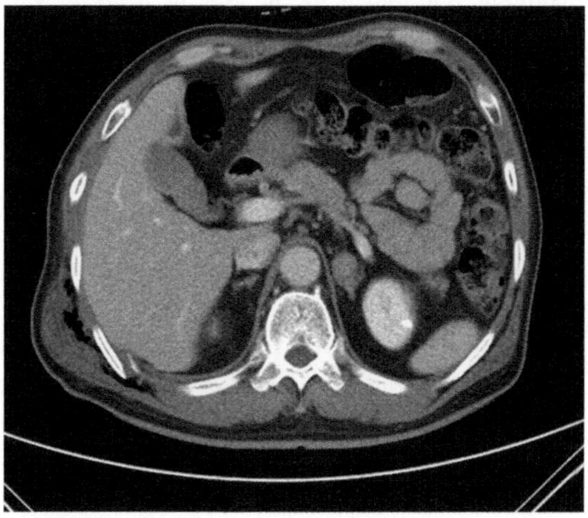

Fig. 39.1 Computed tomography demonstrating adrenal gland adenoma

Supplementary Information The online version contains supplementary material available at [https://doi.org/10.1007/978-981-16-9340-3_39].

D. Oh · D.-W. Seo (✉)
Department of Gastroenterology, University of Ulsan College of Medicine, Asan Medical Center, Seoul, South Korea
e-mail: dwseoamc@amc.seoul.kr

A. Y.B. Teoh et al. (eds.), *Atlas of Interventional EUS*, https://doi.org/10.1007/978-981-16-9340-3_39

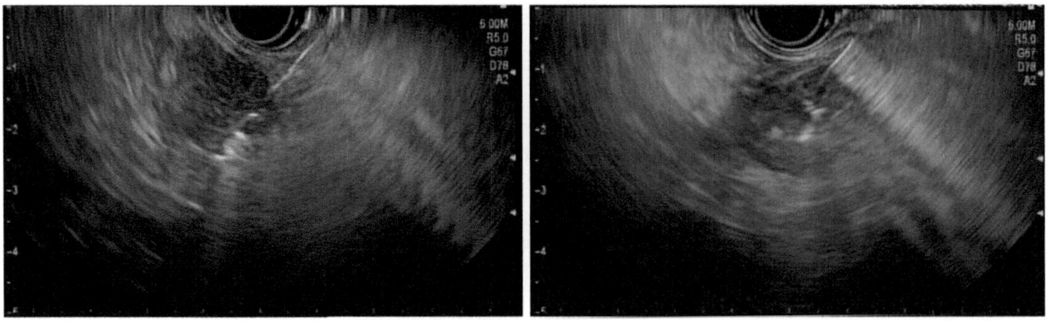

Fig. 39.2 EUS-RFA is performed for adrenal adenoma

39.3 Procedural Plan

RFA usually begins at the right distal part of the mass on the EUS image. After withdrawal of the needle electrode, the needle electrode is reinserted into the tumor, and RFA was repeated at the left side of the previous ablation site (Fig. 39.2). The ablation time duration is related to tissue impedance measured in a real-time manner by the radiofrequency generator. Energy delivery was controlled by an endosonographer using a foot pedal switch. Tumor ablation was repeated until the hyperechoic zone around the electrode sufficiently covered the entire tumor. When treating larger tumor, fanning technique can be used to further ablate multiple sites within the same lesion. Several sizes of the needle are available but the 1-cm needle is used in this patient.

39.4 Description of the Procedure

Before EUS-RFA, prophylactic antibiotics were administered. EUS-RFA was conducted with a 19-G RFA needle and a VIVA radiofrequency generator (Video 39.1). After identification of the tumor, the needle electrode was advanced into the tumor under EUS guidance. The echogenic needle tip was positioned at the far end of the tumor. After insertion of the needle electrode, the radiofrequency generator was activated to deliver 50 W of ablation power. Energy was delivered after the location of the tip of the needle electrode had been confirmed by EUS to be within the margin of the lesion. The radiofrequency generator was activated to deliver 50 W of ablation power. During ablation, bubbles will be seen around the needle tip. The ablation is stopped when an echogenic cloud is seen around the needle. The ablation was repeated until the hyperechoic zone around the electrode tip sufficiently covered the tumor.

39.5 Post-Procedural Management

A simple abdominal radiograph and blood tests are obtained for evaluating potential adverse events on the next day. Diet can be resumed 24 h after the procedure. Other studies can be conducted depending on the clinical signs and symptoms. Initial treatment is evaluated within 1 week after initial EUS-RFA by contrast-enhanced EUS (CE-EUS). During CE-EUS, residual enhancing foci indicate viable tumor. When intratumoral enhancement on CE-EUS is observed, a second session of EUS-RFA is performed (Fig. 39.3). After EUS-RFA, cross-sectional imaging studies, including CT or MRI can be obtained at 3 to 6 months to identify marginal recurrence. For long-term follow-up for evaluation of local or remote relapse, CE-EUS and/or contrast-enhanced CT may be the mainstay imaging tools for follow-up after treatment [5].

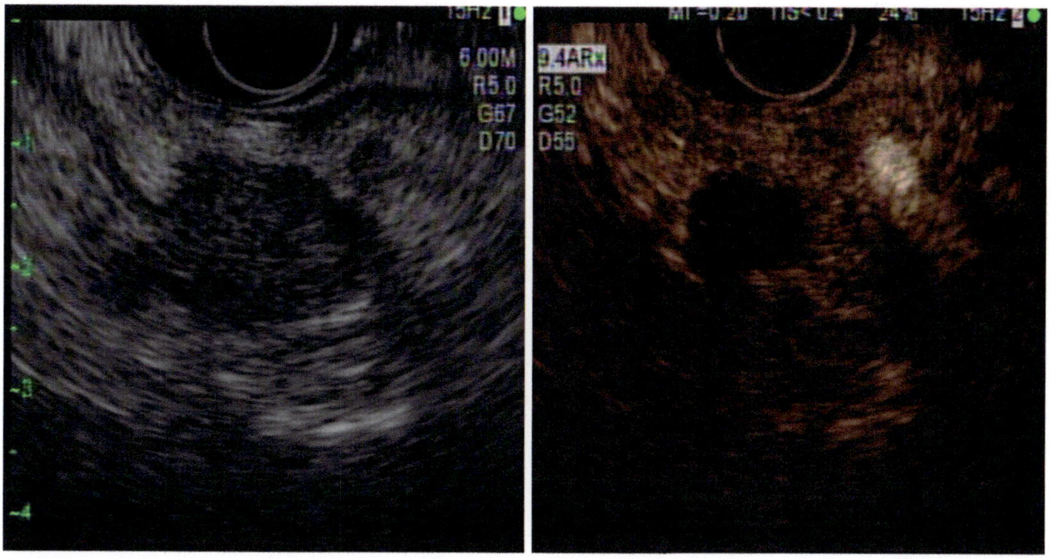

Fig. 39.3 CE-EUS showing viable remnant tumor after EUS-RFA. A second session of RFA is performed to ablate viable tumor

39.6 Potential Pitfalls

The possible adverse events of EUS-RFA are thermal injuries, such as burns of the gastric wall, bowel injury, and peritonitis. RFA-related adverse events are closely associated with the duration of RFA and accurate targeting [2]. For preventing thermal injury to adjacent organs, some technical precautions are required [1]; the maintenance of a 5-mm minimum safety margin from surrounding vessels, and [2] for large lesions larger than 2 cm, a step-up approach is required [6].

For treatment response evaluation, CE-EUS has several advantages over CT scan: [1] the absence of radiation [2], real-time visualization, and detection of viable remnant tumor. A recommended follow-up protocol after ablation suggests the use of CE-EUS within a week to detect remnant tumors. Immediately after ablation, hyperemia is induced around the ablation zone from tissue damage and subsequent inflammatory response. This inflammatory reaction often shows a uniform rim of enhancement which, unlike residual viable tumors, persists throughout the different enhancement phases. Therefore, post-procedure CE-EUS is recommended after a wait of at least 5 to 7 days [5].

References

1. Lakhtakia S, Seo DW. Endoscopic ultrasonography-guided tumor ablation. Dig Endosc JGES. 2017;29(4):486–94.
2. Song TJ, Seo DW, Lakhtakia S, Reddy N, Oh DW, Park DH, et al. Initial experience of EUS-guided radiofrequency ablation of unresectable pancreatic cancer. Gastrointest Endosc. 2016;83(2):440–3.
3. Barthet M, Giovannini M, Lesavre N, Boustiere C, Napoleon B, Koch S, et al. Endoscopic ultrasound-guided radiofrequency ablation for pancreatic neuroendocrine tumors and pancreatic cystic neoplasms: a prospective multicenter study. Endoscopy. 2019;51(9):836–42.
4. Choi JH, Seo DW, Song TJ, Park DH, Lee SS, Lee SK, et al. Long-term outcomes after endoscopic ultrasound-guided ablation of pancreatic cysts. Endoscopy. 2017;49(9):866–73.
5. Choi JH, Seo DW, Song TJ, Park DH, Lee SS, Lee SK, et al. Utility of contrast-enhanced harmonic endoscopic ultrasound for the guidance and monitoring of endoscopic radiofrequency ablation. Gut Liver. 2020;14(6):826–32.
6. Choi JH, Seo DW, Song TJ, Park DH, Lee SS, Lee SK, et al. Endoscopic ultrasound-guided radiofrequency ablation for management of benign solid pancreatic tumors. Endoscopy. 2018;50(11):1099–104.

EUS-Guided Radiofrequency Ablation for Recurrent Lymph Node Metastasis

40

Anthony Y.B. Teoh

40.1 Background

Radiofrequency ablation causes tissue destruction through the application of a high-frequency alternating current, generating local temperatures above 60 °C and leading to coagulative necrosis [1, 2]. The technique has been widely used in many solid organ tumours and has been shown to result in 5-year survival rates comparable to surgery. The application of EUS-guided RFA was first described in the pancreas in 1999 [3]. Since then, there have been significant improvements in the device and EUS-guided RFA is currently under evaluation in humans. In an initial report, EUS-guided RFA was shown to be technically feasible in 6 patients with unresectable pancreatic adenocarcinoma [4]. Two patients suffered from mild abdominal pain but no serious adverse events were reported. Thereafter, the technique has been described in patients suffering from pancreatic neuroendocrine tumour (NET), pancreatic cystic neoplasms, hepatocellular carcinoma, and adrenal metastasis [5–7]. In pancreatic cancer, EUS-guided RFA was able to induce tumour ablation. In pancreatic NET, up to 86% of the patients had complete resolution of the tumour. In pancreatic cystic neoplasms, 64.7% had complete response. However, whether the procedure is associated with improved outcomes as compared to conventional treatment requires further evaluation. In our centre, a research protocol is in place to evaluate the role of EUS-guided RFA in isolated metastatic lymph nodes. The current case is used to illustrate the potential role of EUS-guided RFA in this clinical scenario.

40.2 Case History

A 72-year-old gentleman has a known history of advanced squamous oesophageal carcinoma 29 cm from the incisors. He was planned for neoadjuvant chemoradiation followed by 3 stage oesophagectomy. After neoadjuvant chemoradiation, OGD noted complete resolution of the luminal tumour. Repeated PET-CT noted persistence of multiple hypermetabolic mediastinal lymph nodes. He was then scheduled for 3 stage oesophagectomy. During the operation, he developed repeated desaturation on one lung ventilation and the procedure had to be abandoned. A repeat multidisciplinary meeting noted that further radiotherapy was not possible due to previous

Supplementary Information The online version contains supplementary material available at [https://doi.org/10.1007/978-981-16-9340-3_40].

A. Y.B. Teoh (✉)
Department of Surgery, The Prince of Wales Hospital, The Chinese University of Hong Kong, Shatin, Hong Kong SAR, China
e-mail: anthonyteoh@surgery.cuhk.edu.hk

A. Y.B. Teoh et al. (eds.), *Atlas of Interventional EUS*, https://doi.org/10.1007/978-981-16-9340-3_40

chemoradiation. He was then subjected to surveillance endoscopy and imaging.

A follow-up PET-CT was then performed 4 months after the operation. It reviewed that the previous tumour was no longer present and the hypermetabolic lymph nodes had also resolved or showed a significant decrease in metabolic activity. A follow-up OGD and EUS was then performed. It showed no luminal tumour, but 2 suspicious lymph nodes were noted on EUS and EUS-guided fine needle aspiration cytology confirmed metastatic squamous cell carcinoma. Since the two metastatic lymph nodes were the only residue tumour detected and no further chemo or radiotherapy could be offered, EUS-guided RFA was offered to the patient for ablation of the remaining lymph nodes.

40.3 Procedural Plan

On EUS, the exact location and proximity of the lymph nodes to the oesophageal wall, blood vessels and airway need to be documented as these structures are at risk of thermal injury from the RFA. Furthermore, in the cervical oesophagus, there is a risk of injury to the recurrent laryngeal nerve resulting in vocal cord palsy. If the nodes are located close to these structures, injection of a normal saline–hyaluronic acid mixture around the target node may prevent thermal injury to surrounding structures. In this patient, the two confirmed metastatic nodes were located at 20 cm (1.56 cm) and 30 cm (1.61 cm) (Fig. 40.1) from the incisors at the para-oesophageal region. Hence, they are feasible for EUS-RFA ablation.

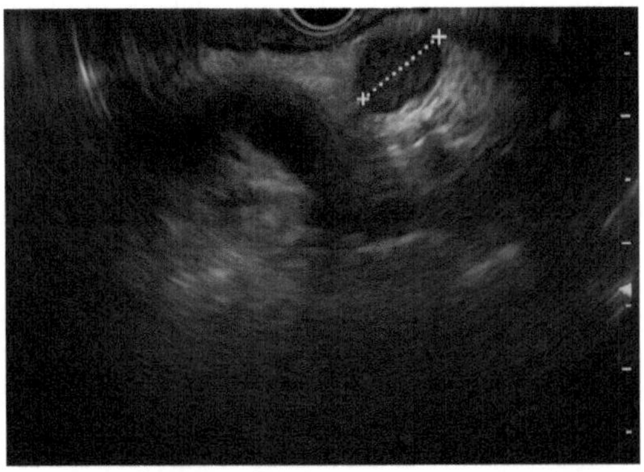

Fig. 40.1 Metastatic lymph node at 30 cm from incisors

40.4 Description of the Procedure

A linear therapeutic endosonoscope was used (GF-UCT260, Olympus Medical, Japan). The two metastatic lymph nodes were identified (Video 40.1). A pre-RFA contrast-enhanced harmonic imaging (CE-EUS) of the nodes was first performed to assess the characteristic of the contrast enhancement (Fig. 40.2). Then EUS-RFA was performed at 50 W power and 70 degrees temperature. The EUS-RFA needle is a 19-gauge needle electrode (STARmed, Seoul, Korea). The RFA probe is located at the terminal 1 cm and the device is connected to a radiofrequency generator. The needle was used to puncture the lymph node directly (Fig. 40.3). The system also features an internal cooling system that allows circulation of cold saline solution through the needle electrode in order to maintain a stable temperature. RFA was then commenced and bubbling would be seen around the needle (Fig. 40.4). Currently, there is no consensus on what the optimal duration of RFA is and our strategy is to ablate until the impedance rises to more than 100 ohm. After complete ablation, a post-RFA CE-EUS was performed to confirm the absence of microvessels in the nodes (Fig. 40.5).

In the current patient, the 20-cm lymph node was ablated 4 times with multiple punctures by the RFA needle. The 30-cm lymph node was ablated 2 times by the RFA needle. A post-RFA OGD was performed and noted suspected mucosal thermal injury at 30 cm. A haemoclip was applied to the site.

40.5 Post-Procedural Management

The patient was allowed oral diet and discharged on the same day. He was followed up one week later for an assessment of presence of complications. A follow-up OGD and EUS was performed 3 months later and showed a decrease in size of

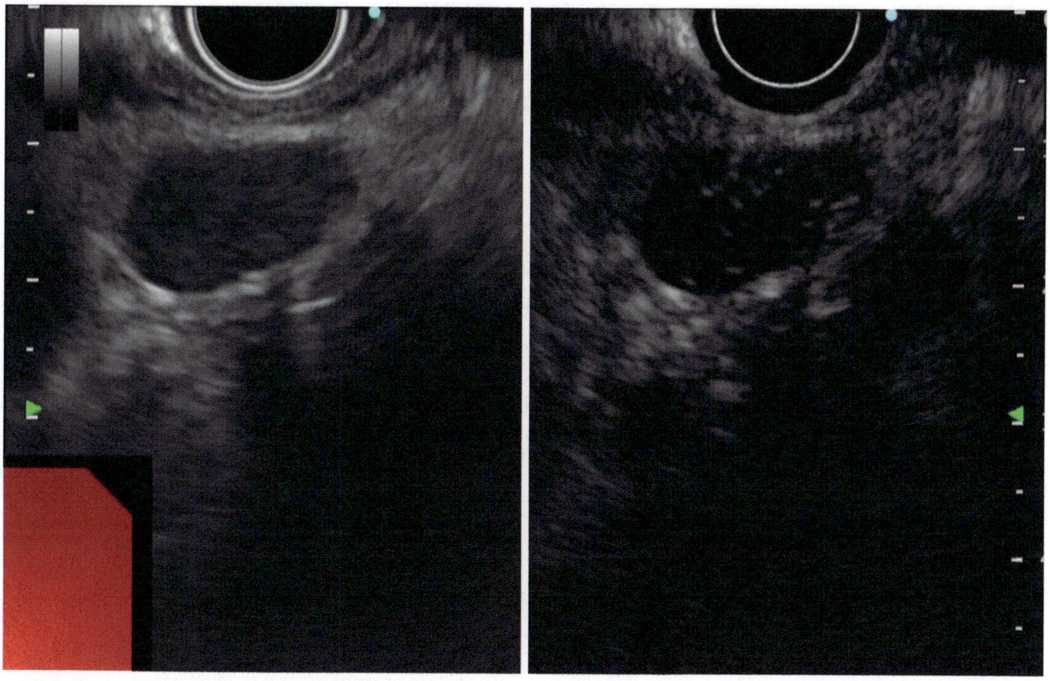

Fig. 40.2 Pre-RFA CE-EUS images of the lymph node

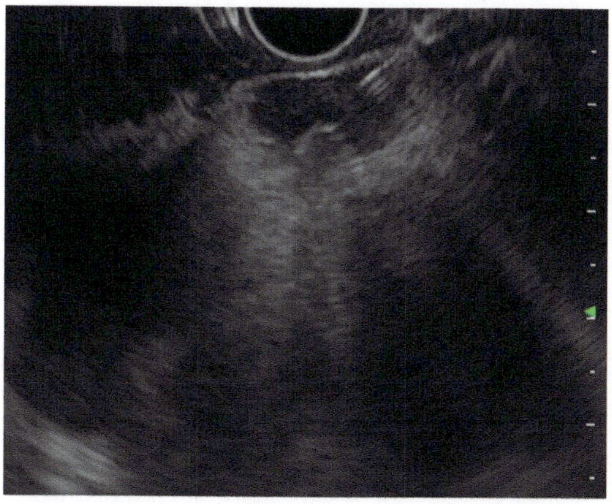

Fig. 40.3 The lymph node punctured by the RFA needle

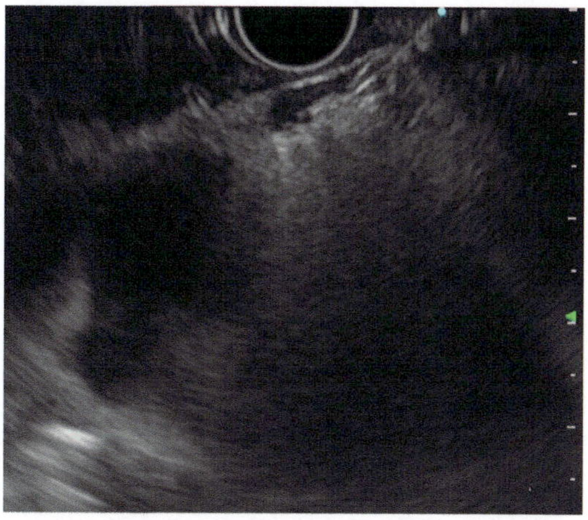

Fig. 40.4 Bubbling around the needle during application of RFA

the 20-cm lymph node to 0.89 cm and the 30 cm lymph node to 1.17 cm.

40.6 Potential Pitfalls

The potential pitfall of this procedure is risk of injury surrounding structures as mentioned. These include blood vessels, the airway and the recurrent laryngeal nerves. If the nodes are located close to these structures, injection of a normal saline–hyaluronic acid mixture around the target node may prevent thermal injury to surrounding structures and also push the node away from these structures. Since after RFA, the lymph node will remain hot for a period of time,

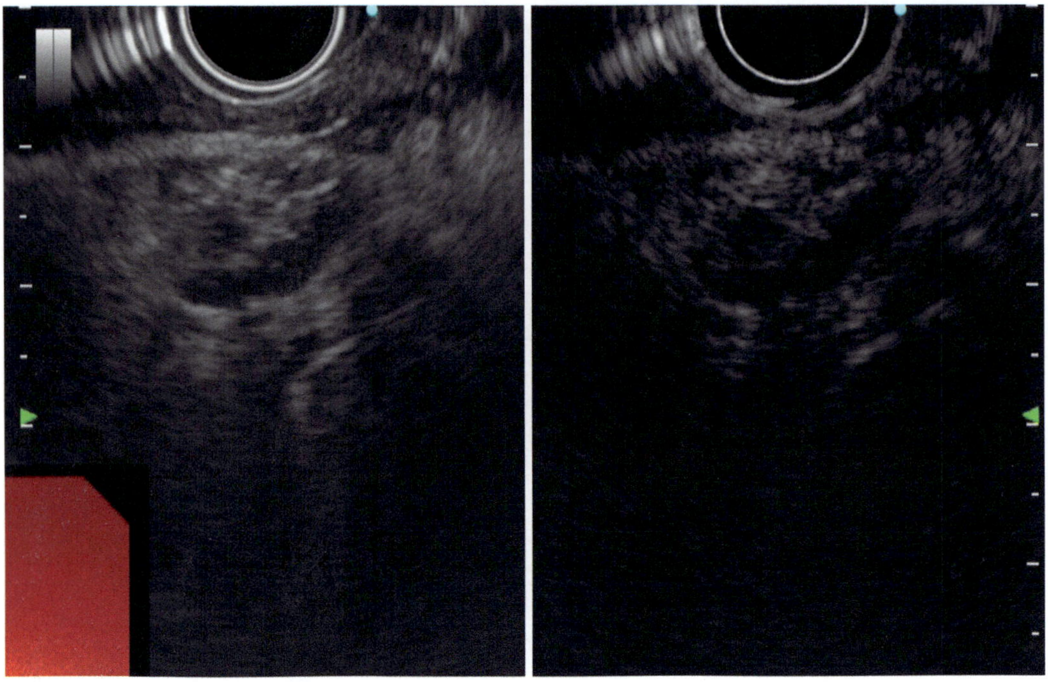

Fig. 40.5 Post-RFA CE-EUS demonstrating absence of microvessels in the lymph node

thermal injury can be delayed and present sometime after the procedure. Hence, it is our routine to follow up with the patients 1 week after EUS-RFA.

References

1. Rossi S, Fornari F, Pathies C, Buscarini L. Thermal lesions induced by 480 KHz localized current field in Guinea pig and pig liver. Tumori. 1990;76(1):54–7.
2. McGahan JP, Browning PD, Brock JM, Tesluk H. Hepatic ablation using radiofrequency electrocautery. Investig Radiol. 1990;25(3):267–70.
3. Goldberg SN, Mallery S, Gazelle GS, Brugge WR. EUS-guided radiofrequency ablation in the pancreas: results in a porcine model. Gastrointest Endosc. 1999;50(3):392–401.
4. Song TJ, Seo DW, Lakhtakia S, Reddy N, Oh DW, Park DH, et al. Initial experience of EUS-guided radiofrequency ablation of unresectable pancreatic cancer. Gastrointest Endosc. 2016;83(2):440–3.
5. Choi JH, Seo DW, Song TJ, Park DH, Lee SS, Lee SK, et al. Endoscopic ultrasound-guided radiofrequency ablation for management of benign solid pancreatic tumors. Endoscopy. 2018;50(11):1099–104.
6. Attili F, Boskoski I, Bove V, Familiari P, Costamagna G. EUS-guided radiofrequency ablation of a hepatocellular carcinoma of the liver. VideoGIE. 2018;3(5):149–50.
7. Inderson A, Slingerland M, Farina Sarasqueta A, de Steur WO, Boonstra JJ. EUS-guided radiofrequency ablation for a left adrenal oligometastasis of an esophageal adenocarcinoma. VideoGIE. 2018;3(5):159–61.

41 EUS-Guided Photodynamic Therapy for Pancreatic Cancer

John DeWitt

41.1 Background

In the USA in 2018, an estimated 55,440 Americans were diagnosed with pancreatic cancer while an estimated 44,330 deaths occurred from the disease [1]. Despite advances in chemotherapy [2, 3], 5-year survival remains under 10% [1].

Photodynamic therapy (PDT) is an oxygen-dependent reaction between a photosensitizing agent and light that produces tissue necrosis. The light is usually given as a laser and is applied after administration of the agent [4]. Percutaneous application of a light fiber is required for use of radiologic assistance. This technique may be uncomfortable for the patient since it requires passage of the fiber from the skin to the primary tumor. Due to the close proximity of the endoscope to the pancreas, EUS may be an alternative to deliver PDT to the pancreas.

In a recent phase 1 study, EUS-PDT for untreated pancreatic cancer using the photosensitizer porfimer sodium was technically feasible, safe, and produced tumor necrosis in selected patients [5]. Furthermore, chemotherapy after EUS-PDT led to tumor downstaging and allowed attempted surgical resection in some patients.

41.2 Case History

A 70-year-old man with a 2-month history of anorexia, abdominal pain, back pain with an associated 50 pound weight loss. Work-up included CT scan that showed a large mass in the body of pancreas encasing the celiac axis (Figs. 41.1 and 41.2). These findings were confirmed by EUS on 12/9/16 which found a 48 mm by 32 mm mixed solid and cystic (cystic component measured 17 mm × 12 mm and was septated) oval mass. The mass invaded the celiac trunk, splenic artery, hepatic artery, and splenic vein. FNA demonstrated adenocarcinoma. No obvious distant metastatic disease was noted on CT scan or EUS confirming locally advanced pancreatic cancer. The patient consented to EUS-guided photodynamic therapy (PDT) on a Phase 1 study.

Supplementary Information The online version contains supplementary material available at [https://doi.org/10.1007/978-981-16-9340-3_41].

J. DeWitt (✉)
Division of Gastroenterology and Hepatology, Indiana University Health Medical Center, Indianapolis, IN, USA
e-mail: jodewitt@iu.edu

A. Y.B. Teoh et al. (eds.), *Atlas of Interventional EUS*, https://doi.org/10.1007/978-981-16-9340-3_41

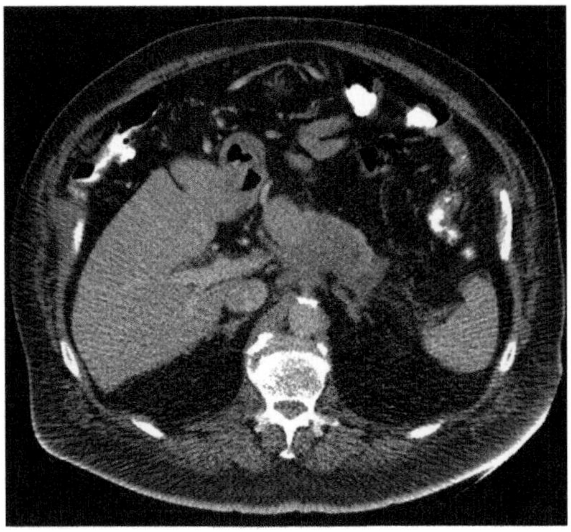

Fig. 41.1 Baseline axial CT scan demonstrating a pancreatic body mass with <5% necrosis

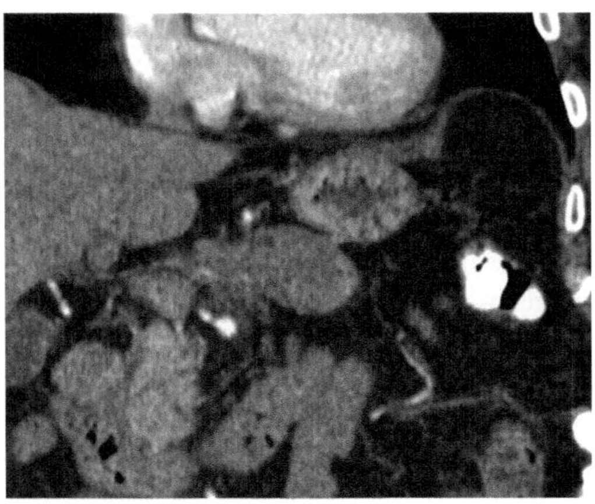

Fig. 41.2 Baseline coronal CT scan demonstrating a pancreatic body mass with <5% necrosis

41.3 Procedural Plan

In this trial, there were four cohorts, which varied by the dose of photosensitizer given and time of light application. Intravenous porfimer sodium (Photofrin, Concordia Laboratories Inc., St. Michael, Barbados) as a photosensitizer was given at a dose of 1 mg/kg (first 6 patients) or 2 mg/kg (last 6 patients) and was considered as day 1 of the study. The current patient received 2 mg/kg of porfimer sodium. For each use of the diffuser, the tumor was illuminated with 30-nm light (Diomed Inc, Andover, Mass). A total light dose of 50 J/cm per needle puncture was used for the first three patients in the first cohort, which increased to 100 J/cm per puncture for the next three patients in the second cohort. A maximum of 3 punctures were made per patient and each treatment (i.e., puncture) site was about 10 mm apart based on the expected region of necrosis produced by each treatment. Treatment application time per site was either 125 or 250 s. Therefore total treatment energy for one or both procedures varied between 150 and 300 joules (Fig. 41.4).

41.4 Description of the Procedure

EUS-PDT (considered day 3 of the study) was performed using a linear echoendoscope.

First, the stylet of a 19-gauge needle (Boston Scientific, Natick, Mass.) was removed, and a plastic locking device was attached to the proximal needle. A small diameter quartz optical fiber with a 1.0-cm cylindrical diffuser (Pioneer Optics, Bloomfield, Conn) was passed through the locking device and needle until about 1.5 cm exited the tip of the FNA needle. The fiber was secured with the locking device and the locking device/fiber combination was withdrawn about 2 to 3 cm proximally inside the needle. The needle was then passed into the endoscope and secured at the accessory channel. The tumor was punctured and the tip passed toward the distal side of the tumor. The needle was then withdrawn 1 to 2 cm proximally inside the tumor and the fiber advanced 1.5 cm into the tumor by advancement of the locking device/fiber combination. The locking device was secured to the proximal end of the FNA needle. The tumor was illuminated with the diffuser fiber for 250 s. The locking device/fiber combination was withdrawn into the needle and the needle was withdrawn from the tumor. The process was repeated twice more, each via a transgastric puncture.

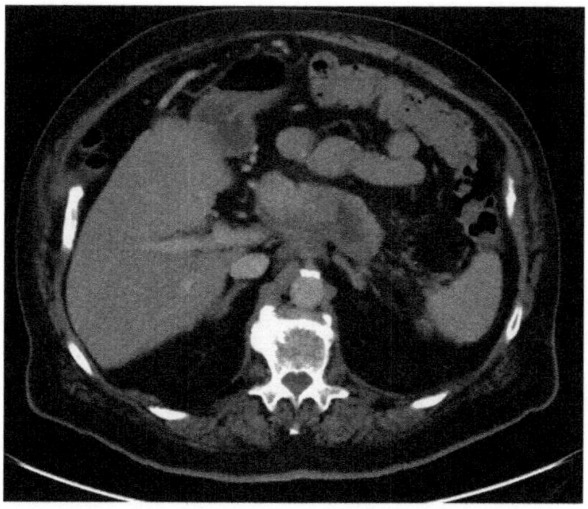

Fig. 41.3 Axial CT scan 3 weeks after EUS-PDT showing 46–50% necrosis within the tumor

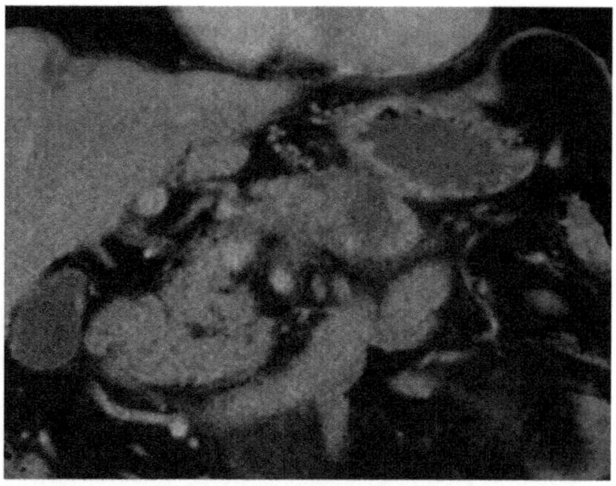

Fig. 41.4 Axial CT scan 3 weeks after EUS-PDT showing 46–50% necrosis within the tumor

41.5 Post-procedural Management

After EUS, the patient remained in recovery without oral intake for 2 hrs. No post-procedure analgesics or antiemetics were required and he was able to resume intake of liquids. Prior to discharge, serum amylase and lipase were normal. Repeat CT scan about 3 weeks after PDT showed 48% necrosis of the tumor that had increased significantly from the baseline scan which had only 2% necrosis (Figs. 41.3 and 41.4). The patient started neoadjuvant therapy with nab-paclitaxel and gemcitabine the following week.

41.6 Potential Pitfalls

This case illustrates one limitation with treatment of locally advanced pancreatic cancer with EUS-directed therapy. Transgastric puncture and fiber delivery to tumors using a 19-gauge needle in the body and tail similar to this patient is technically easier than transduodenal puncture of pancreatic head tumors. Another limitation not illustrated with this case is that imaging of pancreatic head tumors smaller than 35 mm with metallic biliary stents is challenging which makes visualization of the FNA needle puncture and diffuser fiber more difficult. Development of a fiber that may be delivered with a 22-gauge needle would likely make treatment easier.

References

1. Siegel RL, Miller KD, Jemal A. Cancer statistics, 2018. CA Cancer J Clin. 2018;68:7–30.
2. Von Hoff DD, Ervin T, Arena FP, et al. Increased survival in pancreatic cancer with nab-paclitaxel plus gemcitabine. N Engl J Med. 2013;369:1691–703.
3. Conroy T, Desseigne F, Ychou M, et al. FOLFIRINOX versus gemcitabine for metastatic pancreatic cancer. N Engl J Med. 2011;364:1817–25.
4. Sheng C, Pogue BW, Wang E, et al. Assessment of photosensitizer dosimetry and tissue damage assay for photodynamic therapy in advanced-stage tumors. Photochem Photobiol. 2004;79:520–5.
5. DeWitt JM, Sandrasegaran K, O'Neil B, et al. Phase 1 study of EUS guided photodynamic therapy for locally advanced pancreatic cancer. Gastrointest Endosc. 2019;89:390–8.

42 EUS-Guided Ablation with HybridTherm Probe

Sabrina Gloria Giulia Testoni, Gemma Rossi, and Paolo Giorgio Arcidiacono

42.1 Background

EUS-guided local thermal ablation (LTA) is a minimally invasive therapeutic approach [1] increasingly applied in patients with pancreatic cancer (PC), due to the modest survival improvement achieved in the last decade by the new polychemotherapy regimens. The rationale of the use of LTA in PC is the treatment of patients with a locally advanced disease in whom a R0 resection is not obtainable, aiming for local control of the disease and to potentially reduce the chance of metastatic tumor spreading [2, 3]. Several case reports and small series have shown that the EUS-guided approach is associated with fewer adverse events than surgical or percutaneous routes [4, 5]. Recently, a new experimental device, the HybridTherm probe (HTP), combining bipolar radiofrequency ablation and cryotherapy (currently not commercially available), has shown to be feasible and safe in patients with locally advanced pancreatic adenocarcinoma (PDAC) [6].

Supplementary Information The online version contains supplementary material available at [https://doi.org/10.1007/978-981-16-9340-3_42].

S. G. G. Testoni · G. Rossi · P. G. Arcidiacono (✉)
Pancreatico-Biliary Endoscopy & Endosonography Division, Pancreas Translational & Clinical Research Center, San Raffaele Scientific Institute, Vita-Salute San Raffaele University, Milan, Italy
e-mail: testoni.sabrinagloriagiulia@hsr.it; rossi.gemma@hsr.it; arcidiacono.paologiorgio@hsr.it

42.2 Case History

A 71-year-old man, with recent onset of diabetes mellitus type II, was admitted to San Raffaele Scientific Institute for obstructive jaundice. A total body contrast-enhanced computed tomography showed a lesion in the pancreatic head (35 × 30 mm), resulting in dilation of the main pancreatic duct (13 mm) and the biliary tree (Fig. 42.1). No distant metastases were observed. EUS evaluation confirmed the presence of a hypovascular (at Color Doppler and contrast-

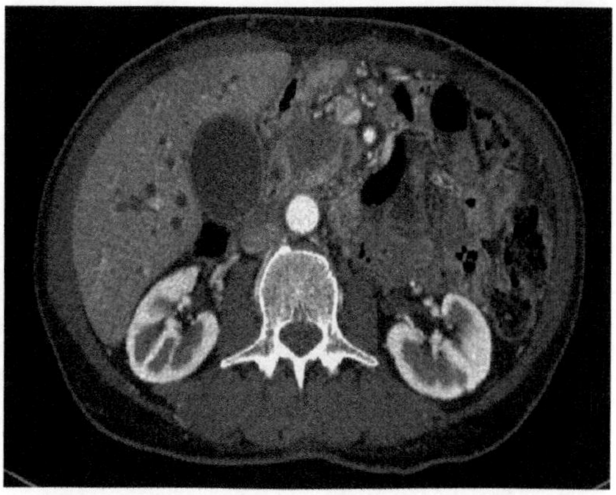

Fig. 42.1 Pancreatic solid lesion at diagnosis CT-scan

A. Y.B. Teoh et al. (eds.), *Atlas of Interventional EUS*, https://doi.org/10.1007/978-981-16-9340-3_42

enhancement evaluation) and rigid (at qualitative and semi-quantitative elastography) lesion in the pancreatic head, 45 mm in size, involving the superior mesenteric vein with a circular extension >180° and with a longitudinal contact with the superior mesenteric artery. Pathologic lymph nodes were observed at the hepatic hilum (Fig. 42.2a, b, c). EUS-fine needle aspiration was performed and pathology report confirmed the diagnosis of PDAC. An ERCP with sphincterotomy and biliary metal stent placement (partially covered, 60 × 10 mm) was performed, with a resolution of jaundice. Serum Ca19.9 at the diagnosis was 2404 U/mL (normal value <34). After a multidisciplinary evaluation, the experimental ablation treatment with HTP under EUS guidance was offered to the patient in addition to chemotherapy, within an approved study protocol (Clinical Trial NCT02336672).

42.3 Technical Characteristics of the HybridTherm Probe

The peculiar characteristic of HTP is the synergistic combination of two thermal technologies, the bipolar radiofrequency ablation (RFA) and cryoablation (CO_2 cryogenic gas). HTP is a 14-gauge EUS "needle-type" probe (diameter of 3.2 mm and length of 1.4 mt), internally cooled by constant flow of carbon dioxide gas (Fig. 42.3a), presenting at the distal tip the electrically active part composed of two electrodes separated by an insulation part (diameter 2.2 mm and length of 26 mm) (Fig. 42.3b). The device can be inserted through the 3.8-mm operative channel of a therapeutic echoendoscope. In this hybrid system, cryotherapy increases the tissue interstitial devitalization induced by bipolar RFA with the need for a lower power and decreasing

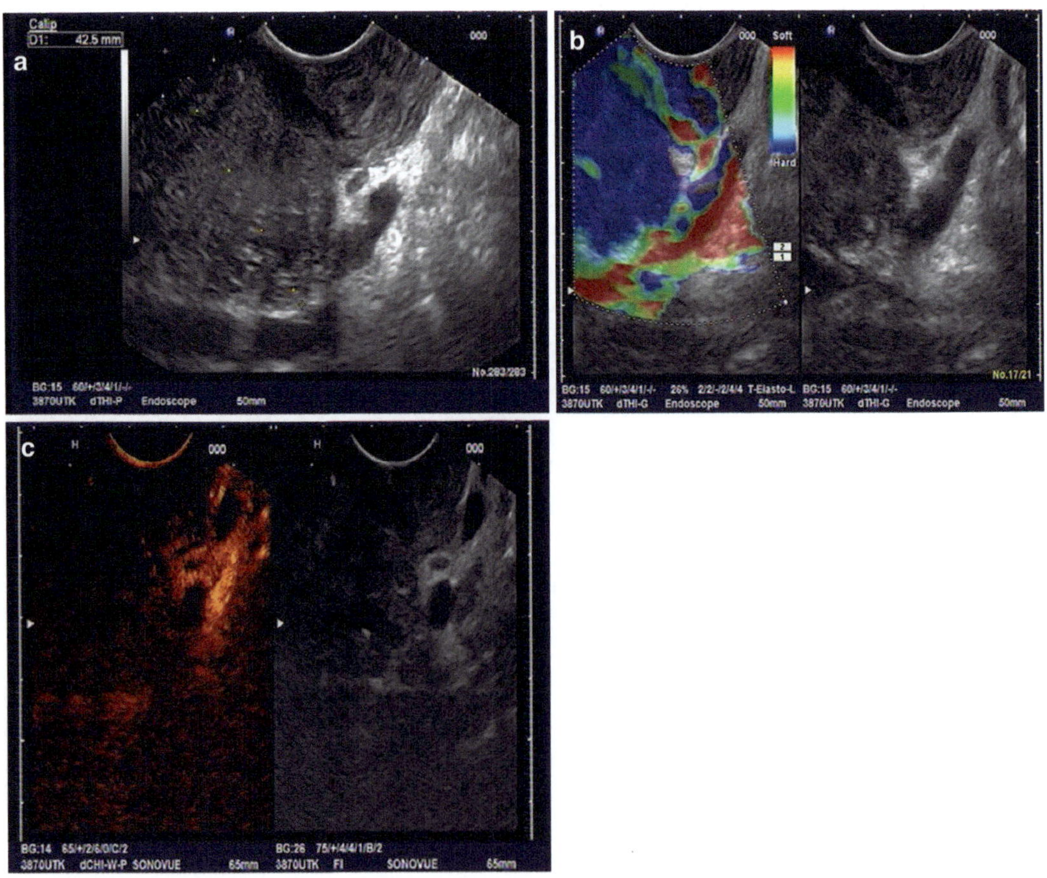

Fig. 42.2 Endoscopic ultrasound aspect of pancreatic cancer: at B-mode (**a**), elastography (**b**), and contrast-enhancement evaluation (**c**)

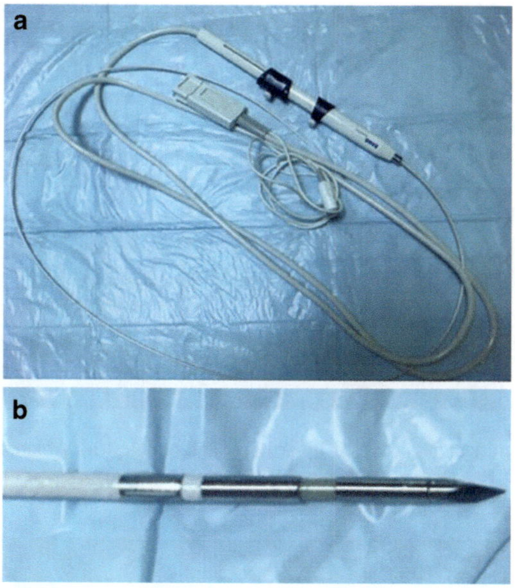

Fig. 42.3 The HybridTherm probe (ERBE, Elektromedizin GmbH, Germany). A 14-gauge endoscopic ultrasound "needle-type" device (length and diameter of 1.4 mt and 3.2 mm, respectively), covered by a protective tube in Teflon for the entire length (**a**). The sharp and stiff distal tip contains the electrically active part (diameter and length of 2.2 mm and 26 mm, respectively), composed of two electrodes separated by an insulation part (**b**)

the risk of thermal injury to the surrounding structures. The energy is delivered by the generator VIO 300D RF-surgery system and the cooling effect is delivered by the ERBECRYO2 system (both ERBE, Elektromedizin GmbH, Tübingen, Germany). The pressure of CO_2 flow, the power setting of the generator, and the duration of application can be regulated independently. Based on preliminary animal and ex vivo human studies [7–9], the ablation parameters were set as follows: fixed RF power of 18 W and fixed pressure of 650 psi, application time ranging from 240 s for a 2-/3-cm mass to 480 s for a >3-cm mass.

42.4 Procedural Plan

The study protocol was planned to perform three EUS-HTP sessions at 1 month interval, depending on the tumor morphological and patient clinical features, along with 6-month chemotherapy based on Nab-paclitaxel + Gemcitabine. The first EUS-HTP session was scheduled 1 week before chemotherapy start. Contrast-enhanced (CE) MDCT scan and MRI were planned 72 h after each ablative procedure to assess the early result of the treatment and eventual procedure-related adverse event.

42.5 Description of the Procedure

With the patient lying on the left side and under deep sedation with propofol, given by an anesthesiologist, EUS-HTP was performed after a preliminary EUS confirming the morphological and tissue features as well as the ideal route for HTP insertion.

In general, EUS-HTP can be performed via a trans-gastric or trans-duodenal approach, depending on the lesion's site (head and body/tail, respectively). In this case, the trans-duodenal approach has been chosen, positioning the tip of the EUS probe in the duodenal bulb. After identifying the safe access to the pancreatic lesion using the Color Doppler evaluation to avoid interposed vessels. The presence of a prepositioned metal biliary stent was not considered a contraindication, because of intrinsic physical characteristics of the HTP (bipolar electrode).

The HTP, connected to the RF generator–cooling system is inserted through the operative channel of a convex linear array echoendoscope. It was then placed directly under real-time EUS guidance into the pancreatic lesion where the thermal energy was delivered. The RF generator–cooling system interface was set to automatically stop the ablation in case of tissue desiccation with an increase of electrical impedance, regardless of the 3-min scheduled time of application, to avoid unnecessary power delivery. During the energy delivery, the firm position of the probe was helpful in controlling the creation of ablation area, under real-time EUS guidance, hyperechoic spots along the hyperechoic needle path were visible, due to the RF energy flowing between the two electrodes (Fig. 42.4a, Video 42.1). At the end of the treatment, the needle probe was retracted into the sheath and then withdrawn and

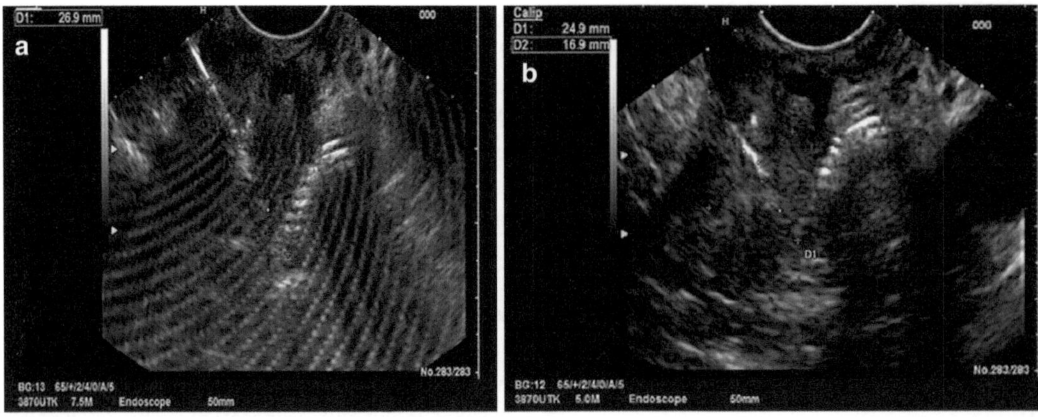

Fig. 42.4 Echoic aspect of the HybridTherm probe treatment: lesion is covered by artifacts and bubbles (**a**). Ablated area size immediately after the first EUS-HTP session (**b**)

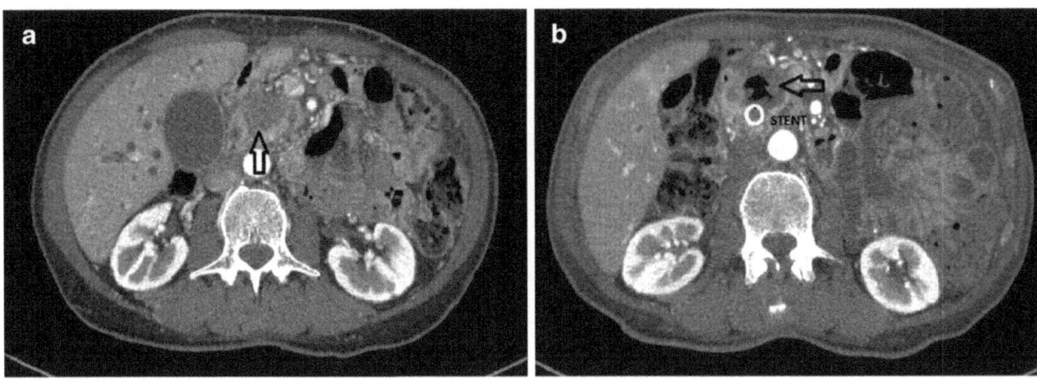

Fig. 42.5 Necrotic area (hypodense area) inside the pancreatic lesion at 72 h CT scan evaluation after the first ablative treatment (**a**). Excavated area inside the lesion after the second ablative session (**b**)

discarded. An immediately post-procedure EUS evaluation was performed in order to assess eventual procedure-related injury to surrounding organs and vessels and determine the size of the ablation-induced necrotic area (Fig. 42.4b).

42.6 Post-Procedural Management

Post procedurally, the patient was scheduled, for a 2-, 4- and 6-month restaging with CE MDCT scan and MRI to assess the response to ablative therapy, consisting on the creation of coagulative necrosis inside the pancreatic lesion.

In this patient, 2 EUS-HTP procedures were performed, both with thermal energy application lasting 3 min. The patient remained asymptomatic after the procedure during the hospital stay, the diet was resumed 24 h after the two ablatives procedure. At 72-h CE MDCT scan and MRI, no signs of acute pancreatitis or other complications were observed following both HTP sessions. After the first EUS-HTP, a central necrotic area in the lesion, adjacent to the metal stent, 30 × 25 mm in size, was seen at radiologic exams (Fig. 42.5a). After the second EUS-HTP session, a central non-enhanced aerated cavitation (36 × 25 mm) with a peripheral hypodense component was observed inside the pancreatic lesion (Fig. 42.5b), in close proximity to the biliary stent, compatible with the induced coagulative necrosis. As a consequence of the local inflammatory reaction to the ablative procedure, a slight

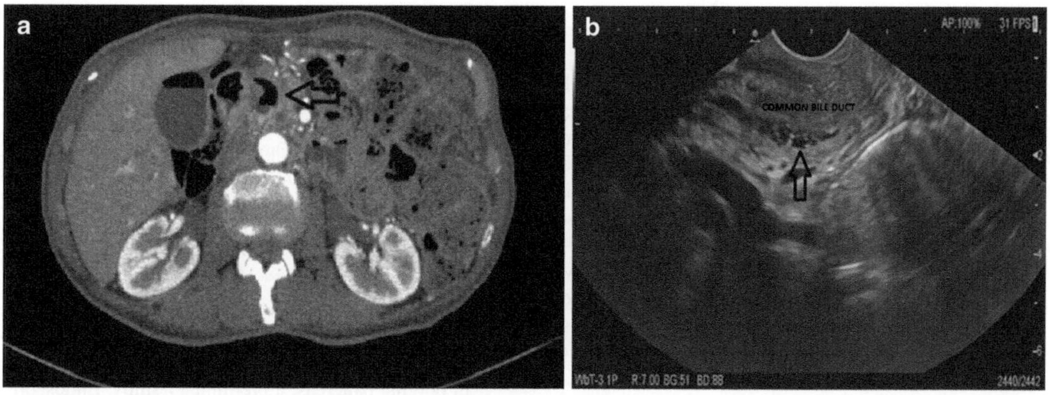

Fig. 42.6 Central excavated alteration at CT scan after 1 month with respect to the second ablative session, with the EUS aspect of common bile duct (**a**), with spontaneous drainage into the duodenal cavity (without biliary metal stent) (**b**)

gastric wall edema and a modest amount of intraperitoneal fluid were observed, without clinical manifestations. The two-month CE MDCT scan and MRI showed a reduction of the lesion (25x21 mm), with persistent hypodense peripheral tissue component and central aerated cavitation (Fig. 42.6a). The subsequent (1 day after CT) EUS evaluation planned to perform the third HTP session evidenced the creation of a pseudo-diverticulum involving the periampullary region and the pancreatic head and directly communicating with a patent common bile duct with a spontaneous migration of the biliary metal stent (Video 42.2, Fig. 42.6b).

The remnant 2-cm pancreatic focal lesion, visible at CT was wrapped around the superior mesenteric vein for less than 180° and no longer affected the superior mesenteric artery. For these reasons, the third EUS-HTP session was not been performed.

Subsequently, after completion of 6-month chemotherapy (225 days after therapy start), the follow-up CT showed stable disease (RECIST1.1) and CA19.9 serum level reduction to 117 U/mL, the patient underwent R0 Whipple pylorus preserving surgery (histology: ypT3N1,G2). He is currently still alive after 1466 days from study enrollment, following adjuvant chemoradiotherapy and actually presents a local disease relapse along the superior mesenteric vein, 18 × 11 mm in size.

42.7 Potential Pitfalls

Potential complications related to LTA are the following: acute pancreatitis, overt bleeding related injury of big vessels, overt bleeding from intestinal wall due to procedure-related injury of parietal vessels or vessels close to the intestinal wall, perforation, pancreatic fistula due to a thermal or direct injury of the main pancreatic duct, pain, gastric, or gut wall burn. The animal and human studies on HTP have not shown any of these.

To prevent the risk of thermal-induced acute pancreatitis and infections, the patient was given rectal indomethacin before the ablation, according to the guidelines for prevention of post-ERCP acute pancreatitis [10].

Other potential pitfalls are related to the caliber of the HTP probe which is thicker in respect to standard EUS needles (14 Gauge versus 19-20-22-25 Gauge) resulting in a rigid ablation device and limiting its movements and reducing the possibility of penetration in stiff lesions.

Moreover, the active distal part of the needle (with the two bipolar electrodes) is quite long (26–27 mm), permitting the use of this local ablative treatment just for large pancreatic solid lesions.

In conclusion, EUS-HTP can offer a new and interesting alternative treatment for local control of pancreatic cancer, but requires an accurate selection of patients in a multidisciplinary contest.

References

1. VanVeldhuisen E, van den Oord C, Brada LJ, Walma MS, Vogel JA, Wilmink JW, et al. Dutch pancreatic cancer group and international collaborative group on locally advanced pancreatic cancer. Locally advanced pancreatic cancer: work-up, staging, and local intervention strategies. Cancers (Basel). 2019;11(7):E976.
2. Shah R, Ostapoff KT, Kuvshinoff B, Hochwald SN. Ablative therapies for locally advanced pancreatic cancer. Pancreas. 2018;41(1):6–11.
3. Han J, Chang KJ. Endoscopic ultrasound-guided direct intervention for solid pancreatic Tumors. Clin Endosc. 2017;50:126–37.
4. Testoni SGG, Healey AJ, Dietrich CF, Arcidiacono PG. Systematic review of endoscopy ultrasound-guided thermal ablation treatment for pancreatic cancer. Endosc Ultrasound. 2020;9(2):83–100.
5. Signoretti M, Valente R, Repici A, Delle Fave G, Capurso G, Carrara S. Endoscopy-guided ablation of pancreatic lesions: technical possibilities and clinical outlook. World J Gastrointest Endosc. 2017;9(2):41–54.
6. Arcidiacono PG, Carrara S, Reni M, Petrone MC, Cappio S, Balzano G, et al. Feasibility and safety of EUS-guided cryothermal ablation in patients with locally advanced pancreatic cancer. Gastrointest Endosc. 2012 Dec;76(6):1142–51.
7. Carrara S, Arcidiacono PG, Albarello L, Addis A, Enderle MD, Boemo C, et al. Endoscopic ultrasound-guided application of a new internally gas-cooled radiofrequency ablation probe in the liver and spleen of an animal model: a preliminary study. Endoscopy. 2008 Sep;40(9):759–63.
8. Carrara S, Arcidiacono PG, Albarello L, Addis A, Enderle MD, Boemo C, et al. Endoscopic ultrasound-guided application of a new hybrid cryotherm probe in porcine pancreas: a preliminary study. Endoscopy. 2008 Apr;40(4):321–6.
9. Petrone MC, Arcidiacono PG, Carrara S, Albarello L, Enderle MD, Neugebauer A, et al. US-guided application of a new hybrid probe in human pancreatic adenocarcinoma: an ex vivo study. Gastrointest Endosc. 2010 Jun;71(7):1294–7.
10. Cotton PB, Eisen GM, Aabakken L, Baron TH, Hutter MM, Jacobson BC, et al. A lexicon for endoscopic adverse events: report of an ASGE workshop. Gastrointest Endosc. 2010;71(3):446–54.

Part IX

EUS-Guided Implantation and Injection Therapy

43 EUS-Guided Radioactive Iodine Seeds Insertion for Pancreatic Cancer

Jiefang Guo and Zhendong Jin

43.1 Background

Radioactive iodine-125 is most commonly used for brachytherapy because of its long half-life and short penetration distance, which is appropriate in targeting rapidly growing tumors such as pancreatic cancer and allows for precise localization of radiation in the tumor itself and the minimization of damage to the surrounding healthy tissues [1–4]. With the development of interventional EUS, EUS-guided radioactive iodine-125 seeds insertion has emerged as a novel therapeutic strategy for the management of patients with advanced unresectable pancreatic cancer as well as those who are inappropriate for or refuse to undergo pancreaticoduodenectomy [1–6]. This procedure has been proved to be a feasible, minimally invasive, and safe technique for interstitial brachytherapy [7–10]. Despite no significant survival benefit, it provides a comparable option for patients with advanced pancreatic cancer because of its good effect on inhibiting tumor growth [8, 9], alleviating cancer-related pain [8–11], improving quality of life [8–10], and prolonging life expectancy as well [8–10], with mild complications.

43.2 Case History

A 75-year-old male patient was admitted for weight loss and epigastric pain radiating to the midback. The level of CA 19-9 was significantly increased (>1200 U/ml; normal, 0–37 U/ml). CT scan showed a hypodense mass measuring 5.0 × 3.2 cm in the pancreatic body, which encased the splenic vein, splenic artery, and celiac truck (Fig. 43.1). Enlarged retroperitoneal lymph nodes were also identified. EUS examination demonstrated a hypoechoic lesion in the pancreatic body, with a well-defined margin.

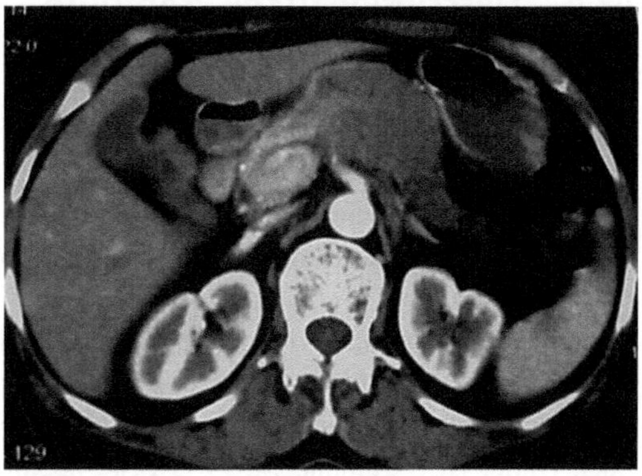

Fig. 43.1 CT image of a hypodense mass in the pancreatic body

Supplementary Information The online version contains supplementary material available at [https://doi.org/10.1007/978-981-16-9340-3_43].

J. Guo · Z. Jin (✉)
Department of Gastroenterology, Changhai Hospital, Naval Medical University, Shanghai, China

A. Y.B. Teoh et al. (eds.), *Atlas of Interventional EUS*, https://doi.org/10.1007/978-981-16-9340-3_43

EUS-guided FNA revealed pancreatic adenocarcinoma. EUS-guided radioactive iodine-125 seeds insertion was then performed in this patient.

43.3 Procedural Plan

A pre-procedural plan was made to determine the number of seeds required for EUS-guided brachytherapy to ensure the adequate treatment dose concentrated on the tumors. Based on the information from CT or MR images of tumor, the tumor volume was calculated and the precise margin of the tumors was outlined by using the treatment planning system(TPS) [9]. Then, the number of seeds needed was calculated by the TPS software or according to the modified Cevec formula [12] as follows:

$$\text{Number of seeds needed} = \frac{[\text{Tumor length} + \text{width} + \text{height in } cm]}{3} \times 5 / \text{the mean activity per seed in } mCi.$$

In practice, to reach the maximum radiation effect, the number of seeds implanted was 15% more than needed. Additionally, a distribution plan map was drawn by the TPS to guide the well-distributed implantation of seeds throughout the tumor in order to avoid the dose "cold spot" which may reduce the radiation effect.

Iodine-125 seeds we used were obtained commercially (Xinke Pharmaceutical Co., Ltd., Shanghai, China). Each seed was 4.5 mm in length and 0.8 mm in diameter with a radioactive half-life of 60.1 days and a penetration depth of 1.7 cm. After the puncture, the seeds were inserted into the lumen of the needle and deployed using a "stylet-pushing" technique.

43.4 Description of the Procedure

EUS-guided iodine-125 seeds insertion was carried out using a linear-array echoendoscope (EG-530UT2; Fujifilm Corp., Tokyo, Japan). The tumor was observed and the maximal diameter of the tumor was measured. The relationship between the tumor and the surrounding vasculature was then identified. The puncture points and paths were determined by color Doppler imaging to avoid intervening blood vessels and pancreatic duct. Under EUS guidance, a 19-G FNA needle (Cook Medical Corporations, Bloomington, USA) was advanced into the tumor, with the tip of the needle positioned at 0.5–1.0 cm from the distal margin inside the tumor, followed by the removal of the stylet and insertion of a radioactive seed into the lumen of the needle. The stylet was then advanced to push the seed forward, and the seed was released and deposited into the tumor. After that, the echoendoscope was withdrawn and the seeds were deployed at intervals of 1.0 cm until the latest implanted seed was positioned at 0.5–1.0 cm from the proximal margin. Additional passes were made at intervals of 10 mm in a parallel array to implant more seeds as the tumor was large. This procedure was repeated until all the seeds were implanted into the tumor according to the treatment plan. In the case we presented here, a total of 30 seeds were deployed through 3 passes. The video showed the procedure of seeds insertion at the second needle pass(vedio). The procedure was well tolerated without any complications.

43.5 Post-Procedural Management

After the procedure, the patients were usually intensively observed for at least 6 h and remained fasting for at least 12 h. Hemostatic drugs and proton pump inhibitors were routinely used to prevent bleeding in the area of puncture. Antibiotics were administered for 3 days. Abdominal X-ray was performed 1 day after the procedure to verify the location and number of the seeds. The patients were followed up at 1 week, 1, 3 months, and then at 3-month intervals thereafter. CT scan was carried out at 1, 3 months, and then at 3-month intervals thereafter. The tumor diameter, general condition, and pain score of patients were monitored and recorded during follow-up. It was then determined whether reimplantation was required or not based on the evaluation of symptom relief as well as the alteration of tumor size.

43.6 Potential Pitfalls

The most common challenge in performing this procedure is that it may be difficult to advance seeds into the tumors in pancreatic head and uncinate process, even some tumors in pancreatic neck, body, or tail, since the currently commercially available iodine-125 seeds have a fixed length that is too long to pass through the tip of the needle if the echoendoscope and needle device are in an acute angle. Therefore, in clinical practice, it is not recommended to perform this procedure in patients with tumors in pancreatic head and uncinate process. As for patients with tumors in pancreatic neck, body, or tail, the applicants should be highly selected. If this difficulty arises, it is recommended to adjust the scope and maintain it in a straight position or another puncture point and path should be considered. Alternatively, a newly developed brachytherapy device, phosphorus-32 microparticles, containing the radioactive β-emitter P-32 inside inactive silicon particles, is available now for use of brachytherapy in pancreatic cancer, which is in a liquid form and thus would overcome this difficulty [12]. Another challenge is that it is difficult to precisely and evenly deploy seeds into the tumor, which represents a three-dimensional space. To overcome this problem, a detailed treatment plan should be rationally made and a distribution map should be carefully analyzed before the procedure.

The potential adverse events after the procedure include seeds loss or migration, which may reduce the tumoricidal effect of brachytherapy. In these cases, the radioactive dose should be re-evaluated. If the actual dose is less than the reference dose set by the original plan, supplementary seeds should be implanted.

Radiation safety is another important concern in the use of iodine-125 seeds. The seed source is packaged in a titanium alloy tube sealed by laser. To minimize the potential harm of radiation, the seeds are sterilized and placed into a specially designed radiation-resistant releasing device before deployment, which was later connected to the needle used in the procedure. The operator and assistants are requested to wear a lead clothing, gloves, and glasses while performing the procedure. After the procedure, the needle and stylet were sterilized and disposed of according to radiation safety guidelines (Figs. 43.2, 43.3, 43.4, and 43.5).

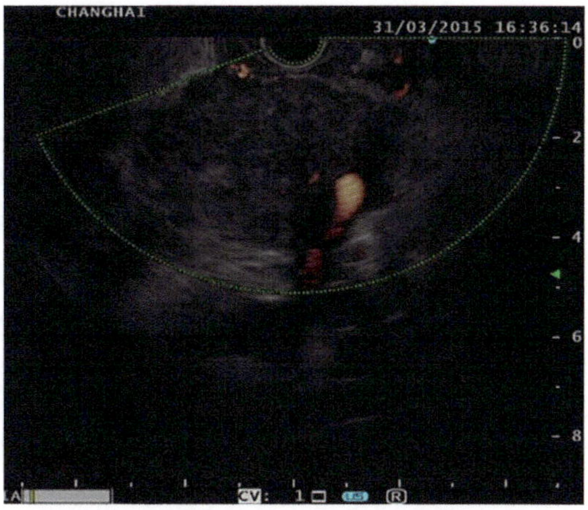

Fig. 43.2 EUS image of a hypoechoic mass in the pancreatic body

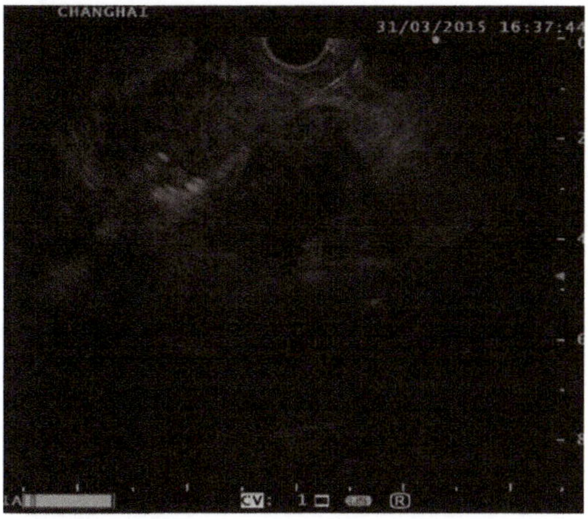

Fig. 43.3 Iodine-125 seeds inserted under EUS guidance

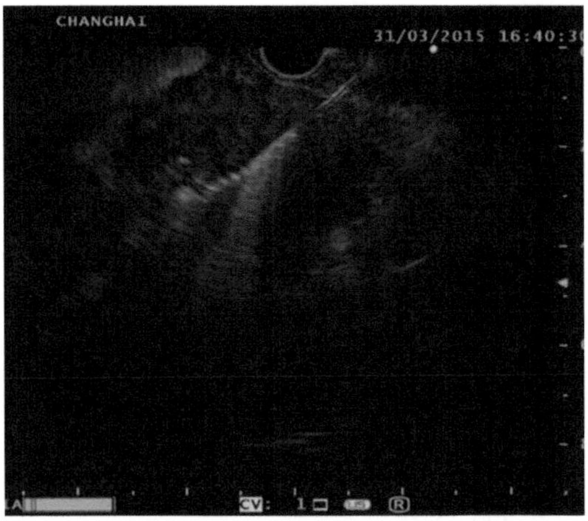

Fig. 43.4 Iodine-125 seeds arranged in a line

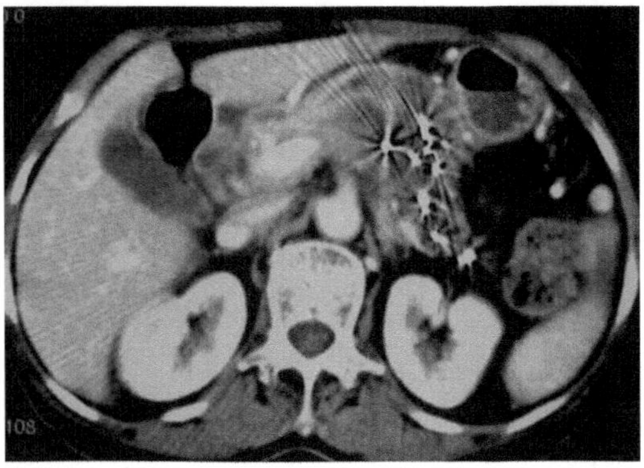

Fig. 43.5 CT image at 1 month after seeds insertion showing a reduced lesion

References

1. Wang AY, Yachimski PS. Endoscopic management of pancreatobiliary neoplasms. Gastroenterology. 2018;154(7):1947–63.
2. Han J, Chang KJ. Endoscopic ultrasound-guided direct intervention for solid pancreatic tumors. Clin Endosc. 2017;50(2):126–37.
3. Du YQ, Li ZS, Jin ZD. Endoscope-assisted brachytherapy for pancreatic cancer:from tumor killing to pain relief and drainage. J Interven Gastroenterol. 2011;1(1):23–7.
4. Oh SY, Irani S, Kozarek RA. What are the current and potential future roles for endoscopic ultrasound in the treatment of pancreatic cancer? World J Gastrointest Endosc. 2016;8(7):319–29.
5. Zhu JW, Jin ZD. Interventional therapy for pancreatic cancer. Gastrointest Tumors. 2016;3(2):81–9.
6. Jin Z, Chang KJ. Endoscopic ultrasound-guided fiducial markers and brachytherapy. Gastrointest Endosc Clin N Am. 2012;22(2):325–31.
7. Sun S, Qingjie L, Qiyong G, Mengchun W, Bo Q, Hong X. EUS-guided interstitial brachytherapy of the pancreas: a feasibility study. Gastrointest Endosc. 2005;62(5):775–9.
8. Sun S, Xu H, Xin J, Liu J, Guo Q, Li S. Endoscopic ultrasound- guided interstitial brachytherapy of unresectable pancreatic cancer: results of a pilot trial. Endoscopy. 2006;38(4):399–403.
9. Jin Z, Du Y, Li Z, Jiang Y, Chen J, Liu Y. Endoscopic ultrasonography-guided interstitial implantation of iodine 125-seeds combined with chemotherapy in the treatment of unresectable pancreatic carcinoma: a prospective pilot study. Endoscopy. 2008;40(4):314–20.
10. Jin Z, Du Y, Li Z. Long-term effect of gemcitabine-combined endoscopic ultrasonography-guided brachytherapy in pancreatic cancer. J Interv Gastroenterol. 2013;3:18–24.
11. Wang KX, Jin ZD, Du YQ, Zhan XB, Zou DW, Liu Y, Wang D, Chen J, Xu C, Li ZS. EUS-guided celiac ganglion irradiation with iodine-125 seeds for pain control in pancreatic carcinoma: a prospective pilot study. Gastrointest Endosc. 2012;76(5):945–52.
12. Bhutani MS, Cazacu IM, Luzuriaga Chavez AA, Singh BS, Wong FCL, Erwin WD, Tamm EP, Mathew GG, Le DB, Koay EJ, Taniguchi CM, Minsky BD, Pant S, Tzeng CD, Koong AC, Varadhachary GR, Katz MHG, Wolff RA, Fogelman DR, Herman JM. Novel EUS-guided brachytherapy treatment of pancreatic cancer with phosphorus-32 microparticles: first United States experience. VideoGIE. 2019;4(5):223–5.

EUS-Guided Ethanol Injection for Pancreatic NET

44

Yu-Ting Kuo and Hsiu-Po Wang

44.1 Background

According to current consensus, surgery is the only known cure for functioning and non-functioning pancreatic neuroendocrine tumors (P-NETs) and the role of endoscopic ablation for P-NETs is still uncertain [1–3]. However, the choice of surgery or observation for small (<2 cm), asymptomatic, low-grade (G1) sporadic P-NETs remains controversial. For these patients or patients unfit for surgery due to high-risk comorbidity or for those who refuse surgical resection, the EUS-guided ethanol injection (EUS-EI) has been reported as a safe and effective alternative treatment [4–6].

For sporadic nonfunctional small P-NETs (<2 cm), the optimal management remains controversial [1–3]. Considering surgical resection for these patients is lack of proven effect on long-term survival [7], observation seems to be safe because the majority of the observed tumors did not show any significant changes during follow-up [8]. However, the natural history of all P-NETs remains highly variable and all P-NETs should be regarded as having malignant potential and the risk of metastasis [9].

EUS is the most sensitive imaging for identifying small pancreatic lesion. Under real-time EUS guidance, EUS-EI is a relatively safe and efficient procedure. There have been a lot of reported studies with good results and low adverse events. EUS-EI achieved complete tumor ablation rate of around 60–90% and only few complications, mostly self-limited acute pancreatitis and abdominal pain, are reported [4–6]. Therefore, EUS-EI appears as an alternative treatment of P-NETs for the patient, who refused surgical resection.

44.2 Case History

A 40-year-old lady with a history of multiple endocrine neoplasia type 1 (MEN-1) received distal pancreatectomy and total parathyroidectomy for pancreatic neuroendocrine tumors and parathyroid hyperplasia 4 years before admission. Because serum chromogranin A level persistently raised from 66.3 ng/ml to 212.2 ng/ml within the last 6 months, EUS was arranged and a 7.1 mm well-defined hypoechoic tumor with the presence of vascularity was found at pancreatic head (Fig. 44.1). Contrast-enhanced harmonic EUS (CEH-EUS) with Sonazoid showed

Supplementary Information The online version contains supplementary material available at [https://doi.org/10.1007/978-981-16-9340-3_44].

Y.-T. Kuo · H.-P. Wang (✉)
Division of Gastroenterology and Hepatology, Department of Internal Medicine, National Taiwan University Hospital, National Taiwan University College of Medicine, Taipei, Taiwan
e-mail: wanghp@ntu.edu.tw

A. Y.B. Teoh et al. (eds.), *Atlas of Interventional EUS*, https://doi.org/10.1007/978-981-16-9340-3_44

the lesion was homogeneously hyperenhanced and the features are compatible with P-NET (Fig. 44.2). Pathological examination obtained by EUS-guided fine needle biopsy (FNB) showed a neuroendocrine tumor with Ki67 index <3%. Because the patient refused surgery, EUS-EI was offered to the patient.

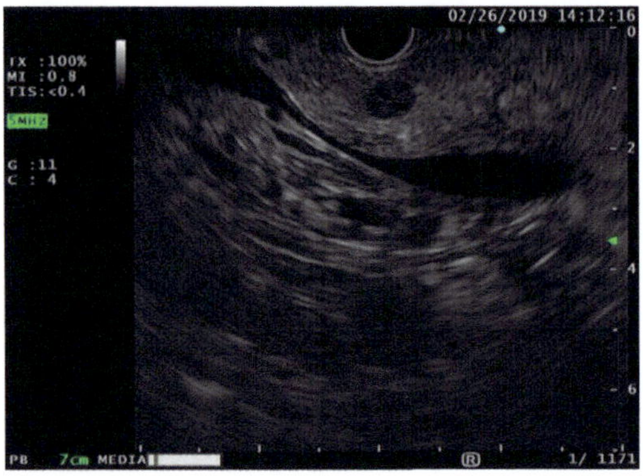

Fig. 44.1 EUS demonstrate a 7.1 mm well-defined hypoechoic tumor at pancreatic head

44.3 Procedural Plan

EUS-EI was performed using a linear array echoendoscopic. Prophylactic antibiotics and rectal non-steroidal anti-inflammatory drug (NSAID) were routinely given before procedure, if there were no contraindications. We preferred to use a 25-gauge conventional needle without side hole (EZ shot3, Olympus Medical, Japan) to perform EUS-EI because the small size needle was easier to target the lesion and precisely control the injection amount. Optimal volume of the amount of ethanol could be roughly calculated according to the size of the tumor [Calculated injection volume = $(4/3)\pi r^3$; r: radius of the tumor] and we suggested to use a 1 ml syringe to prepare the ethanol injection. The puncture site depended on the location of the lesion. For our patient with the pancreatic lesion at the head, transduodenal approach would be preferred. With regards to the pancreatic duct stent placement before EUS-EI,

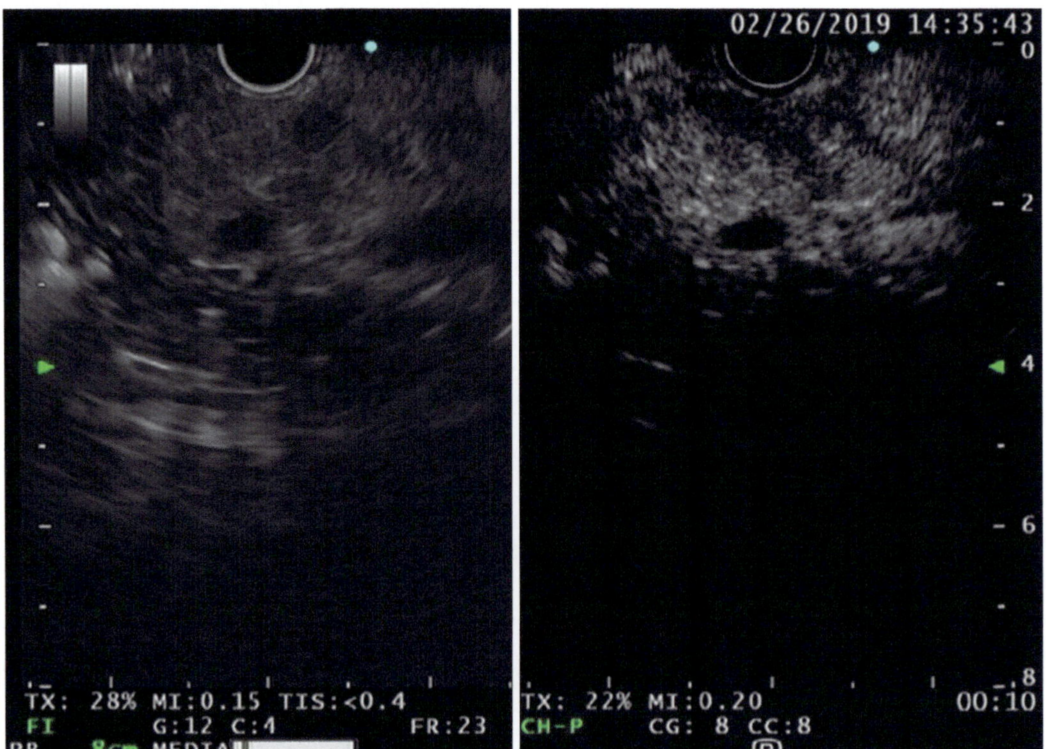

Fig. 44.2 Contrast-enhanced harmonic EUS showed pancreatic head tumor with homogeneously hyperenhancement pattern

prophylactic pancreatic duct stent placement may be considered if the distance between the lesion and main pancreatic duct is very close (<5 mm). In this patient, prophylactic rectal NSAID without pancreatic duct stent placement was planned.

44.4 Description of the Procedure

Before puncturing the lesion, the stylet of the needle was removed first and then the needle was loaded with 99% ethanol to replace the air. After identifying the lesion, the tip of the needle was advanced into the deepest part of the tumor under real-time EUS visualization (Fig. 44.3) (Video 44.1). Then, 99% ethanol was injected slowly with an increment of 0.05 cc while the needle was gently withdrawn from the deep to the proximal part of the tumor. Repeated puncture using fanning technique was performed and the injection was finished when hyperechoic bubble-like appearance was seen inside the whole tumor (Fig. 44.4), and the needle was retrieved. After puncturing, a total amount of 0.6 ml 99% ethanol was injected into the lesion. CEH-EUS with Sonazoid was performed after ablation and no contrast enhancement within the tumor was found (Fig. 44.5).

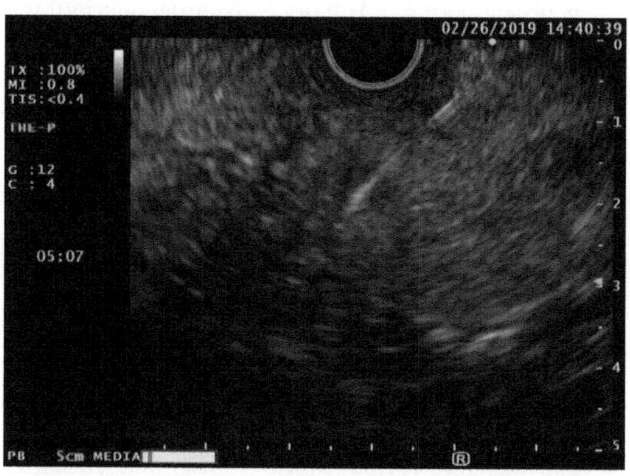

Fig. 44.3 The tip of the needle was advanced into the deepest part of the tumor under real-time EUS guidance

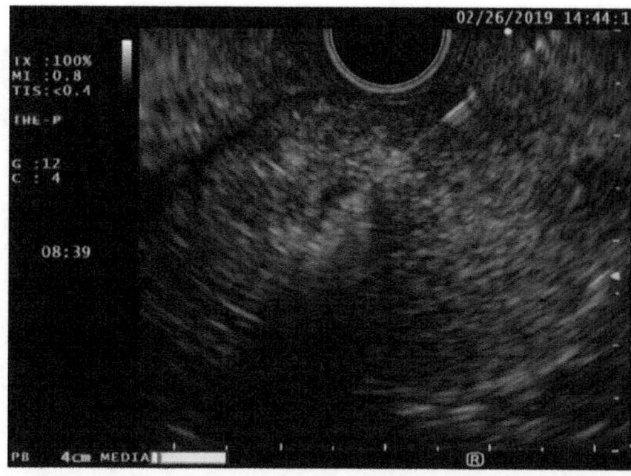

Fig. 44.4 The ethanol injection was finished when hyperechoic blush was seen inside the whole tumor

44.5 Post-Procedural Management

After the procedure, the patients would be fasted for 4 h to closely monitor for possible adverse events, including acute pancreatitis, abdominal pain, bleeding, and infection. If there were no adverse events, patients were discharged 1 day after the procedure. During the first year after the procedure, we will check serum chromogranin A every 3 months and choose the one of following modalities, including CEH-EUS, abdominal multiphasic CT or MRI, to follow up on the patients every 3–6 months. If no local recurrence is noted, we will lengthen image surveillance interval to 6–12 months. In this patient, serum chromogranin A decreased to 118.6 ng/ml and the follow-up EUS showed no local recurrence 1 year after EUS-EI.

44.6 Potential Pitfalls

Severe pancreatitis may occur due to peripancreatic ethanol leakage, especially using the celiac plexus neurolysis (CPN) needle with multiple side holes. Thus, we recommend careful intratumor injection with a small size single-hole needle in

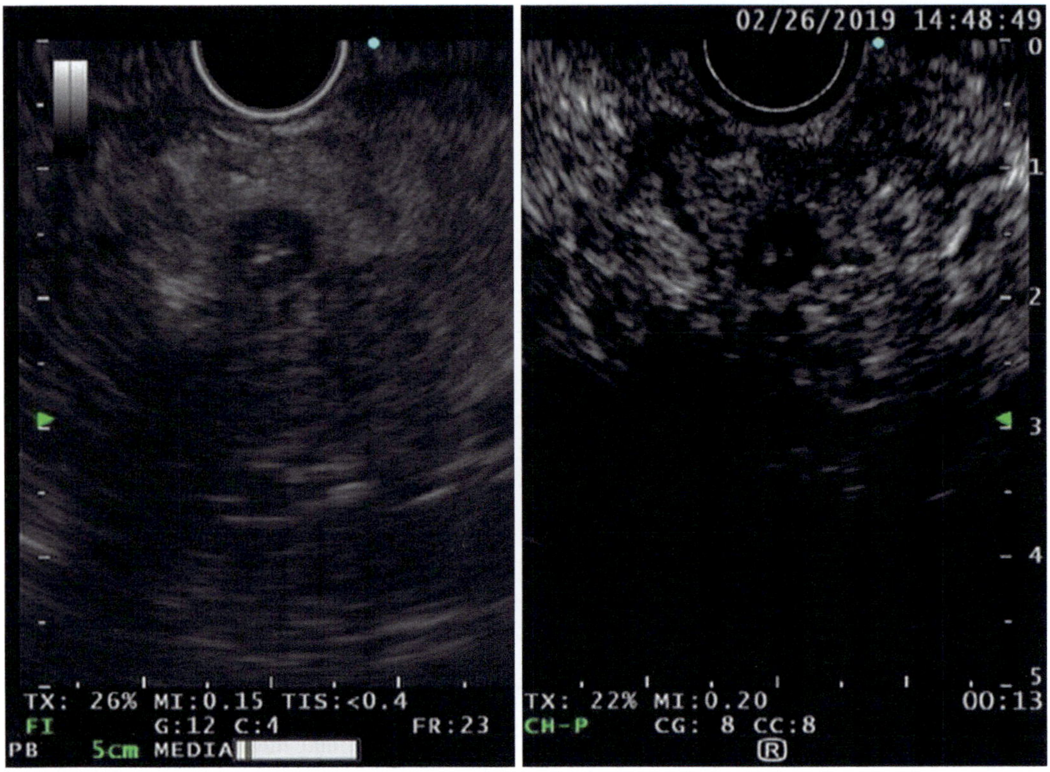

Fig. 44.5 Contrast-enhanced harmonic EUS showed no contrast enhancement within the tumor after procedure

order to minimize the risk of peripancreatic ethanol leakage. In addition, injecting the minimal volume of ethanol required to achieve complete tumor ablation should also prevent procedure-related adverse events. Like endoscopic retrograde cholangiopancreatography (ERCP), rectal diclofenac may be used as recommended before EUS-EI to prevent post-procedure pancreatitis [10]. Pancreatic duct stricture was another potential adverse event that has been reported [11]. If the distance between the lesion and main pancreatic duct was very close (e.g., <5 mm), prophylactic pancreatic duct stent placement may be considered to perform before EUS-EI.

References

1. Kunz PL, Reidy-Lagunes D, Anthony LB, Bertino EM, Brendtro K, Chan JA, et al. Consensus guidelines for the management and treatment of neuroendocrine tumors. Pancreas. 2013;42(4):557–77.
2. Falconi M, Eriksson B, Kaltsas G, Bartsch DK, Capdevila J, Caplin M, et al. ENETS consensus guidelines update for the Management of Patients with functional pancreatic neuroendocrine Tumors and non-functional pancreatic neuroendocrine Tumors. Neuroendocrinology. 2016;103(2):153–71.
3. Shah MH, Goldner WS, Halfdanarson TR, Bergsland E, Berlin JD, Halperin D, et al. NCCN guidelines insights: neuroendocrine and adrenal Tumors, version 2.2018. J Natl Compr Cancer Netw. 2018;16(6):693–702.
4. Paik WH, Seo DW, Dhir V, Wang HP. Safety and efficacy of EUS-guided ethanol ablation for treating small solid pancreatic neoplasm. Medicine (Baltimore). 2016;95(4):e2538.
5. Armellini E, Crinò SF, Ballarè M, Pallio S, Occhipinti P. Endoscopic ultrasound-guided ethanol ablation of pancreatic neuroendocrine tumours: a case study and literature review. World J Gastrointest Endosc. 2016;8(3):192–7.
6. Choi JH, Park DH, Kim MH, Hwang HS, Hong SM, Song TJ, et al. Outcomes after endoscopic ultrasound-guided ethanol-lipiodol ablation of small pancreatic neuroendocrine tumors. Dig Endosc. 2018;30(5):652–8.

7. Mintziras I, Keck T, Werner J, Fichtner-Feigl S, Wittel U, Senninger N, et al. Implementation of current ENETS guidelines for surgery of small (≤2 cm) pancreatic neuroendocrine neoplasms in the German surgical community: an analysis of the prospective DGAV StuDoQ|pancreas registry. World J Surg. 2019;43(1):175–82.
8. Gaujoux S, Partelli S, Maire F, D'Onofrio M, Larroque B, Tamburrino D, et al. Observational study of natural history of small sporadic nonfunctioning pancreatic neuroendocrine tumors. J Clin Endocrinol Metab. 2013;98(12):4784–9.
9. Tsutsumi K, Ohtsuka T, Mori Y, Fujino M, Yasui T, Aishima S, et al. Analysis of lymph node metastasis in pancreatic neuroendocrine tumors (PNETs) based on the tumor size and hormonal production. J Gastroenterol. 2012;47(6):678–85.
10. Barthet M, Giovannini M, Lesavre N, Boustiere C, Napoleon B, Koch S, et al. Endoscopic ultrasound-guided radiofrequency ablation for pancreatic neuroendocrine tumors and pancreatic cystic neoplasms: a prospective multicenter study. Endoscopy. 2019;51(9):836–42.
11. Park do H, Choi JH, Oh D, Lee SS, Seo DW, Lee SK, et al. Endoscopic ultrasonography-guided ethanol ablation for small pancreatic neuroendocrine tumors: results of a pilot study. Clin Endosc. 2015;48:158–64.

45 EUS-Guided Injection of Anti-Tumor Agents for Malignancy

Reiko Ashida

45.1 Background

Over the last few decades, endoscopic ultrasound (EUS) has become an important procedure in both the diagnosis and local treatment of pancreatic cancer (PC). EUS-guided fine-needle injection (EUS-FNI) is a feasible and safe technique that can be applied to numerous local treatments, including anti-tumor agent delivery, radiofrequency ablation, photodynamic therapy, radioactive seed insertion, celiac neurolysis, and fiducial marker placement [1, 2]. EUS-FNI has been used experimentally in human clinical studies for the delivery of anti-tumor agents such as ethanol, virus vectors, dendritic cells, gemcitabine, and paclitaxel [1, 2]. Among the viral vectors, an oncolytic virus has been developed as a novel anti-tumor agent that can kill cancer cells directly and also via immune modulation [3]. This investigational viral product is delivered by intratumoral injection, and its anti-tumor effect has been demonstrated in various tumor types such as recurrent breast cancer, head, and neck cancer, unresectable pancreatic cancer, and melanoma [4–6]. In preliminary clinical studies for the treatment of pancreatic cancer, promising results have been observed with tolerable toxicities when administrated intraoperatively, percutaneously, or endoscopically [7, 8]. Among the various approaches to performing injection of anti-tumor agents for the treatment of pancreatic cancer, the endoscopic approach shows promise for mainstream use in the future because EUS-guided injection is precise, safe, and minimally invasive [8, 9].

45.2 Case History

A 63-year-old male was referred to our hospital with the chief complaint of abdominal pain. Imaging examinations revealed a mass of diameter 4 cm in the body of the pancreas and multiple liver metastases (Fig. 45.1). The patient was diagnosed histologically with stage IV pancreatic cancer by EUS-FNA, and gemcitabine + nab-paclitaxel was administered as a first-line treatment with partial response. CT performed 9 months later revealed exacerbation of the disease, and the patient was diagnosed with progressive disease. Therefore, the patient was enrolled in the Phase 1 trial of EUS-guided local injection of viral product in combination with S-1, an oral

Supplementary Information The online version contains supplementary material available at [https://doi.org/10.1007/978-981-16-9340-3_45].

R. Ashida (✉)
Second Department of Internal Medicine, Wakayama Medical University, Wakayama, Japan

Departments of Cancer Survey and Gastrointestinal Oncology, Osaka International Cancer Institute, Osaka, Japan
e-mail: rashida@goo.jp

A. Y.B. Teoh et al. (eds.), *Atlas of Interventional EUS*, https://doi.org/10.1007/978-981-16-9340-3_45

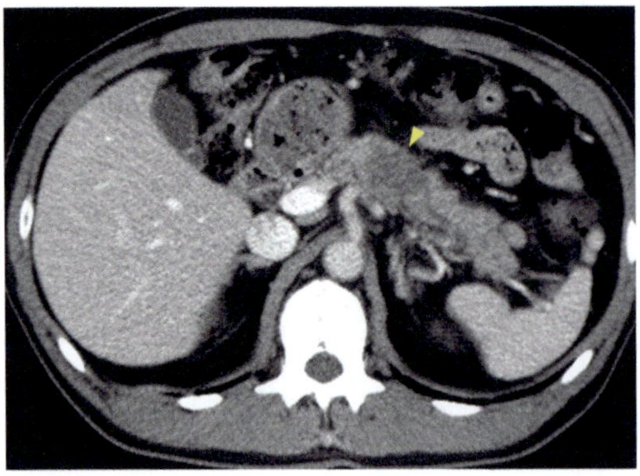

Fig. 45.1 Contrasted CT findings. Contrasted computed tomography reveals a hypo-enhancing mass (*arrowhead*) in the pancreatic body

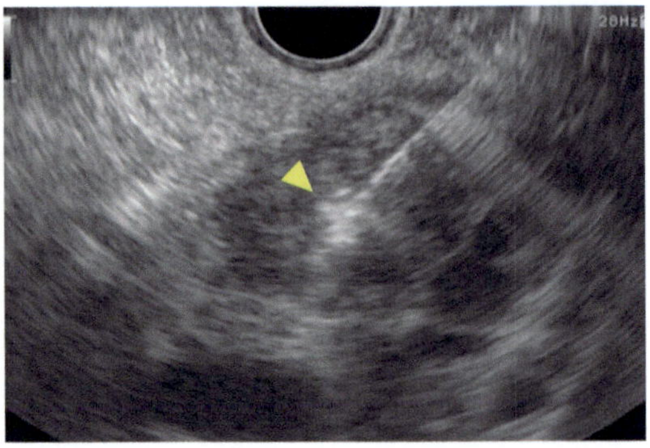

Fig. 45.2 EUS image during viral injection. Hyperechoic change (arrowhead) indicates virus solution injected into the tumor

5-fluorouracil (5-FU) prodrug designed to improve the anti-tumor activity of 5-FU by inhibiting dihydropyrimidine dehydrogenase, the key enzyme of 5-FU catabolism.

45.3 Procedural Plan

EUS-guided virus injection was scheduled at 2-week intervals in combination with oral 60 mg S-1 twice daily for 4 weeks, followed by 2 weeks rest. The virus used for this case is an oncolytic, spontaneous mutant Herpes Simplex Virus type1 [8]. This virus has two anti-cancer effects, such as direct cytotoxic effects by viral replication in the tumor cell and systemic anti-tumor effects by activated cytotoxic T lymphocytes following tumor destruction.

45.4 Description of the Procedure (Video 45.1)

EUS-FNI of viral solution is performed in the outpatient setting. The patient is asked to fast from 9:00 pm the day before the injection. The procedure is performed using a linear-array echoendoscope (GF-UCT 260-AL5; Olympus Corp., Tokyo, Japan) under conscious sedation. The viral solution is prepared as follows, with saline for flushing. First, the stylet is removed from a regular 22G FNA needle and the needle is filled with saline. Under EUS guidance, the lesion is punctured and the needle is advanced as far as possible into the lesion, after which 1 ml of the viral solution is then injected gradually into the tumor (Fig. 45.2). It is important to inject the solution slowly to prevent backflush. While monitoring the spread of the viral solution into the tumor, injection is performed as the FNA needle is gradually withdrawn, so the solution diffuses throughout the tumor. The needle is flushed with saline and retained in the tumor for 15–30 seconds to enable the viral solution to spread throughout the tumor and to prevent leakage of the fluid from the needle puncture site. The needle is then removed and the injected area is checked for the extent of spread of viral solution in the tumor and for possible complications such as bleeding.

45.5 Post-Procedural Management

After the procedure, the patient is observed for 2–4 h in the recovery room. Unless there is abdominal pain or fever, the patient is allowed to return home and to eat a meal. Antibiotics were not prescribed routinely in this study. The following day, the patient was contacted by phone to confirm their general condition and check for any problems related to the procedure.

45.6 Potential Pitfalls

There are two important challenges in EUS-guided local injection therapy for pancreatic cancer: local injection of a drug solution to the entire tumor, and prevention of leakage of the solution from the puncture site. If the virus solution is injected into an area of internal necrosis, which can occur in pancreatic cancer, the biological effects will be minimal. Therefore, it is important to select a viable site and inject as much of the solution into this area as possible. If the drug solution is injected through multiple puncture holes into a solid tumor, the fluid may exit from any of these holes due to intra-tumoral pressure. Therefore, it is important to make only a single puncture in one session, but change the needle position within the tumor so that the drug solution spreads over as wide an area as possible.

In addition, it is important to avoid injecting the solution into areas adjacent to major vessels such as the splenic vein or superior mesenteric vein, which are commonly invaded in pancreatic cancer, to prevent diffusion of viral solution into the blood vessels. The possible procedure-related complications are similar to those for general EUS-FNA, which include bleeding, perforation, pancreatitis, infection, and tumor dissemination. Complications of viral injection may be due to inflammation caused by the virus itself. Complications that have been reported following local injection of viral solution into a pancreatic cancer include pancreatitis, abscess, and thrombus, although these adverse reactions were within acceptable limits [8, 9].

References

1. Ashida R, Chang KJ. Interventional EUS for the treatment of pancreatic cancer. J Hepato-Biliary-Pancreat Surg. 2009;16(5):592–7.
2. Han J, Chang KJ. Endoscopic ultrasound-guided direct intervention for solid pancreatic Tumors. Clinical endoscopy. 2017;50(2):126–37.
3. Hamid O, Ismail R, Puzanov I. Intratumoral immunotherapy-update 2019. Oncologist. 2020;25(3):e423–e38.
4. Kasuya H, Kodera Y, Nakao A, Yamamura K, Gewen T, Zhiwen W, et al. Phase I dose-escalation clinical trial of HF10 oncolytic herpes virus in 17 Japanese patients with advanced cancer. Hepato-Gastroenterology. 2014;61(131):599–605.
5. Andtbacka RH, Ross M, Puzanov I, Milhem M, Collichio F, Delman KA, et al. Patterns of clinical response with Talimogene Laherparepvec (T-VEC) in patients with melanoma treated in the OPTiM phase III clinical trial. Ann Surg Oncol. 2016;23(13):4169–77.
6. Eissa IR, Bustos-Villalobos I, Ichinose T, Matsumura S, Naoe Y, Miyajima N, et al. The current status and future prospects of oncolytic viruses in clinical trials against melanoma. Glioma, Pancreatic, and Breast Cancers Cancers (Basel). 2018;10(10)
7. Nakao A, Kasuya H, Sahin TT, Nomura N, Kanzaki A, Misawa M, et al. A phase I dose-escalation clinical trial of intraoperative direct intratumoral injection of HF10 oncolytic virus in non-resectable patients with advanced pancreatic cancer. Cancer Gene Ther. 2011;18(3):167–75.
8. Hirooka Y, Kasuya H, Ishikawa T, Kawashima H, Ohno E, Villalobos IB, et al. A phase I clinical trial of EUS-guided intratumoral injection of the oncolytic virus, HF10 for unresectable locally advanced pancreatic cancer. BMC Cancer. 2018;18(1):596.
9. Hecht JR, Farrell JJ, Senzer N, Nemunaitis J, Rosemurgy A, Chung T, et al. EUS or percutaneously guided intratumoral TNFerade biologic with 5-fluorouracil and radiotherapy for first-line treatment of locally advanced pancreatic cancer: a phase I/II study. Gastrointest Endosc. 2012;75(2):332–8.

EUS-Guided Implantation of Radioactive Phosphorus (^{32}P) for Locally Advanced Pancreatic Cancer

46

Jeevinesh Naidu and Nam Q. Nguyen

46.1 Background

Up to 80% patients who present with pancreatic ductal adenocarcinoma (PDAC) are not suitable for surgical resection, a treatment that provides the best survival outcome for these patients [1, 2]. A significant proportion of these patients have locally invasive diseases that are classified as "borderline resectable" or "locally advanced" diseases [3]. Neoadjuvant chemotherapy, either FOLFIRINOX or Gemcitabine-Nabpaclitaxel, has been the gold-standard treatment for these patients as it can result in the downstaging of cancer and enable margin-free resection (termed conversion surgery) in approximately 25% of patients [4]. The addition of targeted radiotherapy, in the form of stereotactic body radiotherapy (SBRT), to chemotherapy, has been shown to increase the rate of conversion surgery by up to 60% for the "borderline resectable" and 40% for the "locally advanced" PDAC [5], providing support for the use of combined chemo-radiotherapy for unresectable PDAC.

Another approach to provide targeted radiotherapy is by directly implantation of radioactive material to the pancreatic cancer under endoscopic ultrasound (EUS) guidance, a technique that is known as brachytherapy. The feasibility of EUS-guided ^{125}I radioactive seeds has been reported in 15 patients with locally advanced pancreatic cancer (LAPC) [6]. In order to deliver an adequate but uniform amount of radioactive seeds to the cancer, multiple needle punctures into the pancreatic lesion are often required, and thus, can result in an increase in the risk of pancreatitis, infections, and pseudocyst formation. Fever has been reported in 54% of patients who undergone EUS-guided ^{125}I radioactive seeds insertion [6]. Such limitations can be overcome by an aqueous form of radioactive material, in which the precise amount and location can be injected into the cancer. Recently, a liquid form 32-Phosphorus (^{32}P, known as Oncosil™) has been developed as a form of radioactive material for the treatment of PDAC. In early trials, the use of ^{32}P in combination with chemotherapy has demonstrated a good safety profile and rate of conversion surgery in patients with LAPC [7].

Supplementary Information The online version contains supplementary material available at [https://doi.org/10.1007/978-981-16-9340-3_46].

J. Naidu · N. Q. Nguyen (✉)
Department of Gastroenterology and Hepatology, Royal Adelaide Hospital, Port Road, Adelaide, SA, Australia

School of Health and Medical Sciences, University of Adelaide, Adelaide, SA, Australia
e-mail: QuocNam.Nguyen@sa.gov.au

A. Y.B. Teoh et al. (eds.), *Atlas of Interventional EUS*, https://doi.org/10.1007/978-981-16-9340-3_46

46.2 Case History

A 72-year-old lady presented with painless obstructive jaundice with abdominal computed tomography (CT) scan demonstrated a large mass in the head/neck region of pancreas. This caused biliary obstruction with tumour invasion into the portal vein (Fig. 46.1a and b). ERCP was performed to place a biliary stent to relieve the biliary obstruction, and tissue diagnosis of PDAC was established by EUS-guided biopsy. Disease staging with EUS confirmed that the 3 cm lesion had invaded the splenoportal confluence, making it not suitable for surgery. After discussion in the pancreatico-biliary cancer multidisciplinary team meeting, the patient was advised to have neoadjuvant chemotherapy with FOLFIRINOX and intra-tumoral ^{32}P implantation.

46.3 Pre-Procedural Preparation

In order to ensure the absence of metastatic disease, SPECT and MRI were performed. The total tumour volume was determined from CT scan, using a 3D-geometric computer program, to allow calculation of the amount of ^{32}P for implantation. Based on a previous benchtop study [8], the calculated amount of ^{32}P to deliver 100Gy into the lesion amounted to 8% of the tumour volume. The dose calculation and ^{32}P preparation were processed by our nuclear physicists at the Department of Nuclear Medicine 2–3 days prior to the procedure. This patient's tumour volume was 21.3 cm^3, and thus, 1.7 ml of ^{32}P was the calculated amount to be implanted.

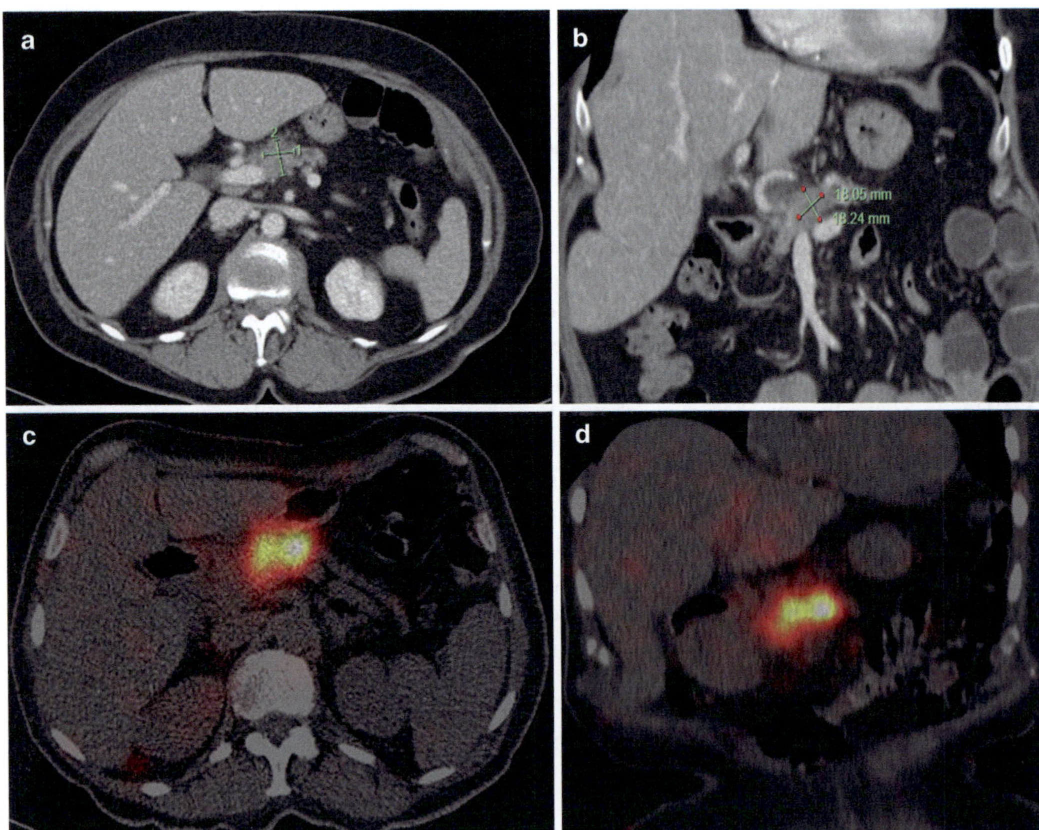

Fig. 46.1 Coronal CT showing a pancreatic head/neck mass invading the portal vein rendering the lesion unresectable (**a** and **b**). Bremsstrahlung Scan showing distribution of 32-P 4 h after the procedure within the pancreas mass (**c** and **d**)

46.4 Description of the Procedure

EUS-guided intra-tumoral implantation of ^{32}P was performed a week after completing the second chemotherapy cycle. In order to reduce the risk of radioactive spill and contamination of the endoscopy suite, the floor space at the implantation location was covered by disposable plastic. Similarly, all involved members of staff were required to wear standard personal protective gear, including impenetrable gowns, visors, masks, and cytotoxic gloves. However, lead gowns were not needed as the emission distance of the radioactive material was only 5 cm. Under propofol sedation guided by a consultant anaesthetist, a detailed EUS evaluation of the pancreatic lesion was performed with a curvilinear echoendoscope, with the aim to delineate the border of the lesion. In this case, EUS contrast study with Definity™ was also used to outline vasculature as well as the hypo-perfused area to increase the accuracy of implantation (Fig. 46.2a). Using Doppler flow to avoid overlying vessels, the lesion was punctured using a 22-gauge fine needle aspiration (22G Echotip Ultra™ FNA needle, Cook Medical, USA) needle, through a transduodenal approach (Fig. 46.2b). Once the tip of the needle was in the correct location, the stylet was removed and liquid ^{32}P was injected into the cancer from a prepared syringe (Fig. 46.3), with a distribution of 25% at the distal edge, 50% in the centre, and 25% at the proximal edge of the lesion. Particular care was taken to avoid injection into blood vessels, the pancreatic duct and the common bile duct. The dead space of the needle was flushed

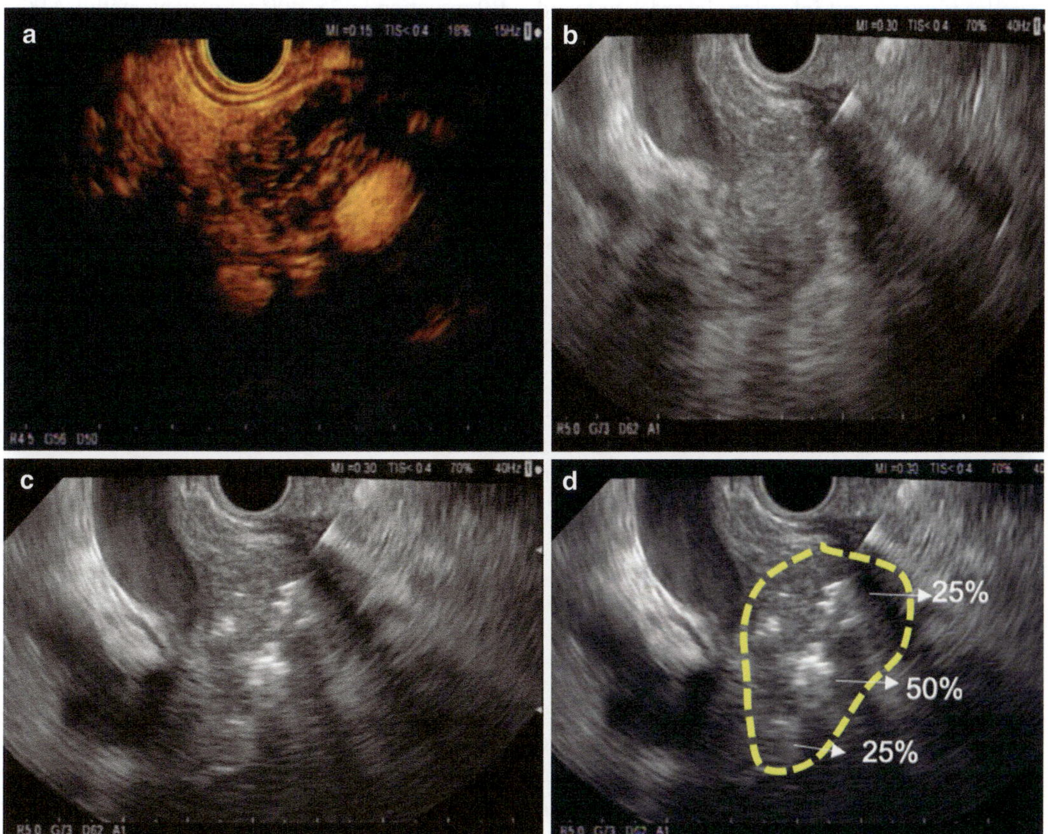

Fig. 46.2 Steps in implantation of radioactive ^{32}P (Oncosil) into the cancer. The malignant lesion was evaluated careful with both regular and contrast EUS study (**a**). Using a 22G FNA needle, the lesion was punctured (**b**), and the Oncosil was injected in a 25–50%–25% distributing pattern (**c** and **d**)

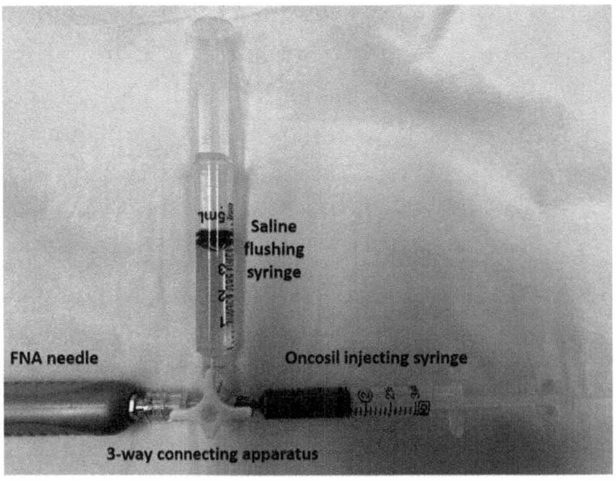

Fig. 46.3 Set up and equipment required for 32-P injection via EUS needle. The three-way Luer-lock secured the attachment of the 32-P (Oncosil) injecting syringe to the saline flushing syringe and the EUS needle

with 1 ml of normal saline before the needle tip was pulled out of the lesion (Fig. 46.2c and d). Similar to histoacryl injection, in order to avoid scope contamination, suction was turned off and the entire needle/sheath complex was withdrawn into the gastric antrum. The needle was flushed with 5 ml of saline before the sheath was extended out of scope to cover the needle tip. The echoendoscope and the needle-sheath complex were then removed from the patient and disposed into a radioactive hazard disposal container for further flushing and cleaning. The entire scope was checked for radioactivity using a Geiger Counter and taken for cleaning only when no abnormal signal was detected. All involved members of staff were scanned for any radioactive contamination in a similar manner, before de-gowning and exiting the room.

46.5 Post-Procedural Management

The patient underwent a SPECT and Bremsstrahlung scan 4 h after implantation to confirm the localisation of ^{32}P implantation and to check for dissemination of the material within the abdomen (Fig. 46.1c and d). The patient was allowed to have clear fluid for 12 h post-procedure, followed by regular diet. She was advised to isolate herself from other human contact in a similar way to radioiodine treatment, which included having a separate bed and toilet for 1 week. Without disruption to her chemotherapy schedule, the patient continued to complete another 6 cycles of FOLFIRINOX chemotherapy after the ^{32}P implantation. The SPECT and Bremsstrahlung scans were repeated 7 days post-procedure to ensure local distribution of ^{32}P within the tumour.

Restaging CT 3 months after chemotherapy showed a 50% reduction in tumour size with minimal portal vein involvement. Surgery was undertaken 5 months after and a R0 margin resection was achieved. The patient is still alive 28 months after implantation of ^{32}P. Preliminary data from our centre and the PANCO study [7] suggest that combined chemotherapy and intratumoral ^{32}P can lead to conversion surgery with R0 resection in 25–40% of patients with LAPC.

46.6 Potential Pitfalls

Due to the potential risk of dissemination of radiation to other body organs, intravascular injection of ^{32}P must be avoided at all cost. This can be achieved by careful sonographic assessment of surrounding vessels, using both Doppler flow and contrast study. The risk of intravascular injection is particularly high in cases when portal and/or splenic vein thrombosis is present, leading to multiple collaterals and varices in the region of the lesion. If in doubt, aspiration the needle for blood prior to ^{32}P injection should be performed.

Given the long half-life of ^{32}P (14.3 days), unrecognized contamination of the echoendoscope can disrupt the EUS/endoscopy service for 2.5 months as it can lead to contamination of the entire scope cleaning system. This is why it is important to repeatedly flush the needle and clean the scope after implantation, as well as to check for any radioactivity prior to returning the scope to the cleaning room. It is critical to have a safety officer from Nuclear Medicine at the implantation to ensure the absence of contamination to the equipment and staff [7].

46.7 Conclusion

Preliminary experience with combined chemotherapy and EUS-guided intra-tumoral ^{32}P implantation suggests the treatment is safe, feasible, well tolerated and can lead to margin-free resection in up to 40% of cases. These findings warrant further evaluation in a larger randomized trial prior to its widespread use.

References

1. Tummala P, Howard T, Agarwal B. Dramatic survival benefit related to R0 resection of pancreatic adenocarcinoma in patients with tumor ≤25 mm in size and ≤1 involved lymph nodes. Clin Transl Gastroenterol. 2013;4:e33.
2. Bray F, et al. Global cancer statistics 2018: GLOBOCAN estimates of incidence and mortality worldwide for 36 cancers in 185 countries. CA Cancer J Clin. 2018; https://doi.org/10.3322/caac.21492.
3. Tempero, M. A. *et al.* Pancreatic adenocarcinoma, version 2.2017: Clinical practice guidelines in Oncology. JNCCN Journal of the National Comprehensive Cancer Network 15, 1028–1061 (2017).
4. Gemenetzis G, et al. Survival in locally advanced pancreatic cancer after neoadjuvant therapy and surgical resection. Ann Surg. 2019;270:340–7.
5. Mellon EA, et al. Long-term outcomes of induction chemotherapy and neoadjuvant stereotactic body radiotherapy for borderline resectable and locally advanced pancreatic adenocarcinoma. Acta Oncol (Madr). 2015;54:979–85.
6. Sun S, et al. Endoscopic ultrasound-guided interstitial brachytherapy of unresectable pancreatic cancer: results of a pilot trial. Endoscopy. 2006;38:399–403.
7. Ross, P. J. *et al.* PanCO: an open-label, single-arm pilot study of phosphorus-32 (P-32; Oncosil) microparticles in patients with unresectable locally advanced pancreatic adenocarcinoma (LAPC) in combination with FOLFIRINOX or gemcitabine + nab-paclitaxel (GNP) chemotherapies. J Clin Oncol. 2019;37:4125–5.
8. Naidu J, Bartholomeusz D, Zobel J, Safaeian R, Hsieh W, Crouch B, Ho K, Calnan D, Singhal N, Ruszkiewicz A, Chen JW, Tan CP, Dolan P, Nguyen NQ. Combined chemotherapy and endoscopic ultrasound-guided intratumoral 32P implantation for locally advanced pancreatic adenocarcinoma: a pilot study. Endoscopy. 2022;54(1):75–80. https://doi.org/10.1055/a-1353-0941.
9. Ross PJ, Wasan HS, Croagh D, Nikfarjam M, Nguyen N, Aghmesheh M, Nagrial AM, Bartholomeusz D, Hendlisz A, Ajithkumar T, Iwuji C, Wilson NE, Turner DM, James DC, Young E, Harris MT. Results of a single-arm pilot study of (32)P microparticles in unresectable locally advanced pancreatic adenocarcinoma with gemcitabine/nab-paclitaxel or FOLFIRINOX chemotherapy. ESMO Open. 2021;7(1):100356. https://doi.org/10.1016/j.esmoop.2021.100356.
10. A Pilot Study of OncoSil™ Given to Patients With Pancreatic Cancer Treated With FOLFIRINOX or Gemcitabine+Abraxane - Full Text View - ClinicalTrials.gov. https://clinicaltrials.gov/ct2/show/NCT03003078. Accessed 11 Aug 2020.

Part X

EUS-Guided Drainage of Abscesses

47 EUS-Guided Drainage of Liver Abscess

Ramon Sanchez-Ocaña
and Manuel Perez-Miranda

47.1 Background

EUS-guided abscess drainage with potential debridement follows the paradigm of EUS-guided pancreatic fluid collection drainage. Postoperative mediastinal or pelvic abscesses are most commonly drained under EUS, because in these locations percutaneous access is difficult or impossible and external drainage catheters are very inconvenient to patients.

Liver abscesses can be drained under EUS based on the close proximity of the liver to the GI tract [1], particularly when percutaneous access is challenging [2, 3]. Plastic pigtail stents or nasocystic catheters were originally used for EUS-guided liver abscess drainage [1–3]; however, use of lumen-apposing [4, 5] or standard biliary covered metal stents [6–8] is increasingly being reported. Through-the-stent intervention for irrigation and debridement is possible with either type of metal stent. EUS-guided liver abscess drainage appears comparable to percutaneous drainage in terms of safety and efficacy, while minimizing patient discomfort [6, 8].

Supplementary Information The online version contains supplementary material available at [https://doi.org/10.1007/978-981-16-9340-3_47].

R. Sanchez-Ocaña · M. Perez-Miranda (✉)
Department of Gastroenterology, Hospital Universitario Rio Hortega, Valladolid, Spain
e-mail: mperezmiranda@saludcastillayleon.es

47.2 Case History

A 49-year-old female with a history of cholecystectomy 20 years before, who was undergoing endoscopic management of bilateral hepatolithiasis with sequential ERCPs, developed a 44 × 62 mm right-lobe liver abscess across segments V and VI. She presented with septic shock and underwent emergency percutaneous abscess drainage. She improved initially after percutaneous drainage while on intravenous antibiotics, but then experienced persistent fever. EUS-guided abscess drainage with a covered biliary metal stent was offered to the patient, with abscess debridement as needed.

47.3 Procedural Plan

Left liver lobe abscesses are easily drained under EUS-guidance from the stomach [1–5]. Transduodenal EUS-guided access to the right liver lobe with successful abscess drainage is also possible [6–8]. The large-caliber metal stents (10 or 15-mm in diameter) that can be placed using a linear echoendoscope allow more efficient abscess drainage than the thinner plastic catheters placed percutaneously. As drainage is a temporary measure in the setting of benign disease, stent removal after abscess resolution is anticipated. Fully covered biliary metal stents can easily be removed once drainage is complete [4–8]. The type of cov-

A. Y.B. Teoh et al. (eds.), *Atlas of Interventional EUS*, https://doi.org/10.1007/978-981-16-9340-3_47

ered metal stent chosen is based on the distance between the GI tract and the abscess. When this distance is less than 1-cm, lumen-apposing metal stents with one-step delivery systems can be used [4, 8], just as in EUS-guided drainage of the gallbladder or pancreatic walled-off necrosis. However, when the distance between the abscess and the GI wall is more than 1-cm, fully covered biliary metal stents need to be used instead [6–8].

Prior to stent placement, transhepatic EUS-guided abscess needle puncture is customarily performed for microbiological sampling. Contrast can be injected to outline the abscess cavity. Depending on the size and contents of the abscess cavity and on initial treatment response, follow-up sessions can occasionally be scheduled for debridement.

47.4 Description of the Procedure

With the linear echoendoscope in the duodenal bulb, the right-lobe liver abscess is imaged and punctured with a 19G needle under EUS (Video 47.1). Pus is aspirated for culture and contrast is injected to outline the abscess cavity under fluoroscopy (Fig. 47.1). A guidewire is passed through the needle and coiled into the abscess. The punc-

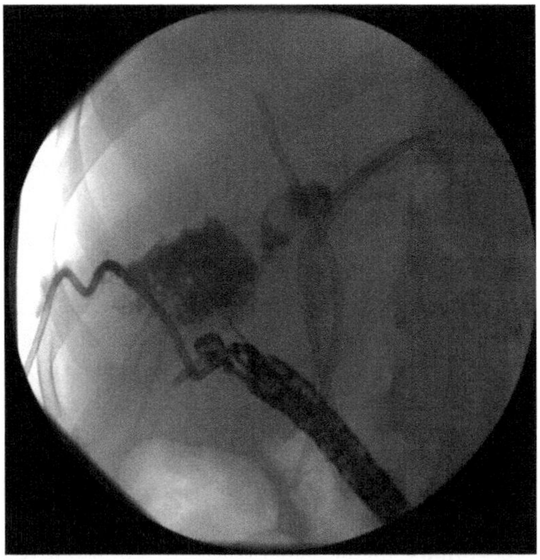

Fig. 47.1 Transduodenal EUS-guided puncture and contrast injection into right-lobe liver abscess. Percutaneous drainage catheter and bilateral biliary stents in place

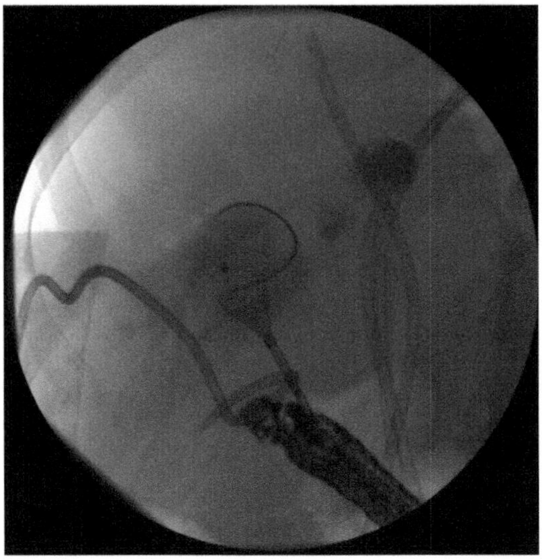

Fig. 47.2 Transduodenally inserted fully covered biliary metal stent is deployed inside the liver abscess under fluoroscopy

ture tract is balloon dilated over the wire with a 6-mm balloon catheter and a 40 × 10 mm fully covered biliary metal stent is then inserted into the abscess over the wire. The stent is next deployed under combined fluoroscopy (Fig. 47.2), EUS, and endoscopy. Pus is seen draining into the duodenum endoscopically and immediate contrast emptying from the abscess on fluoroscopy (Fig. 47.3). The stent is clipped to the duodenal wall to prevent inward migration. CT scan 1 week later shows partial abscess resolution and proper stent placement (Fig. 47.4). Three weeks later a thin-caliber upper endoscope is passed through the transduodenal stent into the abscess. Stone fragments are washed out and removed with forceps into the duodenum.

47.5 Post-Procedural Management

Following EUS-guided liver abscess drainage, defervescence occurs a median of 1 day later. The patient should be kept on intravenous antibiotics until clinical resolution. Stents should be removed in patients without underlying malignancy, although timing of stent removal is not established and typically varies between one to several

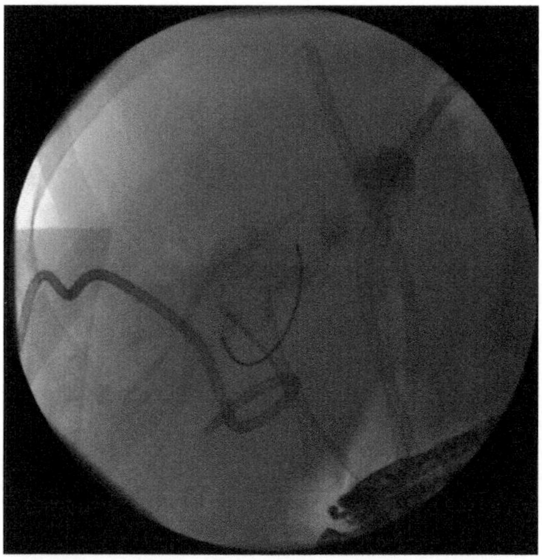

Fig. 47.3 Immediate contrast drainage following balloon expansion of the transduodenal biliary metal stent

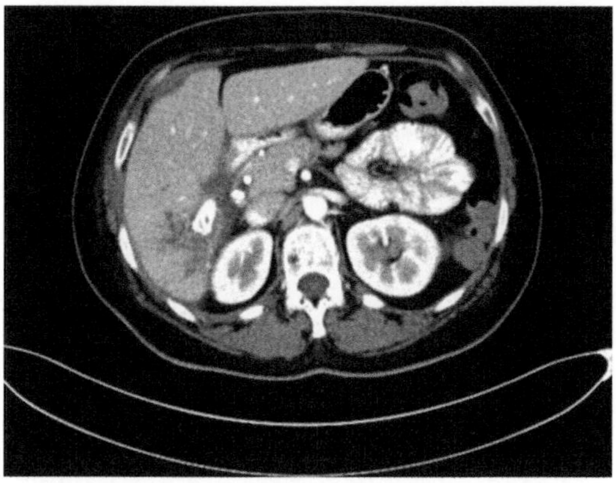

Fig. 47.4 Computed tomography 1-week following EUS-guided abscess drainage. Metal stent coursing medially and inferiorly towards the duodenum

weeks after initial placement. In addition to clinical and laboratory assessment of the treatment response, computed tomography or transabdominal ultrasound is helpful before stent removal.

47.6 Potential Pitfalls

EUS-guided abscess drainage with plastic pigtail stents may be less efficient because of clogging. Nasocystic catheter drainage is possible, but not liked by patients. Covered metal stents carry a small but real risk of migration [6]. Anchoring strategies for covered metal stents are advisable, such as using lumen-apposing metal stents if the abscess is within close range of the GI wall or inserting a coaxial plastic pigtail through a covered biliary metal stent if otherwise [7]. Hemoclips proved useful in our case; however, based on high migration rates observed with covered biliary metal stents in hepaticogastrostomy despite clipping [9], additional anchorage beyond clips should perhaps be considered. Leaving an extra length of the stent inside the GI tract is a relatively simple measure and may also help prevent migration.

Competing Interests Dr. Manuel Perez-Miranda is a consultant for Boston Scientific, Olympus, Medtronic and M.I.Tech.

References

1. Seewald S, Imazu H, Omar S, et al. EUS-guided drainage of hepatic abscess. Gastrointest Endosc. 2005;61:495–8.
2. Noh SH, Park DH, Kim YR, et al. EUS-guided drainage of hepatic abscesses not accessible to percutaneous drainage (with videos). Gastrointest Endosc. 2010;71:1314–9.
3. Keohane J, Dimaio CJ, Schattner MA, Gerdes H. EUS-guided transgastric drainage of caudate lobe liver abscesses. J Interv Gastroenterol. 2011;1:139–41.
4. Alcaide N, Vargas-Garcia AL, De La Serna-Higuera C, et al. EUS-guided drainage of liver abscess by using a lumen-apposing metal stent (with video). Gastrointest Endosc. 2013;78:941–2.
5. Kawakami H, Kawakubo K, Kuwatani M, et al. Endoscopic ultrasound-guided liver abscess drainage using a dedicated, wide, fully covered self-expandable metallic stent with flared ends. Endoscopy. 2014;46:E982–3.
6. Tonozuka R, Itoi T, Tsuchiya T, et al. EUS-guided drainage of hepatic abscess and infected biloma using short and long metal stents (with videos). Gastrointest Endosc. 2015;81:1463–9.
7. Ogura T, Masuda D, Saori O, et al. Clinical outcome of endoscopic ultrasound-guided liver abscess drainage using self expandable covered metallic stent (with video). Dig Dis Sci. 2016;61:303–8.
8. Carbajo AY, Brunie Vegas FJ, et al. Retrospective cohort study comparing endoscopic ultrasound-guided and percutaneous drainage of upper abdominal abscesses. Dig Endosc. 2019;31:431–8.
9. Miranda-García P, Gonzalez JM, Tellechea JI, et al. EUS hepaticogastrostomy for bilioenteric anastomotic strictures: a permanent access for repeated ambulatory dilations? Results from a pilot study. Endosc Int Open. 2016;4:E461–5.

EUS-Guided Drainage of Splenic Abscess

48

Ahmed Mohammed Elmeligui,
Ameya Deshmukh, Enad Dawod, and Jose Nieto

48.1 Background

Splenic abscess is an uncommon clinical infection with an estimated incidence of 0.5% [1]. The diagnosis of this condition could be missed resulting in a very high mortality of more than 70%. With proper treatment, the mortality could be reduced to less than 1%. Prompt assessment with a CT scan could rapidly diagnose the condition and help with treatment planning on the aspiration or drainage of the splenic collection [2–4]. Hematogenous spread from another infected area in the body is the most common source of splenic abscess. While in some cases, a pancreatic abscess and diverticulitis may sometimes extend and involve the spleen [5]. EUS-guided drainage of splenic abscess using lumen apposing metal stent is an emerging novel procedure and it can be an appropriate alternative in patients who cannot tolerate surgery.

Supplementary Information The online version contains supplementary material available at [https://doi.org/10.1007/978-981-16-9340-3_48].

A. M. Elmeligui
Department of Gastroenterology, Hepatology and Endoscopy, Kasr Alainy Hospital, Cairo University, Giza, Egypt
e-mail: Ahmed.elmeligui@kasralainy.edu.eg

A. Deshmukh
Department of Internal Medicine, Saint Louis University – School of Medicine, St. Louis, MO, USA
e-mail: ameya.deshmukh@health.slu.edu

E. Dawod
NYP/Weill Cornell Medical Center, New York, NY, USA

J. Nieto (✉)
Division of Gastroenterology, Hepatology and Endoscopy, Baptist Medical Center Jacksonville, Borland Groover Clinic, Jacksonville, FL, USA

48.2 Case History

A 44-year-old male has a past medical history of hypertension and necrotizing pancreatitis that was treated in our center after an episode of syncope at home. He was admitted 3 months ago for abdominal pain. During that time, he had an ERCP performed, developed pancreatic necrosis and underwent drainage. He also underwent abdominal surgeries for abdominal compartment syndrome. The patient reported that on the day of admission, he developed low-grade fever and had syncope. He also had recurrent abdominal pain that was similar to his previous admissions. The abdomen was soft, mildly distended, with tenderness on palpation in the left and right lower quadrants. CT of the abdomen revealed a gastric drainage catheter extending into a complex splenic collection (Fig. 48.1) with soft tissue stranding and fluid tracking throughout the abdomen. The images were similar to the scans from his previous admission. Blood cultures were positive for ESBL and the patient was started on anti-

A. Y.B. Teoh et al. (eds.), *Atlas of Interventional EUS*, https://doi.org/10.1007/978-981-16-9340-3_48

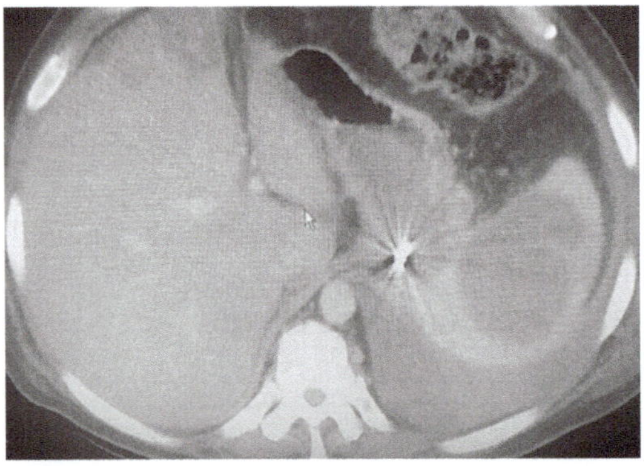

Fig. 48.1 CT abdomen illustrates the splenic abscess

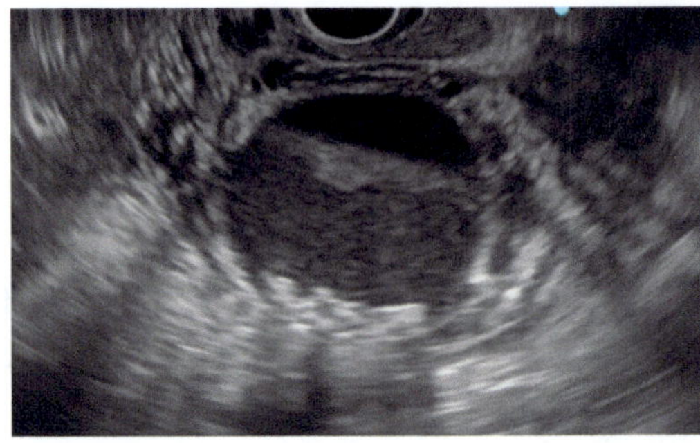

Fig. 48.2 EUS view of the splenic collection

biotics. EUS was performed and showed a splenic abscess measuring 59 mm x 65 mm. EUS-guided splenic abscess drainage was planned using a lumen apposing metal stent (LAMS).

48.3 Procedural Plan

EUS-guided splenic abscess drainage can be performed through a transgastric approach. In this case we preferred this approach as the abscess was in close proximity to the stomach wall. In addition, the large size of the abscess made it suitable and convenient to use a lumen apposing metal stent 10x10mm (Axios, Boston Scientific, Marlborough, USA) rather than double pigtail plastic stents. The use of LAMS can also reduce the chance of leakage and stent migration. A cautery enhanced catheter system can directly puncture the abscess cavity in a single stage and hence reduce the time of the procedure and the need for exchange of devices. The LAMS will also provide a larger draining diameter and less risk of obstruction than when using the smaller double pigtail plastic stent. Yet, when using LAMS through the transgastric approach, we need to be wary that there is a chance of food impaction. The alternative would be to perform percutaneous CT guided drainage [6]. Despite the above considerations, a randomized controlled study is needed to evaluate the efficacy and effectiveness of EUS-guided splenic abscess drainage using LAMS.

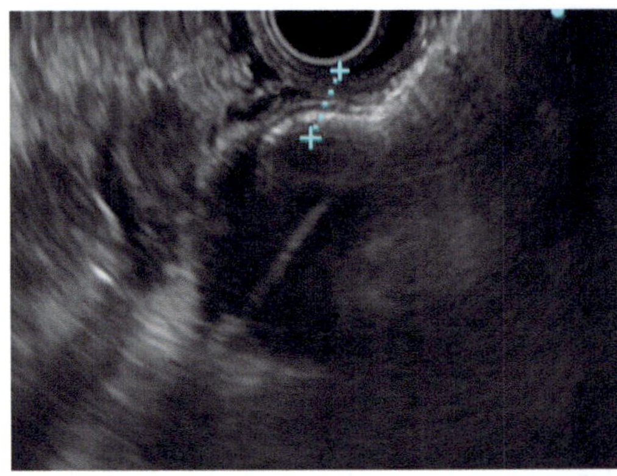

Fig. 48.3 EUS-guided placement of LAMS (Distal flange)

48.4 Description of the Procedure

Splenic abscess drainage was achieved using single stage cautery enhanced lumen apposing metal stent via a transgastric approach using linear echo-endoscope. The splenic abscess was identified through the stomach and measured 51 mm × 65 mm (Fig. 48.2) (Video 48.1). The splenic abscess was directly punctured using cautery enhanced delivery system. The distal flange was deployed inside the abscess cavity under the guidance of echo-endoscope (Fig. 48.3). Then, the stent was pulled back to appose the cavity of the splenic abscess with the lumen of the stomach. The proximal flange was then deployed under endoscopic guidance (Fig. 48.4) and the pyogenic content was drained.

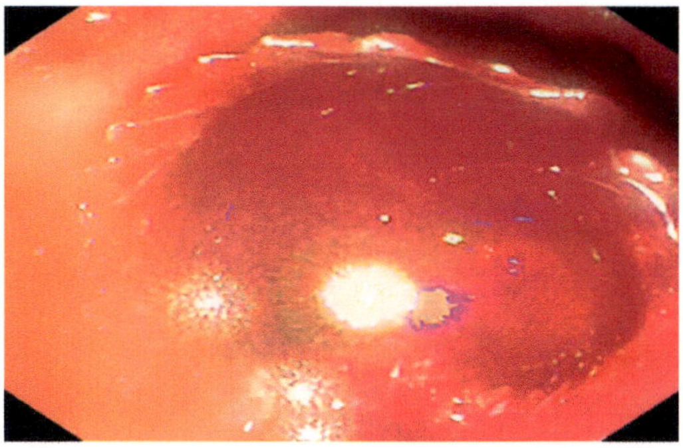

Fig. 48.4 Endoscopic view of LAMS (Proximal flange)

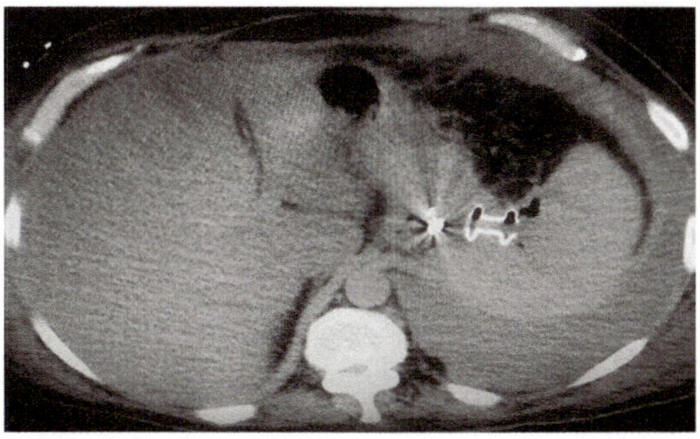

Fig. 48.5 CT abdomen showing complete resolution of splenic abscess during follow up

48.5 Post-Procedural Management

Low residue diet was resumed as fever and pain subsided. Antibiotics were continued for about 10 days after the procedure. Repeat EGD for debridement and lavage using hydrogen peroxide solution was performed 1 week post-procedure and the LAMS was replaced with a double pigtail stent to ensure proper and complete drainage of the abscess cavity and to avoid buried stent syndrome. Follow up CT scan performed 1 month after the procedure revealed complete splenic abscess resolution (Fig. 48.5). A repeat EGD was done to remove the double pigtail stent. Six-month post-procedural CT scan showed no abscess recurrence.

48.6 Potential Pitfalls

The early adverse events of EUS-guided splenic abscess drainage includes mis-deployment, migration, self-limited bleeding after stent insertion, delayed bleeding, perforation, infection and buried stent syndrome. In case of stent mis-deployment, management can be achieved by adjusting the stent position using gastroscope and pediatric biopsy forceps. If it is not feasible, then a fully covered self-expandable metal stent or another LAMS can be deployed through the mis-deployed LAMS in order to connect the two lumens to drain the abscess in a proper way [7]. Buried stent syndrome can be avoided by early removal of the stent usually after 1 week and replacement with double pigtail plastic stent. Concerning stent migration, if the fistula is still present, then another plastic stent or LAMS can be reinserted. However, if the fistula tract is absent, then a repeat EUS-guided drainage or percutaneous CT guided abscess drainage may be required.

Conflicts of Interest Ahmed Mohammed Elmeligui: None. Javier Tejedor-Tejada: None. Ameya Deshmukh: None. Enad Dawod: None. Jose Nieto: Consultant for Boston Scientific.

References

1. Nieto J, Nguyen A, Dawood E. Splenic abscess management with a lumen apposing metal stent: case report. Am J Gastroenterol. 2019;114(Supplement) https://doi.org/10.14309/01.ajg.0000598040.83460.34.
2. Lee MC, Lee CM. Splenic abscess: an uncommon entity with potentially life-threatening evolution. Can J Infect Dis Med Microbiol. 2018;2018:8610657.
3. Sahu M, Kumar A, Nischal N, Bharath BG, Manchanda S, Wig N. Splenic abscess caused by salmonella typhi and co-infection with Leptospira. J Assoc Physicians India. 2017 Dec;65(12):95–7.
4. Chen H, Hu ZQ, Fang Y, Lu XX, Li LD, Li YL, Mao XH, Li Q. A case report: splenic abscess caused by Burkholderia pseudomallei. Medicine (Baltimore). 2018;97(26):e11208.
5. Splenic Abscess. Definitions. 2020. https://doi.org/10.32388/1cfh03.

6. Thanos L, Dailiana T, Papaioannou G, Nikita A, Koutrouvelis H, Kelekis DA. Am J Roentgenol. 2002;179(3):629–32.
7. Hsueh W, Shah-Khan SM, Stemple M, Nasr JY. Salvage of a misdeployed 20-mm lumen-apposing metal stent by use of a through-the-scope esophageal stent. VideoGIE. 2019;4(5):200–2. https://doi.org/10.1016/j.vgie.2019.01.011.

Part XI

EUS-Guided Fiducial Marker Insertion

49 EUS-Guided Fiducial Marker Insertion for Esophageal Cancer

Shannon Melissa Chan
and Anthony Y.B. Teoh

49.1 Background

Chemoirradiation (CRT) therapy plays a vital role in the curative treatment of esophageal cancer. The primary objective of esophageal cancer radiotherapy (RT) is to deliver the highest radiation dose to the target volume while minimizing toxicity to the adjacent organs. In esophageal cancer, the target volume is notoriously difficult to define, especially in a non-obstructive tumor with a collapsed esophagus. This inaccuracy can lead to an overestimation or underestimation of the tumor extent, thus leading to an over-treatment or under-treatment of the disease. There are sparse case series describing the use of fiducial marker insertion for esophageal cancer, and the optimal technique of insertion of these markers has not been investigated. Machiels et al. performed a study on the delineation variation of esophageal tumors in the gross tumor volume (GTV) [1]. The inter- and intraobserver generalized conformity index were significantly larger in the series with markers than in the series without markers ($p < 0.001$), especially in the longitudinal direction. The authors concluded then, that the use of fiducial markers is indicated for esophageal cancer patients with radiotherapy planned. The original method of insertion was extrapolated from methods used for pancreatic tumors. However, we observed that the fiducial marker migration rate was high. Therefore, we developed an alternative way of inserting the fiducial markers into the submucosa after the creation of a submucosal pocket with injection of solution. A retrospective comparative study conducted by our center showed that the submucosal insertion method was associated with a lower fiducial marker migration rate [2]. The optimal method, however, still needs further studies to define.

49.2 Case History

An 75-year-old gentleman was diagnosed with a mid-esophageal squamous cell carcinoma. Staging PET-CT showed hypermetabolic lesions at the mid esophagus together with mildly hypermetabolic left paraesophageal lymph nodes suspicious of early nodal metastases. The radiological staging was T3N1. The patient enjoyed good past health and has an excellent functional status. He was therefore planned for neoadjuvant chemoirradiation, followed by 3 staged esophagectomy.

Supplementary Information The online version contains supplementary material available at [https://doi.org/10.1007/978-981-16-9340-3_49].

S. M. Chan · A. Y.B. Teoh (✉)
Department of Surgery, The Prince of Wales Hospital, The Chinese University of Hong Kong, Shatin, Hong Kong SAR, China
e-mail: shannonchan@surgery.cuhk.edu.hk; anthonyteoh@surgery.cuhk.edu.hk

A. Y.B. Teoh et al. (eds.), *Atlas of Interventional EUS*, https://doi.org/10.1007/978-981-16-9340-3_49

Narrow-band magnifying endoscopy and EUS-guided fiducial marker placement were planned before RT planning.

49.3 Procedural Plan

For all patients with esophageal cancer, we routinely examine the esophagus with a high-definition gastroscope (EGD) under white light and narrow-band imaging to assess the extent of the tumor and to look for synchronous skip lesions. The proximal and distal extent of the tumor was noted endoscopically and fluoroscopically. Locations of any skip lesions were also recorded. The next step of the procedure depends on whether the tumor is obstructive or non-obstructive. For non-obstructive tumors where a linear echoendoscope (GF-UCT260, Olympus Medical, Japan) could traverse the tumor, a 22-gauge fiducial needle preloaded with fiducials (EF) were used (EchoTip, Cook Medical, USA). According to our previous study, it is our routine practice to place the markers submucosally. The submucosa was first raised under EUS guidance with a mixture of hyaluronic acid and normal saline (3:7 ratio) using a 19G needle, followed by the insertion of the fiducial markers. In obstructing tumors, the tumor was first traversed with a 5.4 mm ultrathin gastroscopy (GIF-XP290, Olympus Medical, Japan). A guidewire was then inserted for insertion of a endobronchial ultrasound to look for the presence of submucosal extension of tumor and metastatic lymph nodes. The submucosa was first raised after puncture with a 22G needle, then the fiducial marker was inserted by puncturing with the same needle. The fiducial markers were backloaded into the needle and fixed in position with bone wax. The proximal and distal markers were placed so that they include the metastatic lymph nodes. The final positions of the fiducial markers were confirmed by fluoroscopy and EUS.

49.4 Description of the Procedure

Patient was put on left lateral position. Linear echoendoscope was introduced. A staging EUS was first performed, examining the T and N staging. The scope was then passed to the distal end of the tumo (Figs. 49.1, 49.2, 49.3, 49.4, and 49.5). A more extensive submucosal involvement was found at the distal end, and therefore the insertion of fiducial marker was planned at the most distal end of the submucosal involvement. The location of the marker should include the presence of paraesophageal lymph nodes. After the location of the distal marker was decided, a submucosal bleb was created with a mixture of hyaluronic acid and normal saline (ratio 3:7) with a 19G needle. The needle was inserted to pass point the adventitia and subsequently pulled back into the submucosal with the solution injected. The EchoTip was

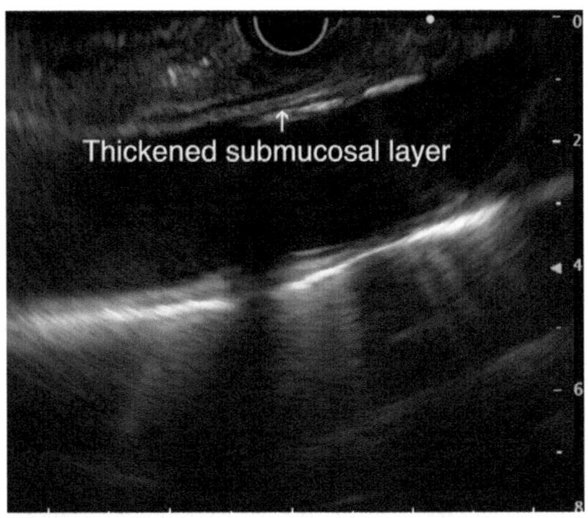

Fig. 49.1 Submucosal involvement of the distal end of the tumor

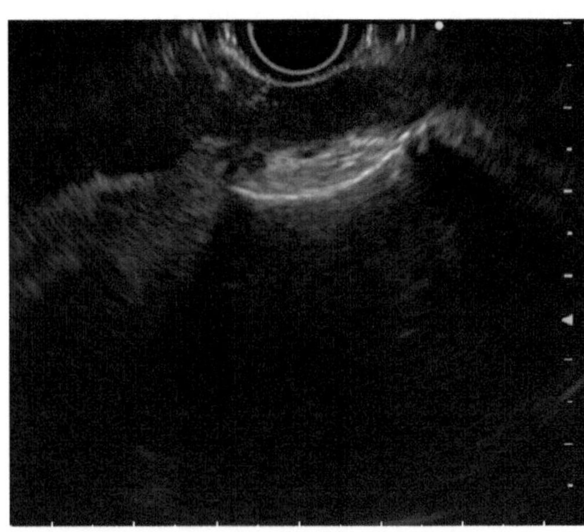

Fig. 49.2 Tumor invaded to adventitia layer

then introduced. Under EUS and fluoroscopy guidance, the fiducial marker was deployed. Normal saline was also flushed to ensure the security of the marker. The endoscope was then pulled back to the proximal end. The absence of paraesophageal lymph nodes was confirmed.

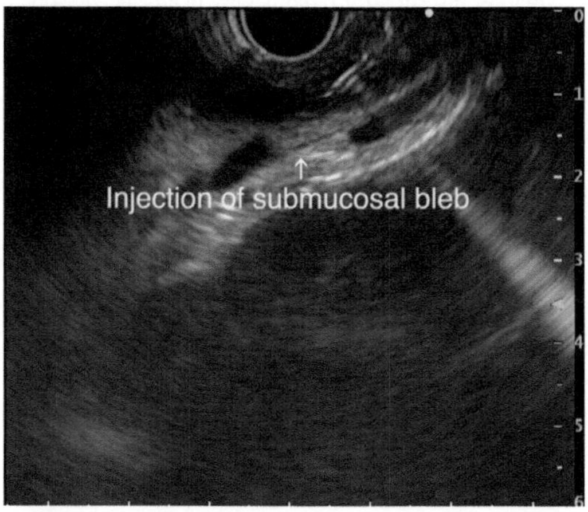

Fig. 49.3 Submucosal bleb injection at the distal end

The submucosal bleb was again created, and the proximal fiducial marker was inserted in the same way. The location of both markers was confirmed on fluoroscopy.

49.5 Post-Procedural Management

Patient can be discharged on the same day, followed by RT planning.

49.6 Potential Pitfalls

This is a relatively safe procedure. The thin submucosal layer may sometimes be difficult to inject. The technique is to overshoot a little and pull back, inject the mixed solution bit by bit, and once a small submucosal bleb was created, the needle was adjusted to inject more solution into the bleb. The technique is more cumbersome when the tumor is obstructive (details described in procedural plan).

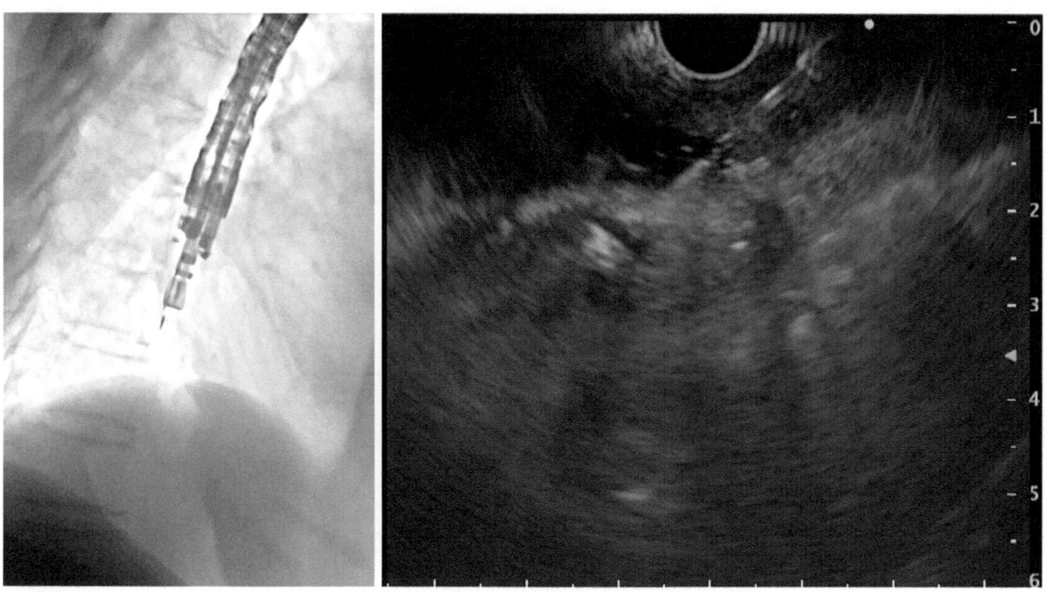

Fig. 49.4 Fiducial marker insertion in both endoscopy and fluoroscopy view

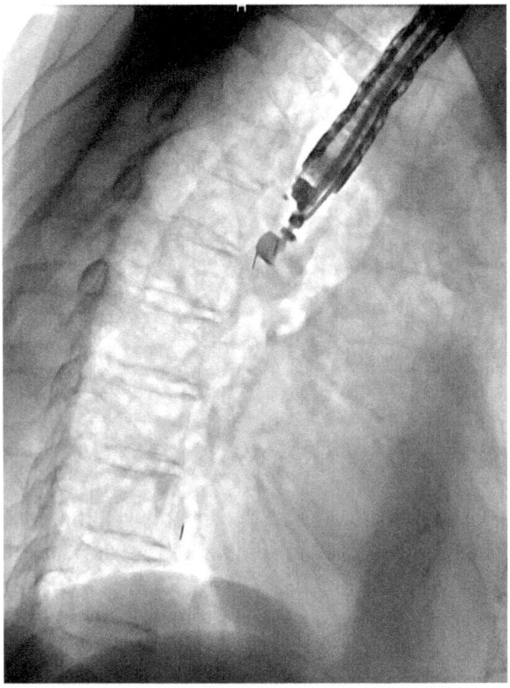

Fig. 49.5 Fluoroscopy view of both distal and proximal markers at the end of the procedure

References

1. Machiels M, Jin P, van Hooft JE, Gurney-Champion OJ, Jelvehgaran P, Geijsen ED, et al. Reduced inter-observer and intra-observer delineation variation in esophageal cancer radiotherapy by use of fiducial markers. Acta Oncol. 2019;58(6):943–50.
2. Chan SM, Tse T, Yip HC, Chan DL, Lam DCM, Chiu PWY, Ng EKW, Teoh AYB. EUS-guided fiducial marker insertion for radiotherapy in advanced esophageal carcinoma: submucosal insertion may lead to less migration when compared to intratumoral insertion. Surg Endosc. 2022;36(2):1666–74. https://doi.org/10.1007/s00464-021-08711-8. Epub 2021 Sep 15. PMID: 34528128.

50 EUS-guided Fiducial Marker Placement for Pancreatic Cancer

Reiko Ashida

50.1 Background

Chemoradiation therapy (CRT) is increasingly being applied for localized pancreatic cancer (LPC) [1, 2]. In image-guided radiation therapy (IGRT), such as intensity-modulated radiation therapy (IMRT) and respiration synchronization, fiducial markers must be placed to maximize the efficacy of CRT and reduce its toxicity. Fiducial marker placement is also mandatory to reduce adverse events in high-dose radiation therapy techniques such as stereotactic body radiation therapy (SBRT) and heavy particle therapy. In the past, fiducial markers were placed percutaneously or intraoperatively under US or CT guidance. However, the markers can now be placed endoscopically by endoscopic ultrasound-guided fiducial marker placement (EUS-FP), using the safe and precise approach developed by Pishvaian in 2006 [3]. In this technique, the marker is loaded into the FNA needle by the back-loading method. A recent meta-analysis concluded that EUS-FP is feasible for GI malignancy and has a high technical success rate (98%), low adverse event (4%) and low fiducial migration rates (3%) [4].

Supplementary Information The online version contains supplementary material available at [https://doi.org/10.1007/978-981-16-9340-3_50].

R. Ashida (✉)
Second Department of Internal Medicine, Wakayama Medical University, Wakayama, Japan

Departments of Cancer Survey and Gastrointestinal Oncology, Osaka International Cancer Institute, Osaka, Japan
e-mail: rashida@goo.jp

50.2 Case History

A 74-year-old male had histologically proven stage IIA pancreatic cancer that was considered suitable for neoadjuvant chemo radiation therapy (Fig. 50.1). The patient was referred for EUS-FP for localization of the tumor by cone-beam computed tomography (CBCT) during daily radiation therapy.

50.3 Procedural Plan

EUS-FP was scheduled a few days prior to the radiation planning CT. The number of fiducial markers and the marker locations are decided depending on the type of radiation therapy and tumor size. Since resectable pancreatic cancer is relatively mobile, marker placement is especially recommended before preoperative chemoradiation [5]. A single marker is sufficient for confirming tumor location on a daily basis; however, when the tumor location must be recognized in real time, as for CyberKnife irradiation or for

A. Y.B. Teoh et al. (eds.), *Atlas of Interventional EUS*, https://doi.org/10.1007/978-981-16-9340-3_50

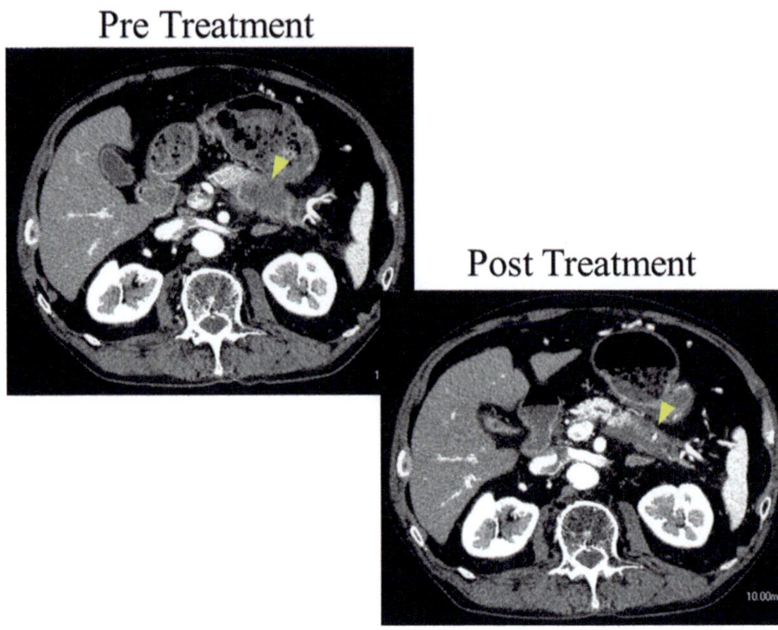

Fig. 50.1 CT findings before and after chemoradiation therapy. A pancreatic tumor (arrowhead) shows a decrease in size after chemoradiation therapy. The gold marker within the tumor appears as a white dot in the post-treatment image

synchronization with respiration, at least three markers at different locations must be placed. Because accurate puncture can be difficult in EUS-FP with a 19G FNA needle, a 22G needle is most suitable for pancreatic lesions.

50.4 Description of the Procedure (Video 50.1)

EUS-FP was performed using a linear-array echoendoscope (GF-UCT 260-AL5; Olympus Corp., Tokyo, Japan) under conscious sedation. A single marker was placed for daily confirmation of the target lesion position. A gold marker (Gold Anchor™; Naslund Medical AB, Huddinge, Sweden) measuring 0.28 × 10 mm was implanted using a 22G FNA needle (EXPECT: 22G; Boston Scientific, United States).

Prior to the procedure, a fiducial marker device designed for percutaneous insertion was backloaded directly into the FNA needle and the marker was inserted into the needle. (Fig. 50.2) The needle tip was sealed with bone wax to prevent the marker from falling out during the procedure. The loaded FNA needle was then advanced through the operating channel. After insertion of the needle into the target lesion, the marker was deployed by advancing the stylet under EUS guidance (Fig. 50.3). Abdominal radiography was performed after the procedure to confirm successful placement and identify the location of the marker, although this is not mandatory.

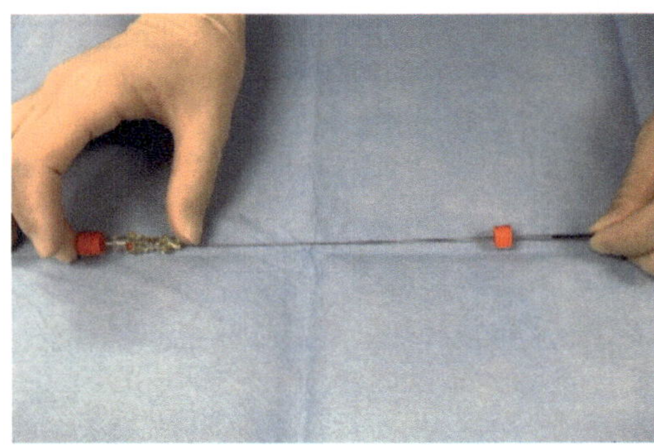

Fig. 50.2 Preparation for EUS-FP. A gold marker is backloaded into an FNA needle using the pusher of a percutaneous needle

50.5 Post-Procedural Management

The patient was admitted and monitored overnight for fever, abdominal pain, and nausea, and was allowed a meal the next day after

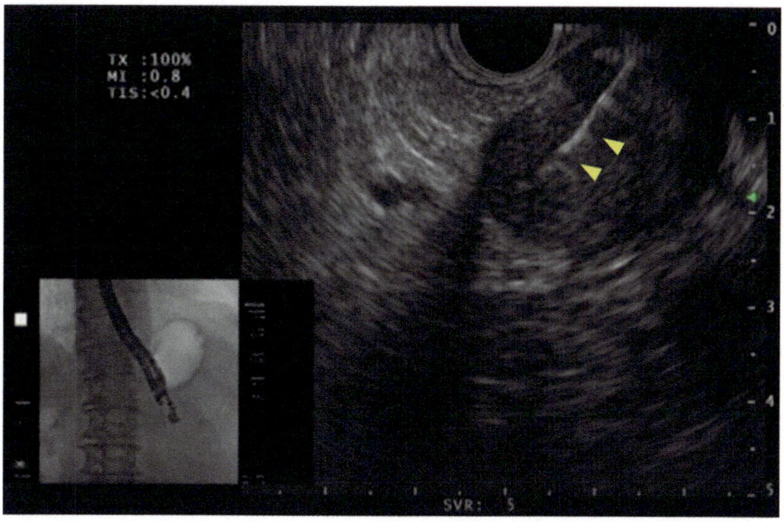

Fig. 50.3 EUS and fluoroscopic images during EUS-FP. A Gold Anchor™ marker was inserted in a straight fashion (arrowheads) into the middle of the tumor

infection and bleeding had been ruled out by blood test results. Intravenous antibiotics (Sulperazone, 1 g × 2 d) were administered prophylactically on the day of the procedure and the following day, although administration of peri-procedural prophylactic antibiotics remains controversial [6].

50.6 Potential Pitfalls

Potential procedure-related adverse events of EUS-FP include bleeding, perforation, infection, and tumor seeding, similar to those of regular EUS-FNA. Spontaneous fiducial migration can occur during passage of the needle or because of tumor necrosis due to treatment, although no migration-related adverse events have yet been reported for EUS-FP. Marker shape is crucial for preventing migration. Conventional markers are straight; however, recent markers designed to avoid migration include a coiled marker that lodges firmly in the tumor, and a notched coil that forms a ball or linear shape depending on the insertion technique.

The following geometrical conditions are recommended for tumor localization in real time: at least three fiducials, minimum interfiducial distance >2 cm, minimum interfiducial angle >15° degrees, and noncollinear placement in the imaging plane.

References

1. de Geus SWL, Eskander MF, Kasumova GG, Ng SC, Kent TS, Mancias JD, et al. Stereotactic body radiotherapy for unresected pancreatic cancer: A nationwide review. Cancer. 2017;123(21):4158–67.
2. Takahashi H, Ohigashi H, Gotoh K, Marubashi S, Yamada T, Murata M, et al. Preoperative gemcitabine-based chemoradiation therapy for resectable and borderline resectable pancreatic cancer. Ann Surg. 2013;258(6):1040–50.
3. Pishvaian AC, Collins B, Gagnon G, Ahlawat S, Haddad NG. EUS-guided fiducial placement for CyberKnife radiotherapy of mediastinal and abdominal malignancies. Gastrointest Endosc. 2006;64(3):412–7.
4. Coronel E, Cazacu IM, Sakuraba A, Luzuriaga Chavez AA, Uberoi A, Geng Y, et al. EUS-guided fiducial placement for GI malignancies: a systematic review and meta-analysis. Gastrointest Endosc. 2019;89(4):659–70, e18.
5. Ashida R, Fukutake N, Takada R, Ioka T, Ohkawa K, et al. Endoscopic ultrasound-guided fiducial marker placement for neoadjuvant chemoradiation therapy for resectable pancreatic cancer. World J Gastrointest Oncol. 2020;12(7):768–81.
6. Chandnani M, Faisal MF, Glissen-Brown J, Sawhney M, Pleskow D, Cohen J, et al. EUS-guided fiducial placement for pancreatobiliary malignancies: safety, infection risk, and use of peri-procedural antibiotics. Endoscopy International Open. 2020;8(2):E179–e85.

Part XII

EUS-Guided Liver Biopsy and Portal Vein Pressure Gradient Measurement

51 EUS-Guided Liver Biopsy in Nonalcoholic Fatty Liver Disease

Ameya Deshmukh, Ahmed Mohammed Elmeligui, Javier Tejedor-Tejada, and Jose Nieto

51.1 Background

Liver biopsy is the gold standard in the evaluation of hepatic disease. It is extremely effective in assessing the histologic degree of fibrosis. Traditional sampling methods can be quite invasive and pose serious risks to the patient. Transjugular, percutaneous and other biopsy methods carry the risk of bleeding, pain and damage to the surrounding organs [1, 2]. The emergence of EUS-guided liver biopsy (EUS-LB) allows the endoscopist to offer a sampling method with decreased risk of adverse events and robust advantages such as decreased pain, increased safety from continuous ultrasound guidance, easily acquisition of multiple samples with a widened view of the organ in one session, and performance in the outpatient setting [2, 3]. EUS-LB accurately evaluates fibrosis in patients with fatty liver disease [4]. Several studies showcase diagnostic yields ranging from 91–100% [5–7].

51.2 Case History

A 56-year-old female with multiple comorbidities including obesity, hypertension and diabetes mellitus type 2 presented with right upper abdominal discomfort and worsening fatigue. She denies alcohol use. The patient was found to have mild hepatomegaly with RUQ pain. In addition, a comprehensive metabolic panel revealed moderately elevated aminotransferases. There was high clinical suspicion of nonalcoholic fatty liver disease due to the combination of her physical exam findings, abnormal LFTs and radiographic findings. EUS-guided liver biopsy was offered to this patient.

51.3 Procedural Plan

A linear EUS endoscope is advanced into the duodenum at the location of the duodenal bulb. In this position, the right hepatic lobe can be biop-

Supplementary Information The online version contains supplementary material available at [https://doi.org/10.1007/978-981-16-9340-3_51].

A. Deshmukh
Department of Internal Medicine, Saint Louis University – School of Medicine, St. Louis, MO, USA
e-mail: ameya.deshmukh@health.slu.edu

A. M. Elmeligui
Department of Gastroenterology, Hepatology and Endoscopy, Kasr Alainy Hospital, Cairo University, Giza, Egypt
e-mail: Ahmed.elmeligui@kasralainy.edu.eg

J. Tejedor-Tejada
Department of Gastroenterology, Hospital Universitario Rio Hortega, Valladolid, Spain

J. Nieto (✉)
Division of Gastroenterology, Hepatology and Endoscopy, Baptist Medical Center Jacksonville, Borland Groover Clinic, Jacksonville, FL, USA

A. Y.B. Teoh et al. (eds.), *Atlas of Interventional EUS*, https://doi.org/10.1007/978-981-16-9340-3_51

sied. The left hepatic lobe can then be biopsied through the proximal stomach or through the oesophagus. Avoiding splenic puncture is necessary by differentiating the left and right hepatic lobe from the spleen, as both can have similar echotextures on ultrasound. Generally, a 19-gauge needle is utilized for liver biopsies, with wet suction being the preferred method.

51.4 Description of the Procedure

The linear echoendoscope was advanced into the duodenum and was stopped at the position of the proximal bulb in order to locate the liver and nearby structures on endoscopic ultrasound (EUS) (Fig. 51.1) (Video 51.1). EUS examination of the liver found areas of increased echogenicity (Fig. 51.2). The 19-gauge needle was then prepared and the stylet removed. The needle was flushed with normal saline. After, a needle trajectory of approximately 5 cm was chosen, avoiding large vessels. A transmural approach was taken for the needle path, as it was penetrating through the duodenal wall into the liver. One pass was made through the liver tissue. Subsequently, the needle was withdrawn with the 20 cc suction opened. Suction was stopped once the sample is obtained. The collected specimen was then directly placed into the formalin solution from the needle. Then, the needle was passed through the liver with two passes before removal with a needle trajectory of 5.41 cm (Fig. 51.3).

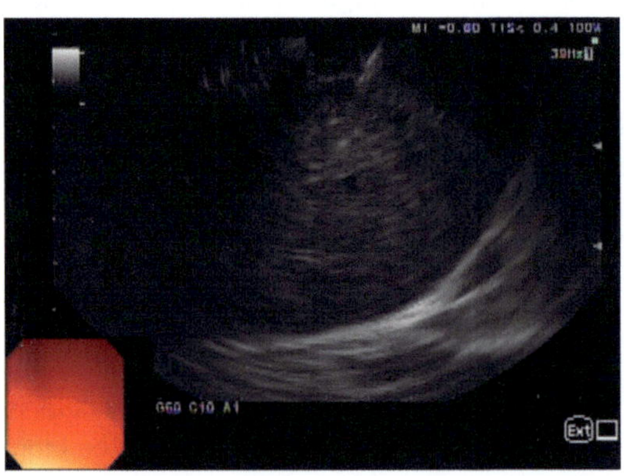

Fig. 51.1 EUS visualization of the liver

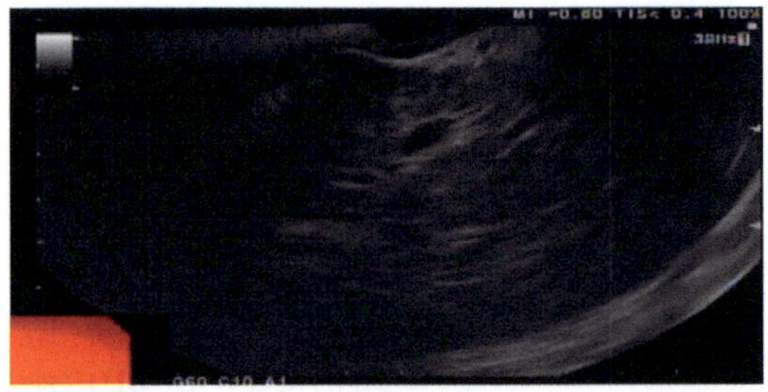

Fig. 51.2 EUS displaying increased areas of hepatic echogenicity suggestive of NAFLD

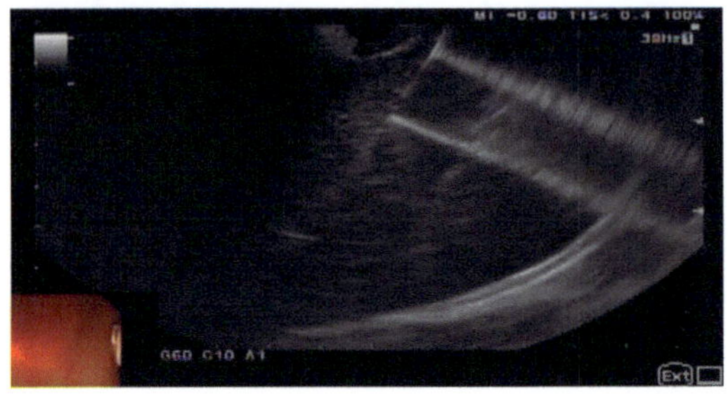

Fig. 51.3 19-gauge needle advancing through the liver using one pass to obtain optimal viable tissue sample

51.5 Post-Procedural Management

Patients were monitored for approximately 30 min to 1 h after the procedure. Patients who developed pain were observed for a longer period of time. Analgesics were given as needed. Patients were recommended to have follow up clinic visits at two- and four-weeks post-procedure for evaluation of any adverse events.

51.6 Potential Pitfalls

Due to the similar visual nature of the liver and spleen on EUS, a misidentified spleen can result in an adverse bleeding complication. Additionally, tissue sample yield can be dependent on the endoscopist's technical skill with this complex procedure. An inexperienced endoscopist may not be able to yield enough usable sample compared to more traditional methods of liver biopsy (Fig. 51.4).

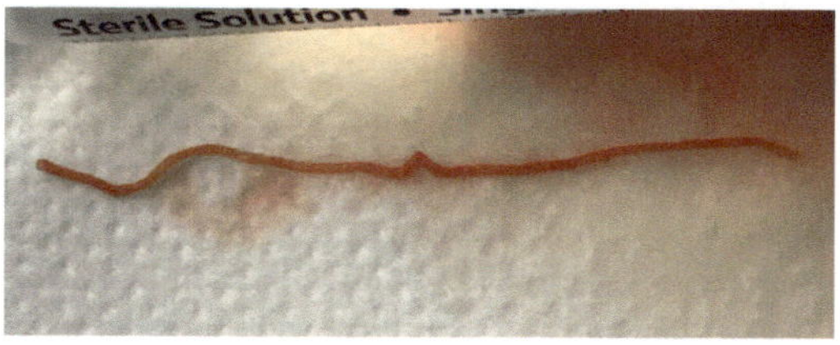

Fig. 51.4 Live view of parenchymal tissue obtained via EUS

Conflicts of Interest Ameya Deshmukh: None. Ahmed Mohammed Elmeligui: None. Javier Tejedor-Tejada: None. Jose Nieto: Consultant for Boston Scientific.

References

1. Shiha GIA, Helmy A. Asian-Pacific Association for the Study of the liver (APASL) consensus guidelines on invasive and non-invasive assessment of hepatic fibrosis: a 2016 update. Hepatol Int. 2017;11:1–30.
2. Johnson KD, Laoveeravat P, Yee EU, Perisetti A, Thandassery RB, Tharian B. Endoscopic ultrasound guided liver biopsy: recent evidence. World Journal of Gastrointestinal Endoscopy. 2020;12(3):83–97.
3. Diehl DL. Endoscopic ultrasound-guided liver biopsy. Interventional Endoscopic Ultrasound. June 2018:83–94.
4. Saab SPJ, Jimenez MA, et al. Endoscopic ultrasound liver biopsies accurately predict the presence of fibrosis in patients with fatty liver. Clin Gastroenterol Hepatol. 2017;15:1477–8.
5. Shah N, Baron T. Taking a poke at the liver: which way is best? Endoscopy International Open. 2019;07(01)
6. Campos S, Poley J-W, Driel LV, Bruno MJ. The role of EUS in diagnosis and treatment of liver disorders. Endoscopy International Open. 2019;07(10)
7. Saraireh HA, Bilal M, Singh S. Role of endoscopic ultrasound in liver disease: where do we stand in 2017? World J Hepatol. 2017;9(24):1013.

EUS-Guided Portal Pressure Gradient Measurement

52

Kenneth J. Chang and David K. Imagawa

52.1 Background

Portal hypertension (PH) is a known complication of liver cirrhosis and is caused by increased resistance to blood flow in the hepatic sinusoids. Once PH develops, the clinical manifestations may include esophageal and gastric varices, portal hypertensive gastropathy, ascites, splenomegaly, and thrombocytopenia. Assessing the intravascular pressure of the portal vein (relative to the hepatic vein) has been useful in determining the stage, progression, prognosis of cirrhosis, as well as the risk for developing hepatocellular carcinoma in individual patients with liver disease. While the hepatic vein can be directly measured using a trans-jugular approach (called the free hepatic venous pressure, or FHVP), the portal vein pressure is assessed indirectly from the wedged hepatic venous pressure (WHVP). In cirrhosis, the WHVP closely reflects portal (sinusoidal) pressure, as the catheter with balloon occlusion creates a continuous fluid column between the catheter, the blood in the hepatic vein, the sinusoidal tract and the portal vein. The difference or gradient between the FHVP and the WHVP is known as the hepatic venous pressure gradient (HVPG). The HVPG accurately reflects the degree of PH in all forms of sinusoidal and post-sinusoidal causes of PH, but not in pre-sinusoidal PH. A portal pressure gradient (PPG) measurement of 0–5 mmHg is considered within the normal range, while 6–9 mmHg is considered portal hypertension, ≥10 mmHg is considered "clinically significant" portal hypertension and associated with the development of esophageal varices [1], and finally, a PPG of ≥12 mmHg is associated with variceal hemorrhage [2]. Reduction of PPG by 20% or to below 12 mmHg with pharmacotherapy has been shown to decrease risk of future bleeding or rebleeding episodes [3, 4].

Author contributions: Chang KJ designed the overall concept, outline of this manuscript and was responsible for writing, and editing of the manuscript. Imagawa DK was responsible for reviewing and editing the manuscript.

Supplementary Information The online version contains supplementary material available at [https://doi.org/10.1007/978-981-16-9340-3_52].

K. J. Chang (✉)
Digestive Health Institute, Gastroenterology Division, University of California, Irvine, Orange, CA, USA
e-mail: kchang@uci.edu

D. K. Imagawa
Digestive Health Institute, Department of Surgery, Division of Hepatobiliary and Pancreas Surgery, University of California, Irvine, Orange, CA, USA
e-mail: dkimagaw@uci.edu

A. Y.B. Teoh et al. (eds.), *Atlas of Interventional EUS*, https://doi.org/10.1007/978-981-16-9340-3_52

The procedure most often used to diagnose portal hypertension in clinical practice is the trans-jugular approach. This percutaneous approach is relatively invasive, requires radiation exposure, intravenous contrast, and only indirectly measures the portal vein pressure. The procedure is done by placing a catheter into the right jugular vein and advancing it into one of the hepatic vein branches under fluoroscopic guidance. A frcc hepatic vein pressure is obtained, followed by a wedged hepatic vein pressure, and the HVPG is estimated by calculating the difference between the two means. This may be inaccurate (e.g., false negative) in cases of pre-hepatic or pre-sinusoidal portal hypertension, which includes possible portal vein thrombosis, primary biliary cholangitis, primary sclerosing cholangitis, polycystic liver disease, myeloproliferative disorders, malignancy, and idiopathic non-cirrhotic portal hypertension [5, 6].

We first developed Endoscopic Ultrasound (EUS) guided porto-systemic pressure gradient (PPG) measurement using a 25 gauge needle and a novel compact manometer in porcine model [7], demonstrating excellent accuracy and strong correlation with pressure values obtained by standard trans-jugular wedged and free hepatic venous pressure measurements by Interventional Radiology. We then went on to conduct the first human pilot study confirming safe and accurate direct portal pressure gradient measurements in the clinical setting. A total of 28 subjects underwent EUS-PPG manometry in this study and pressure measurements were successfully achieved in all subjects. EUS-PPG values ranged from 1.5–19 mmHg with an average of 8.2 mmHg. 15/28 (57.1%) had evidence of PH on EUS-PPG of which 10/15 (66.7%) had clinically significant portal hypertension (CSPH). 11 of 28 subjects had endoscopic evidence of either gastric or esophageal varices with all 11 (100%) having PH and 10 of 11 (90.9%) patients having CSPH based on EUS-PPG measurement [8, 9]. This series demonstrated that EUS-PPG measurement using a 25G needle and compact manometer is feasible and appears safe in humans. A more recent abstract with 51 patients undergoing EUS-PPG was published, again showing 100% technical success, no adverse events, with PPG range of 0–27 mmHg with again strong correlation compared to clinical markers of portal hypertension [10]. We also reported a series of patients who underwent both EUS-PPG with concurrent EUS-guided liver biopsy, showing that the two procedures could be conveniently combined during a single session [11]. EUS-PPG can also overcome the issue of inaccurate diagnosis of pre-sinusoidal portal hypertension (by HVPG)—by measuring the pressure in the portal vein directly. This case illustrates the advantage of EUS-PPG compared to the trans-jugular approach.

52.2 Case History

The patient is a 64-year old female with a recently diagnosed left renal cell carcinoma, undergoing pre-operative work-up. She has a past medical history significant for type 2 diabetes, Lynch Syndrome, myelodysplastic syndrome, monoclonal gammopathy or undetermined significance. She also has a history of upper GI bleeding requiring 4 units of blood transfusion with upper endoscopy showing three columns of esophageal varices which were treated with band ligation over three sessions until near complete obliteration. CT of the abdomen showed an enlarged spleen, normal appearing liver and no ascites. Labs were as follows: Albumin 3.7, Bilirubin 0.6, Total Protein 8.7, ALT 17, AST 32, AP 153, Hb 8.4, Hct 27.4, WBC 0.7, plts 167,000, PT 14.4, Hepatitis serologies negative. Given the documented UGI bleed and esophageal varices, a pre-operative trans-jugular liver biopsy with hepatic venous pressure gradient (HVPG) was performed by interventional radiology. The HVPG was 6 mmHg, and the liver biopsy showed portal and periportal fibrosis with focal bridging and associated numerous dilated portal veinous radicals, absent to minimal portal inflammation, and less than 1% steatosis. The findings were suggestive of idiopathic non-cirrhotic portal hypertension. The patient was then referred for EUS-guided portal pressure gradient measurement for further confirmation.

52.3 Procedural Plan

The equipment used for EUS-guided PPG measurement utilized a linear echoendoscope (GF-UC140P-AL5, Olympus, Tokyo, Japan), a 25G FNA needle (Cook Medical, Winston-Salem, NC, USA), and a compact manometer with non-compressible tubing (Cook Medical, Bloomington, IN, USA). All pertinent vessels were first identified and assessed with pulse wave Doppler.

52.4 Description of the Procedure

The middle hepatic vein (MHV) was first accessed by advancing the EUS needle through the gastric wall and liver parenchyma and directly puncturing the vein (Fig. 52.1). Once in the vessel, a small amount (less than 0.5 ml) of saline with dilute heparin was flushed through the FNA needle to prime the entire set-up prior to each manometric reading. Following 30–60 sec of pressure equilibration, the number on the display was recorded. Three separate readings per vessel were performed and a mean pressure was calculated. The MHV pressures were 8, 8, and 7 mmHg (mean = 7.66 mmHg). Next, the left portal vein (LPV) was targeted (Fig. 52.2). The LPV pressures were 20, 20, and 19 mmHg (mean = 19.66). Thus, the EUS-PPG gradient as 12 mmHg (19.66–7.66), which is consistent with clinically significant portal hypertension (Fig. 52.3).

52.5 Post-Procedural Management

The patient then underwent arterial embolization of both the splenic artery and left renal artery by interventional radiology, followed by open left nephrectomy and splenectomy along with wedge biopsy of the liver. The liver biopsy again showed minimal to mild periportal fibrosis with rare bridging and minimal interstitial chronic inflammation with no steatosis. The spleen showed diffuse vascular congestion and hemorrhage and evidence of extramedullary hematopoiesis.

Although trans-jugular measurement of HVPG is considered the gold standard in diagnosing portal hypertension, it has certain limitations. Trans-jugular measurement of the portal venous pressure is an indirect measurement, whereas EUS-PPG directly measures the pressure in the portal vein. The indirect measurement of the portal vein is done by wedging the trans-jugular balloon catheter within the hepatic vein (wedged hepatic venous pressure, or WHVP). WHVP correlates well with portal venous pressure and is elevated in patients with sinusoidal

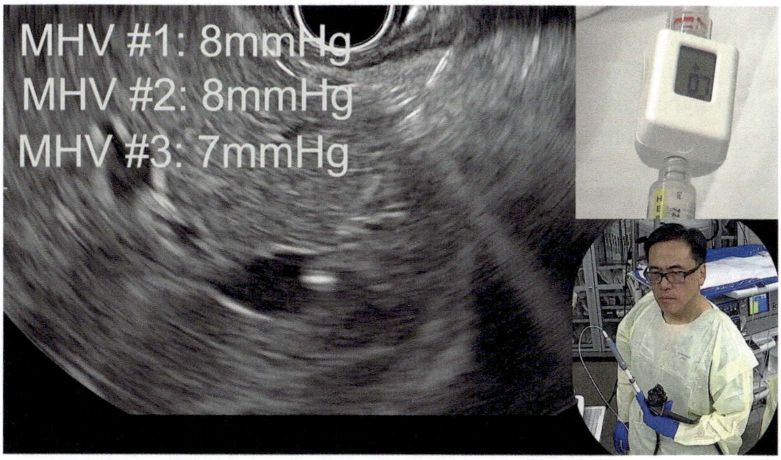

Fig. 52.1 Needle placed in the middle hepatic vein (MHV) with manometric pressures measurements 1, 2, and 3

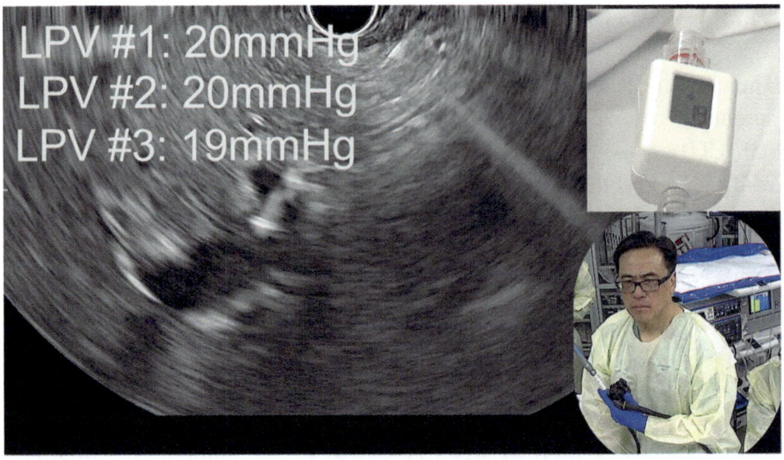

Fig. 52.2 Needle placed in the left portal vein (LPV) with manometric pressures measurements 1, 2, and 3

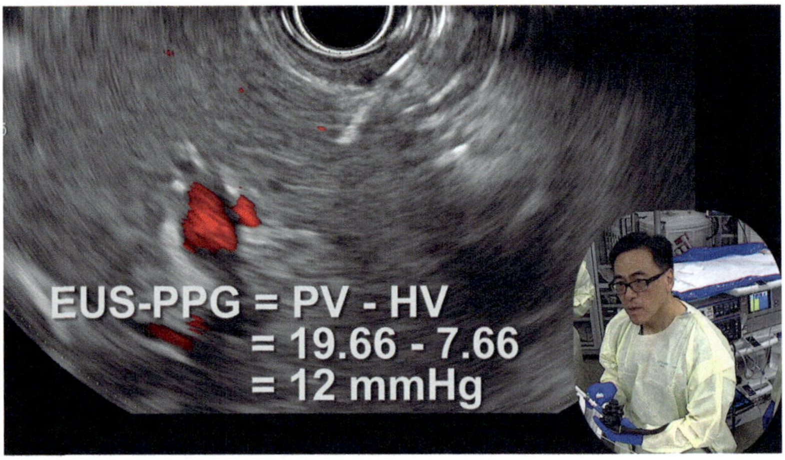

Fig. 52.3 EUS-PPG complete with needle withdrawn through liver parenchyma. Final porto-systemic pressure gradient = 12 mmHg, which is consistent with clinically significant portal hypertension

portal hypertension. However, this correlation does not hold in patients with pre-sinusoidal portal hypertension, as we saw in this case. The final clinical diagnosis was idiopathic non-cirrhotic portal hypertension treated with splenectomy at the time of nephrectomy.

52.6 Potential Pitfalls

Potential complications of EUS-PPG include bleeding, infection, and perforation. Bleeding is minimized by the following: (1) use of a 25G needle (2) excluding patients with platelet count less than 50,000 or INR greater than 2.0 (3) advancing the needle through liver parenchyma before entering the vessel—leveraging the fact that the liver parenchyma will tamponade the puncture site of the vessel (4) using Color Doppler to make sure there is no flow in the needle track prior to completely withdrawing the needle from the liver. If there is remaining blood flow in the needle tack, the following strategies can be employed: (a) maintain the needle in the liver as a "stopper," (b) slowly retract the needle in a zig-zag path to create further pinch points to flow, and (c) advance the sheath forward to put pressure on the liver puncture site as the needle is withdrawn into the sheath.

Infection is minimized by the use of prophylactic antibiotics and avoiding going through ascites fluid. Perforation is minimized with the use of a 25G needle, and avoiding scope torque will the needle is in the liver. Potential pitfalls to avoid erroneous manometric readings include (a) movement of the manometer (changing height) during the measurement, (b) presence of air bubbles in the manometer, needle, or tubing, (c) taking measurements with the needle against the vessel wall.

Conflict of Interest Dr. Chang has served as consultant for Apollo Endosurgery, Cook, Erbe, Endogastric Solutions, Mauna Kea, Mederi, Medtronics, Olympus, Ovesco, and Pentax.

References

1. Bosch J, Garcia-Pagan JC, Berzigotti A, et al. Measurement of portal pressure and its role in the management of chronic liver disease. Semin Liver Dis. 2006;26:348–62.
2. Groszmann RJ, Bosch J, Grace ND, et al. Hemodynamic events in a prospective randomized trial of propranolol versus placebo in the prevention of a first variceal hemorrhage. Gastroenterology. 1990;99:1401–7.
3. Albillos A, Banares R, Gonzalez M, et al. Value of the hepatic venous pressure gradient to monitor drug therapy for portal hypertension: a meta-analysis. Am J Gastroenterol. 2007;102:1116–26.
4. D'Amico G, Garcia-Pagan JC, Luca A, et al. Hepatic vein pressure gradient reduction and prevention of variceal bleeding in cirrhosis: a systematic review. Gastroenterology. 2006;131:1611–24.
5. Nakhleh RE. The pathological differential diagnosis of portal hypertension. Clin Liver Dis (Hoboken). 2017;10:57–62.
6. Yan M, Geyer H, Mesa R, et al. Clinical features of patients with Philadelphia-negative myeloproliferative neoplasms complicated by portal hypertension. Clin Lymphoma Myeloma Leuk. 2015;15:e1–5.
7. Huang JY, Samarasena JB, Tsujino T, et al. EUS-guided portal pressure gradient measurement with a novel 25-gauge needle device versus standard transjugular approach: a comparison animal study. Gastrointest Endosc. 2016;84:358–62.
8. Huang JY, Samarasena JB, Tsujino T, et al. EUS-guided portal pressure gradient measurement with a simple novel device: a human pilot study. Gastrointest Endosc. 2017;85:996–1001.
9. Samarasena JB, Huang JY, Tsujino T, et al. EUS-guided portal pressure gradient measurement with a simple novel device: a human pilot study. VideoGIE. 2018;3:361–3.
10. Samarasena JB, Han J, Patel A, et al. EUS-guided portal pressure gradient measurement: a single center experience. Gastrointest Endosc. 2018;87:AB107.
11. Tsujino T, Huang JY, Samarasena JB, et al. Safety and feasibility of combination EUS-guided portal pressure gradient measurement and liver biopsy: the realization of endo-hepatology. Gastrointest Endosc. 2016;83:AB415–6.

Part XIII

EUS-Guided Portal Vein Aspiration

EUS-Guided Portal Vein Aspiration for Circulating Tumour Cells in Colorectal Cancer

53

Anthony Y.B. Teoh

53.1 Background

Circulating tumour cells (CTC) are cells that are fundamental to the process of tumour metastasis. The presence of these cells in the peripheral blood has been shown to be associated with metastatic relapse and progression of tumours in breast, prostate, lung and colorectal cancer [1–4]. CTC's are currently included in the 2010 TNM staging for breast cancer, and interventional studies based on enumeration of CTC's to guide chemotherapy are underway [5]. In metastatic CRC, patients with three or less CTCs after the initiation of chemotherapy are also shown to have better progression-free survival and overall survival [6].

However, CTCs identified in peripheral blood are extremely rare. The use of endoscopic ultrasound (EUS) to acquire portal venous blood for CTC enumeration can avoid the process of hepatic filtration. Recently, the use of EUS-guided portal venous aspiration (PVA) for enumerating CTC in pancreatic cancer has been described [7]. CTC was obtained in 100% of PVA samples vs. 18% in peripheral blood. The mean yield of CTC from PVA was 100 times that in peripheral blood. In colorectal cancer, we have also found that PVA CTC yield was significantly greater as compared to peripheral blood sample [4.5 (2.9) vs. 2.5 (2.3), $P < 0.001$] [8]. The procedure may also help predict which patient may be at higher risk of metastasis.

53.2 Case History

A 79-year-old lady presented with two-month history of per rectal bleeding associated with tenesmus. Per rectal examination noted a rectal mass. Colonoscopy reviewed a half circumferential tumour 5 cm from the anal verge. Biopsy confirmed adenocarcinoma. Carcinoembryonic Antigen was 11 ug/l. Positron emission computed tomography (PET-CT) demonstrated a 3.3×4.9 cm hypermetabolic mass in the rectum with 3–4 tiny nodes without tracer uptake in the mesorectum (Fig. 53.1). Magnetic resonance imaging (MRI) showed a T2N0 tumour. She was planned for laparoscopic total mesorectal excision with end colostomy. EUS-PVA for enumeration of CTC was offered to the patient as part of a research protocol for further stratification of prognosis.

The peripheral blood and portal vein CTC counts were 0 and 3, respectively. The pathology

Supplementary Information The online version contains supplementary material available at [https://doi.org/10.1007/978-981-16-9340-3_53].

A. Y.B. Teoh (✉)
Department of Surgery, The Prince of Wales Hospital, The Chinese University of Hong Kong, Shatin, Hong Kong SAR, China
e-mail: anthonyteoh@surgery.cuhk.edu.hk

A. Y.B. Teoh et al. (eds.), *Atlas of Interventional EUS*, https://doi.org/10.1007/978-981-16-9340-3_53

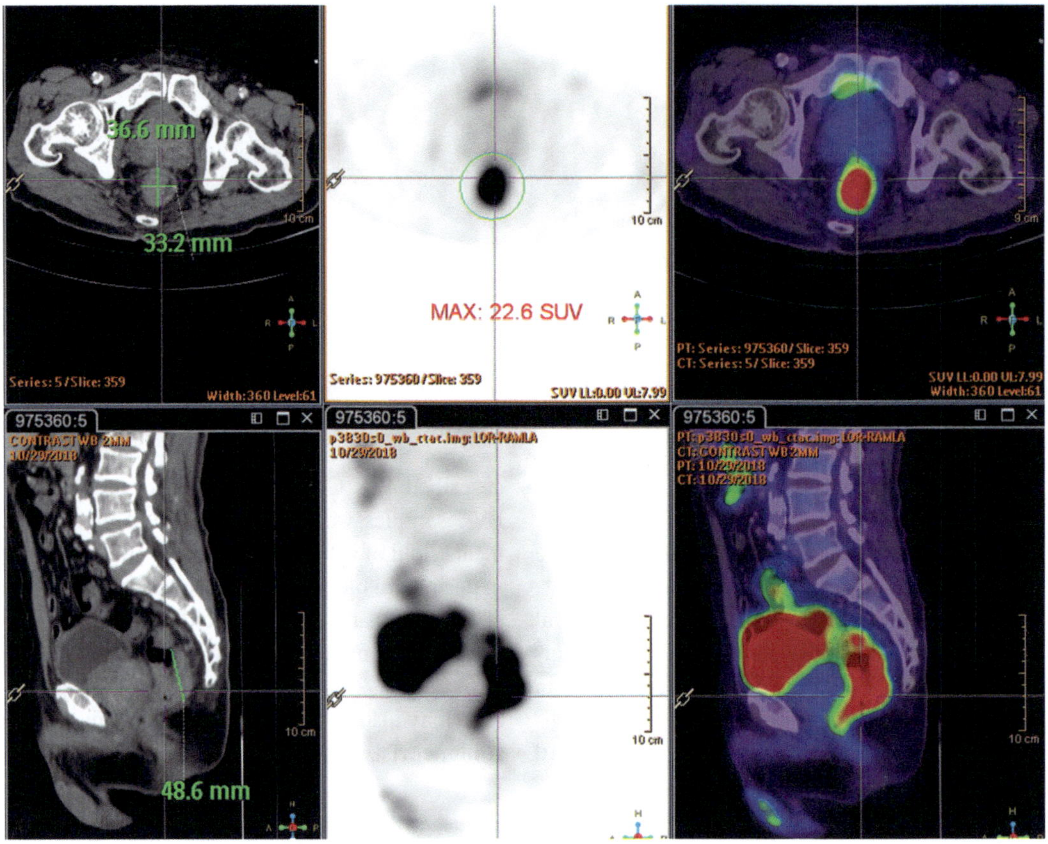

Fig. 53.1 PET-CT of a hypermetabolic mass in the rectum

of the resected tumour was T2N0. Carcinoembryonic Antigen was 9 ug/l after the operation. No adjuvant chemotherapy was given. Follow-up PET-CT 3 months later noted a new 6.7 mm left lung lower lobe lesion with a SUVmax of 1.7 suspicious of lung metastasis (Fig. 53.2). Video-assisted thoracoscopic wedge resection of the lung was performed and confirmed metastatic adenocarcinoma of colorectal primary. EUS-PVA for CTC assessment may be useful in selecting patients at higher risk of recurrence.

53.3 Procedural Plan

We would offer EUS-PVA for CTC assessment in patients with stage 2–4 colorectal carcinomas on pre-operative workup. Second generation cephalosporin would be given prior to the procedure. EUS-PVA is usually performed in the stomach with transhepatic puncture of the main portal vein. If adequate view of the main portal vein could not be obtained from the stomach, the left portal vein could also be punctured. If this is still not possible, another option would be to puncture the right portal vein from the duodenum. Since the vein is punctured with a transhepatic approach, the liver will act as a tamponade to prevent bleeding from the puncture site.

Since CTC is not part of a normal workup for these patients, collaboration with a local partner that is fluent in CTC analysis is essential. The following criteria are used in our institution for a positive CTC to be identified in a blood sample: (1) cytokeratin 8 and 18 positive, (2) CD 45 negative, (3) cell size at least

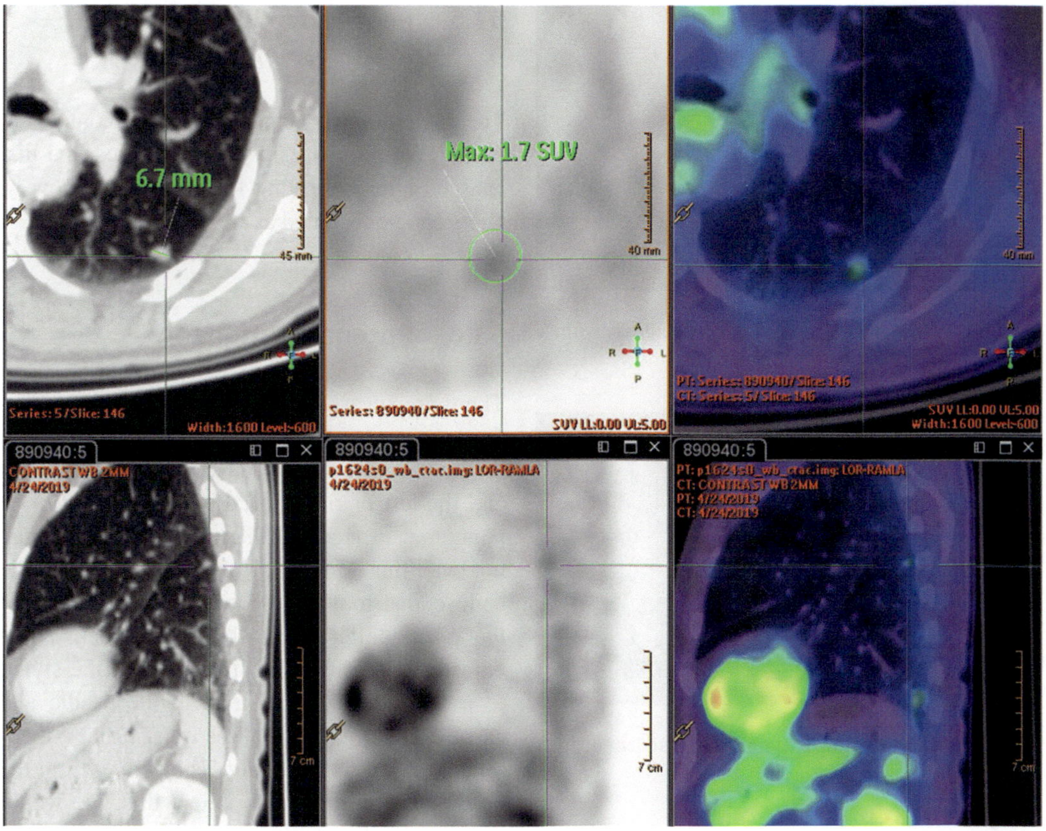

Fig. 53.2 PET-CT showing a 6.7 mm left lung lower lobe lesion with an SUV max of 1.7 suspicious of lung metastasis

1.5 times than that of a lymphocyte. All CTCs are examined under a microscope at 200x magnification and must be quantified by two independent assessors who are blinded from the patient's clinical information.

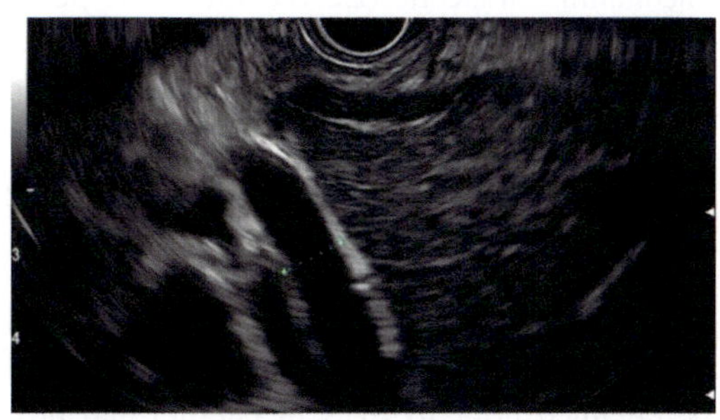

Fig. 53.3 The main portal vein as seen from the stomach under EUS

53.4 Description of the Procedure

The liver would be assessed for the presence of occult metastasis from the duodenum (right lobe) and also the stomach (left lobe). The main portal vein would be identified (Fig. 53.3) (Video 53.1). A 19-gauge nitinol needle would be used for aspiration, the needle is primed with heparin. After verifying flow signal by Doppler ultrasound, the 19-gauge EUS-FNA needle would be advanced trans-hepatically into the main portal vein (Fig. 53.4). The first 10 ml of blood would be discarded as it may be contami-

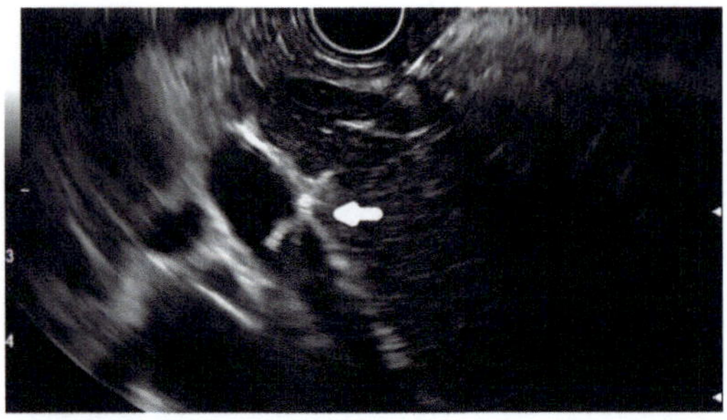

Fig. 53.4 The main portal vein punctured with a 19-gauge needle

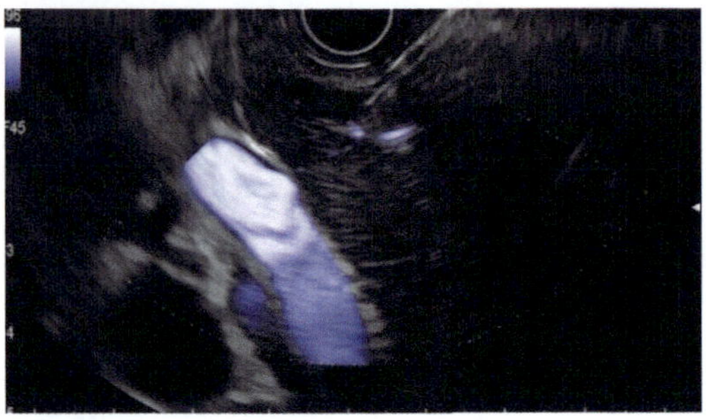

Fig. 53.5 The needle is withdrawn under doppler ultrasound

nated by liver tissue that may interfere with CTC analysis. 20 ml aliquots of portal vein blood would be aspirated and placed in an ethylenediaminetetraacetic (EDTA) tube. The puncture site would then be monitored under doppler EUS for 1 min to observe for any bleeding before the needle is withdrawn (Fig. 53.5). In the unlikely occurrence of bleeding along the needle track, it could be controlled first by pushing out the clot in the needle with the style, followed by injection of histoacryl glue. A paired peripheral blood sample for CTC analysis would be obtained prior to EUS in parallel and processed identically. Recruited patients would have one 10 ml of peripheral blood collected prior to the EUS procedure. The patient would then undergo EUS-PVA and 20 ml of portal venous blood collected.

53.5 Post-Procedural Management

The procedure can be performed on an outpatient basis. Post-procedurally, the patient can be discharged after observing for 2 h in the recovery. Diets can be resumed as well.

53.6 Potential Pitfalls

There are several potential pitfalls to the procedure. As mentioned above, the main portal vein may not be always visualised from the stomach and the left or right portal vein may need to be punctured instead. Furthermore, the needle may not enter the vein after a single puncture, and the endoscopist may need to adjust the position of the needle after removal of the stylet. When adjusting the needle position without the stylet, liver tissue may be trapped in the needle and cause contamination. On the other hand, a theoretical risk of the procedure is bleeding from the needle puncture site. To detect this, we would monitor the puncture site by doppler ultrasound after needle withdrawal. However, in our cohort and published studies, none of the patients suffered from bleeding.

References

1. Zhang L, Riethdorf S, Wu G, Wang T, Yang K, Peng G, et al. Meta-analysis of the prognostic value of circulating tumor cells in breast cancer. Clin Cancer Res. 2012;18(20):5701–10.
2. Scher HI, Jia X, de Bono JS, Fleisher M, Pienta KJ, Raghavan D, et al. Circulating tumour cells as prognostic markers in progressive, castration-resistant prostate cancer: a reanalysis of IMMC38 trial data. Lancet Oncol. 2009;10(3):233–9.
3. Hou JM, Krebs MG, Lancashire L, Sloane R, Backen A, Swain RK, et al. Clinical significance and molecular characteristics of circulating tumor cells and circu-

lating tumor microemboli in patients with small-cell lung cancer. J Clin Oncol Off J Am Soc Clin Oncol. 2012;30(5):525–32.
4. Aggarwal C, Meropol NJ, Punt CJ, Iannotti N, Saidman BH, Sabbath KD, et al. Relationship among circulating tumor cells, CEA and overall survival in patients with metastatic colorectal cancer. Ann Oncol. 2013;24(2):420–8.
5. Bidard FC, Fehm T, Ignatiadis M, Smerage JB, Alix-Panabieres C, Janni W, et al. Clinical application of circulating tumor cells in breast cancer: overview of the current interventional trials. Cancer Metastasis Rev. 2013;32(1–2):179–88.
6. Cohen SJ, Punt CJ, Iannotti N, Saidman BH, Sabbath KD, Gabrail NY, et al. Relationship of circulating tumor cells to tumor response, progression-free survival, and overall survival in patients with metastatic colorectal cancer. J Clin Oncol Off J Am Soc Clin Oncol. 2008;26(19):3213–21.
7. Catenacci DV, Chapman CG, Xu P, Koons A, Konda VJ, Siddiqui UD, et al. Acquisition of portal venous circulating tumor cells from patients with pancreaticobiliary cancers by endoscopic ultrasound. Gastroenterology. 2015;149(7):1794–803.e4.
8. UEG Week 2019 Oral Presentations. United European Gastroenterol J. 2019;7(8_suppl):10–188.

Part XIV

EUS-Guided Variceal Intervention

54 EUS-Guided Esophageal Varices Ablation with Cyanoacrylate

Rafael Romero-Castro
and Angel Caunedo-Alvarez

54.1 Background

Portal hypertension leads to the development of collateral and perforant vessels and the formation of gastroesophageal varices. Bleeding from gastroesophageal varices is the leading cause of mortality in cirrhotic patients [1]. Nowadays, endoscopic variceal ligation (EVL) combined with vasoactive drugs is the first-line therapy [2]. In case of failure, endoscopic injection of CYA could be a bridge therapeutic option while a definitive treatment is available.

Endoscopic injection of CYA could be indicated when massive bleeding precludes EVL. Because of the quick polymerization and hardening of CYA in contact with blood, initial hemostasis rates are superior to 90% [3, 4]. Adverse events could be chest pain, dysphagia, ulcers, glue embolism, sepsis, and damage to the endoscope.

EUS accurately predicts the risk of rebleeding from esophageal varices by displaying patent perforating feeding veins [5]. The inability to reach these perforating with EVL could explain the lower rate of variceal recurrence after endoscopic sclerotherapy [6].

Two studies reporting EUS-guided sclerotherapy of perforating and collateral veins of esophageal varices have been reported [7, 8]. One case series of five patients employed sodium morrhuate injections [7]. In one controlled study with 50 patients 2.5% diluted ethanolamine oleate was used to compare with EUS-guided injection of sclerotherapy [8]. Both studies showed safety and accuracy of EUS-guided injection with a tendency to a lesser rate of recurrence in the EUS-guided group [8].

54.2 Case History

A 68-year old male with severe chronic obstructive pulmonary disease, metastatic lung cancer, alcoholic liver cirrhosis with Child-Pugh B class and, previously diagnosed with large esophageal varices was admitted for hematemesis and hemodynamic instability.

54.3 Procedural Plan

EVL and endoscopic sclerotherapy were not feasible because of poor field of endoscopic vision. Balloon tamponade was not used because of potential severe adverse events [9]. Esophageal covered metal stents have shown greater efficacy

Supplementary Information The online version contains supplementary material available at [https://doi.org/10.1007/978-981-16-9340-3_54].

R. Romero-Castro (✉) · A. Caunedo-Alvarez
Gastroenterology Division, Virgen Macarena University Hospital, Seville, Spain

A. Y.B. Teoh et al. (eds.), *Atlas of Interventional EUS*, https://doi.org/10.1007/978-981-16-9340-3_54

in control of hemorrhage and less adverse events when compared to balloon tamponade [10], however, the device was not available when this patient was admitted. Interventional radiology and surgery were contraindicated.

Hence, a EUS-guided injection of CYA was offered to the patient as the procedure can overcome the issue of poor endoscopic visibility due to massive bleeding.

54.4 Description of the Procedure

The patient was immediately moved from the standard endoscopic room to the adjacent endoscopic suite equipped with EUS and fluoroscopy. We used a EUS-guided approach that was first reported by our group treating gastric varices by injecting CYA and lipiodol in their perforating feeding vessels [11]. Under deep sedation administered by anesthesiologist, a linear-array therapeutic echoendoscope (Video 54.1) is positioned in the fundus and cardia. With slight up and down and clockwise/counter-clockwise movements, two perforating feeding vessels to the esophageal varices were identified (Figs. 54.1 and 54.2). After instilling povidone-iodine in the working channel, a 22-gauge needle was used to puncture each feeder vessel (Fig. 54.3) injecting 1 mL of a mixture (1:1) of CYA (N-butyl-2-cyanoacrylate:

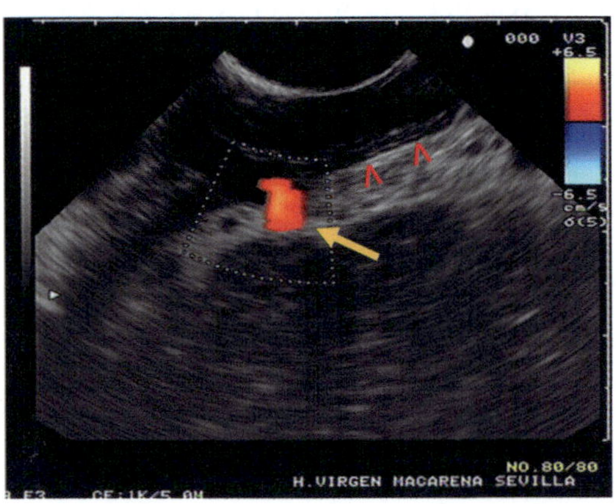

Fig. 54.1 EUS image showing a perforating feeding vein (yellow arrow) penetrating the esophageal wall (red arrowheads)

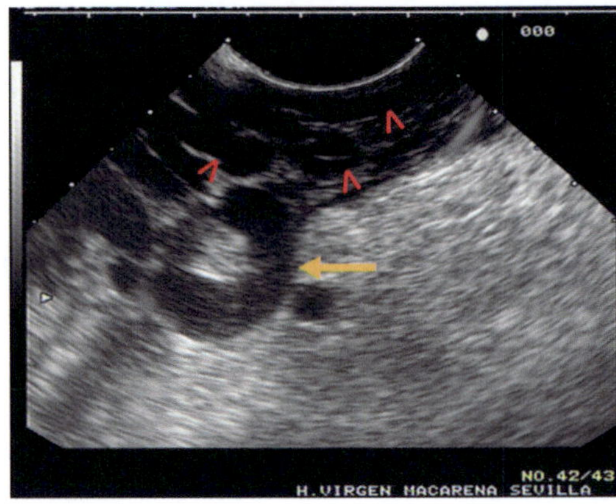

Fig. 54.2 EUS appearance of the feeder vessel (yellow arrow) and the esophageal varices (red arrowheads)

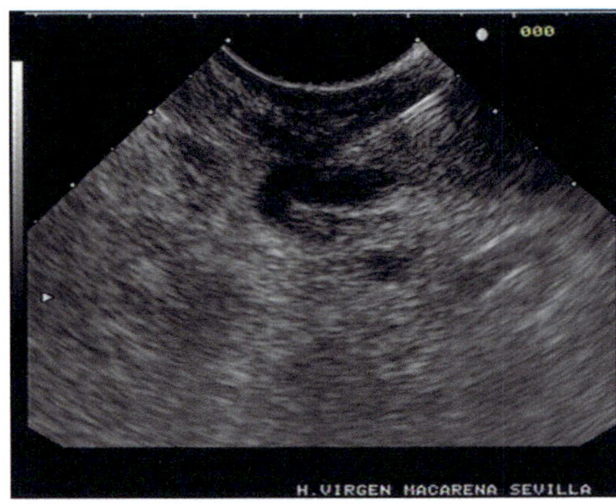

Fig. 54.3 EUS-guided injection of CYA mixed with lipiodol with a 22-gauge needle at the level of the perforating feeding vessel to the esophageal varices

histoacryl®) and lipiodol followed by flushing 2 mL of distilled water to remove the remained glue (Figs. 54.4 and 54.5).

54.5 Post-Procedural Management

Hemostasis was obtained and hemodynamic stability achieved. Antibiotics were continued. The clinical outcome was uneventful and the patient was discharged following scheduled secondary prophylaxis with EVL. The patient died five months later due to the progression of metastatic lung cancer.

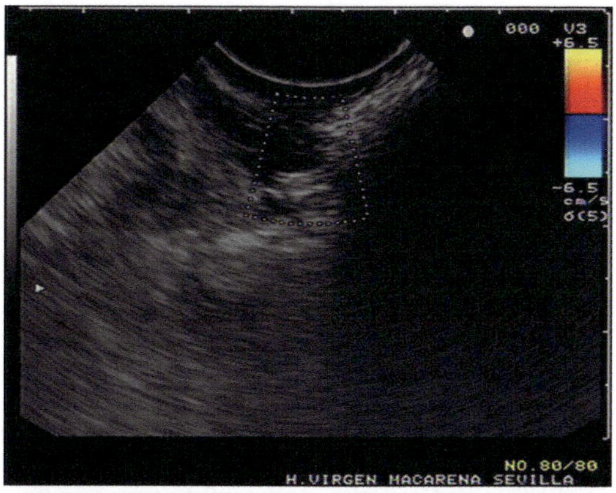

Fig. 54.4 Endosonographic image without blood flow displaying the cast formed after the EUS-guided injection of the mixture of CYA and lipiodol

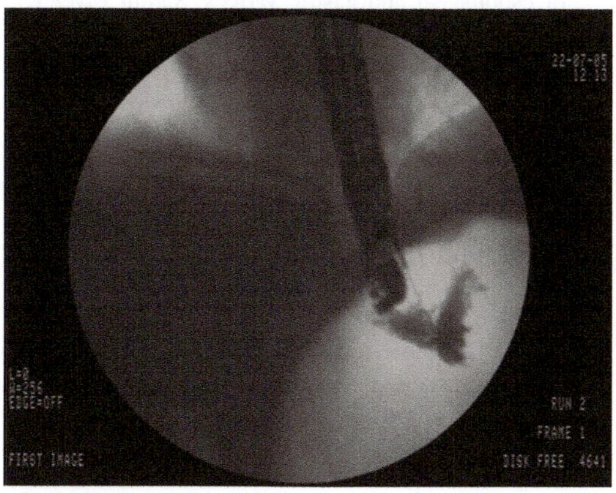

Fig. 54.5 Fluoroscopic image showing the cast of CYA and lipiodol

54.6 Potential Pitfalls

The main pitfalls are related to the glue injection. Adverse events could be systemic (embolism and septicemia) and local (ulcers). However, EUS-guided injection of CYA requires lesser amounts of CYA than conventional endoscopic injection [11] minimizing the risk of embolism. Nevertheless, a high rate of asymptomatic glue embolism of 47% [12] and 50% [13] after EUS-guided injection of CYA of gastric varices has been reported. Moreover, the risk of injection of the esophageal wall and further ulceration and rebleeding from a non-fully obliterated varix is minimized by the real-time injection into the feeding vein. The echoendoscope should be in a straight and stable position to prevent tear the vessel.

EUS-guided therapy requires a skilled endosonographer, well-trained auxiliary personnel and facilities with the appropriate equipment. Fluoroscopy is advisable to ascertain that the target vessel is from the afferent feeding vessel. This can be confirmed after injecting contrast to delineate the blood flow direction. Fluoroscopy also helps in checking if the echoendoscope is in a straight position.

The theoretical risk of damage to the echoendoscope due to the glue is much lesser than in conventional endoscopic injections for two reasons. Firstly, the needle is withdrawn into its outer sheath after injecting the glue. Secondly, it is much easier to have problems with the injector during a conventional endoscopy in a cumbersome retroflexion position with the fundus full of blood.

Esophageal varices are usually formed by several perforating feeding vessels [14]. On the contrary as esophageal varices, collaterals and perforating are easily identified by EUS. Therefore, therapy should be aimed at treating every displayed perforating to obliterate all esophageal varices. Despite the lack of strong scientific levels of evidence there is a growing experience in EUS-guided vascular therapy [15–21].

We report this anecdotal case performed as far as in 2005, in a patient with limited therapeutic options to show the potential advantages of this EUS-guided procedure. Its main drawback, although amenable, would be the lack of widespread availability outside referral centers with local expertise. EUS-guided vascular interventions are another step forward in endoscopy in achieving hemostasis, in a safe and accurate way to treat a wide spectrum of dire clinical situations, avoiding more invasive procedures.

Acknowledgments We thank Ms. Ursula Feore for her kind revision of the English manuscript and Dr. Francisco Pellicer-Bautista for his magistery.

References

1. de Franchis R, Primignani M. Natural history of portal hypertension in patients with cirrhosis. Clin Liver Dis. 2001;5(3):645–63.
2. de Franchis R. Expanding consensus in portal hypertension: report of the Baveno VI consensus workshop: stratifying risk and individualizing care for portal hypertension. J Hepatol. 2015;63(3):743–52.
3. Ibrahim M, El-Mikkawy A, Abdel Hamid M, Abdalla H, Lemmers A, Mostafa I, et al. Early application of haemostatic powder added to standard management for oesophagogastric variceal bleeding: a randomised trial. Gut. 2019;68(5):844–53.
4. Elsebaey MA, Tawfik MA, Ezzat S, Selim A, Elashry H, Abd-Elsalam S. Endoscopic injection sclerotherapy versus N-Butyl-2 cyanoacrylate injection in the management of actively bleeding esophageal varices: a randomized controlled trial. BMC Gastroenterol. 2019;19(1):23.
5. Irisawa A, Saito A, Obara K, Shibukawa G, Takagi T, Shishido H, et al. Endoscopic recurrence of esophageal varices is associated with the specific EUS abnormalities: severe periesophageal collateral veins and large perforating veins. Gastrointest Endosc. 2001;53(1):77–84.
6. Boregowda U, Umapathy C, Halim N, Desai M, Nanjappa A, Arekapudi S, et al. Update on the management of gastrointestinal varices. World J Gastrointest Pharmacol Ther. 2019;10(1):1–21.
7. Lahoti S, Catalano MF, Alcocer E, Hogan WJ, Geenen JE. Obliteration of esophageal varices using EUS-guided sclerotherapy with color Doppler. Gastrointest Endosc. 2000;51(3):331–3.
8. de Paulo GA, Ardengh JC, Nakao FS, Ferrari AP. Treatment of esophageal varices: a randomized controlled trial comparing endoscopic sclerotherapy and EUS-guided sclerotherapy of esophageal collateral veins. Gastrointest Endosc. 2006;63(3):396–402. quiz 63
9. Panes J, Teres J, Bosch J, Rodes J. Efficacy of balloon tamponade in treatment of bleeding gastric and esophageal varices. Results in 151 consecutive episodes. Dig Dis Sci. 1988;33(4):454–9.
10. Escorsell A, Pavel O, Cardenas A, Morillas R, Llop E, Villanueva C, et al. Esophageal balloon tamponade versus esophageal stent in controlling acute refractory variceal bleeding: a multicenter randomized, controlled trial. Hepatology. 2016;63(6):1957–67.
11. Romero-Castro R, Pellicer-Bautista FJ, Jimenez-Saenz M, Marcos-Sanchez F, Caunedo-Alvarez A, Ortiz-Moyano C, et al. EUS-guided injection of cyanoacrylate in perforating feeding veins in gastric varices: results in 5 cases. Gastrointest Endosc. 2007;66(2):402–7.
12. Romero-Castro R, Ellrichmann M, Ortiz-Moyano C, Subtil-Inigo JC, Junquera-Florez F, Gornals JB, et al. EUS-guided coil versus cyanoacrylate therapy for the treatment of gastric varices: a multicenter study (with videos). Gastrointest Endosc. 2013;78(5):711–21.
13. Lobo MRA, Chaves DM, DE Moura DTH, Ribeiro IB, Ikari E, DE Moura EGH. Safety and efficacy of EUS-guided coil plus cyanoacrylate versus conventional cyanoacrylate technique in the treatment of gastric varices: a randomized controlled trial. Arq Gastroenterol. 2019;56:99–105.
14. Arakawa M, Masuzaki T, Okuda K. Pathomorphology of esophageal and gastric varices. Semin Liver Dis. 2002;22(1):73–82.
15. Ryozawa S, Fujita N, Irisawa A, Hirooka Y, Mine T. Current status of interventional endoscopic ultrasound. Dig Endosc. 2017;29(5):559–66.
16. Hall PS, Teshima C, May GR, Mosko JD. Endoscopic ultrasound-guided vascular therapy: the present and the future. Clin Endosc. 2017;50(2):138–42.
17. Siddiqui UD, Levy MJ. EUS-guided transluminal interventions. Gastroenterology. 2018;154(7):1911–24.
18. Levy I, Binmoeller KF. EUS-guided vascular interventions. Endosc Ultrasound. 2018;7(4):228–35.
19. Oleas R, Robles-Medranda C. Insights into the role of endoscopic ultrasound-guided vascular therapy. Ther Adv Gastrointest Endosc. 2019;12:2631774519878282.
20. Mohan BP, Chandan S, Khan SR, Kassab LL, Trakroo S, Ponnada S, et al. Efficacy and safety of endoscopic ultrasound-guided therapy versus direct endoscopic glue injection therapy for gastric varices: systematic review and meta-analysis. Endoscopy. 2020;52(4):259–67.
21. McCarty TR, Bazarbashi AN, Hathorn KE, Thompson CC, Ryou M. Combination therapy versus monotherapy for EUS-guided management of gastric varices: a systematic review and meta-analysis. Endosc Ultrasound. 2020;9(1):6–15.

55 EUS-Guided Venography in Gastric Varices: Anatomic and Hemodynamic Aspects

Rafael Romero-Castro
and Victoria Alejandra Jimenez-Garcia

55.1 Background

Since the first report of EUS-guided therapy of Dieulafoy lesions [1] to the puncture of right atrial masses [2], EUS-guided vascular interventions are applied in a widening spectrum of vascular disorders. Life-threatening hemorrhage from GV requires immediate, safe, and accurate hemostatic therapy. There are several therapeutic options, including endoscopic, interventional vascular radiology and surgical procedures. Direct endoscopic injection of cyanoacrylate (CYA) reported by Soehendra [3] has been the recommended procedure due to its efficacy in obtaining initial hemostasis [4, 5]. Nevertheless, serious life-threatening adverse events, mainly glue embolism, preclude its generalized use in the USA.

To minimize adverse events, lower the rate of rebleeding and to overcome several flaws of direct endoscopic injection of CYA, EUS-guided injection of CYA [6] or EUS-guided deployment of coils in gastric [7] or ectopic varices [8] were developed. Since then, there has been a worldwide growing experience supporting the use of EUS-guided therapy of GV [9]. A recent meta-analysis of 23 studies encompassing 851 patients concluded EUS-guided therapy of GV was clinically effective regarding obliteration, recurrence and long-term rebleeding and being superior to endoscopic injection of CYA with fewer adverse events [10].

The anatomical classifications of GV by Sarin [11] (Table 55.1) and Arakawa [12] (Table 55.2)

Table 55.1 Classification of gastric varices of Sarin [11]

Type		Description
Gastroesophageal varices	Type 1 (GOV1)	Gastric varices located in the lesser curvature, continuing with esophageal varices.
	Type 2 (GOV2)	Gastric varices that extend through the fundus, the greater curvature, continuing with esophageal varices.
Isolated gastric varices	Type 1 (IGV1)	Isolated gastric varices located in the fundus, excluding those caused by thrombosis of the splenic vein.
	Type 2 (IGV2)	Isolated gastric varices in locations other than the gastric fundus.

Note: It is based on the presence or absence of concomitant esophageal varices and on the topographic location of gastric varices in the stomach

Supplementary Information The online version contains supplementary material available at [https://doi.org/10.1007/978-981-16-9340-3_55].

R. Romero-Castro (✉) · V. A. Jimenez-Garcia
Gastroenterology Division, Virgen Macarena University Hospital, Seville, Spain

A. Y.B. Teoh et al. (eds.), *Atlas of Interventional EUS*, https://doi.org/10.1007/978-981-16-9340-3_55

Table 55.2 Morphological classification of gastric varices of Arakawa [12]

Type	Description
Localized varices Type I	Gastric varices are formed by one single vessel with a uniform caliber, nourished by an afferent feeding vein that penetrates the muscular layer of the gastric wall and winds up into the submucosal layer. This single vessel emerges from the gastric wall formed by a single efferent vessel, draining generally in the left renal vein, establishing a gastrorenal shunt.
Diffuse varices Type II	Varices formed by a net of vessels with multiple interconnections between them and receiving the blood supply within the stomach from different veins.

are keys to treatment and provide prognostic information. GOV1 are treated as esophageal varices with band ligation. However, GOV2, IGV1, and IGV2 should be treated with other methods as band ligation could be harmful. The localized type I GV (Fig. 55.1, Video 55.1) has lower rates of rebleeding and mortality than diffuse type II (Fig. 55.2). While, the rate of blood flow is also directly related to the increased diameter of GV [13].

There are different approaches to EUS-guided therapy of GV and the type of GV amenable for EUS-guided treatment are shown in Table 55.3.

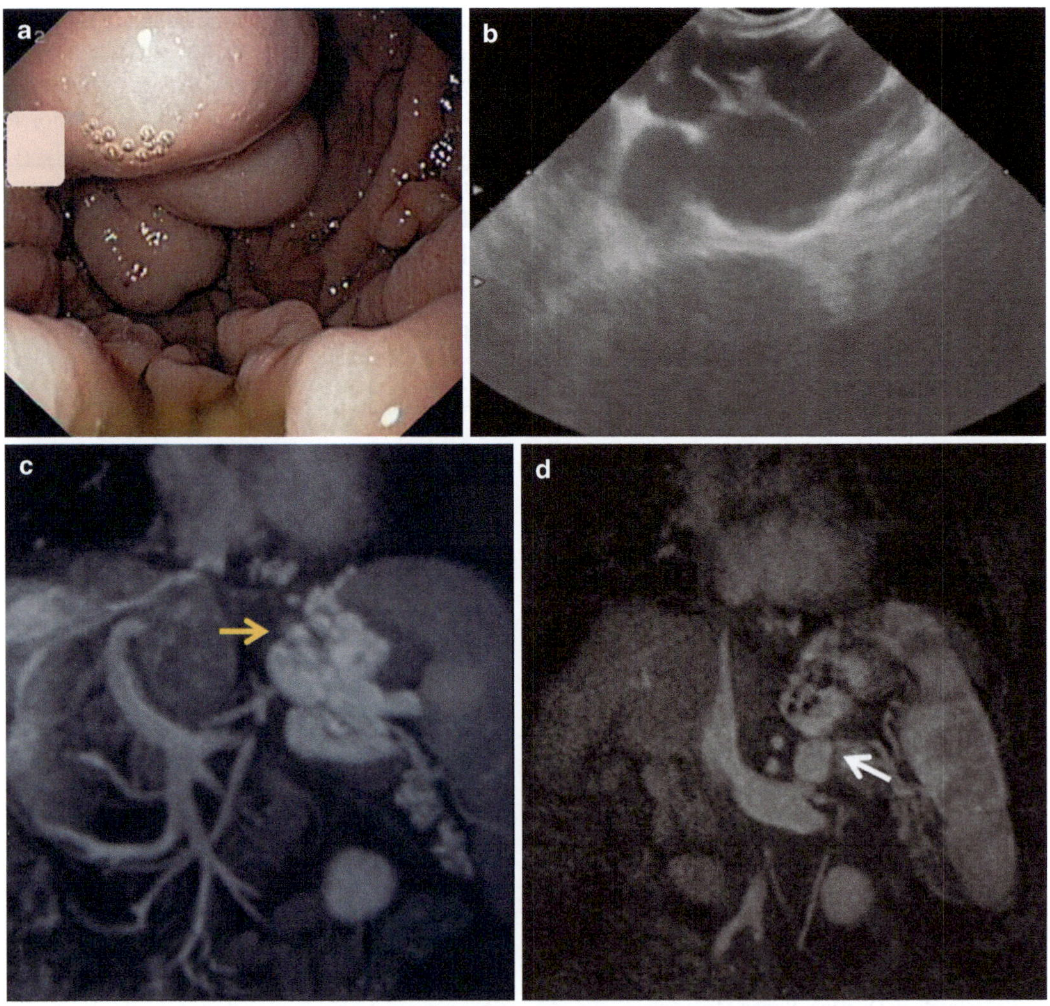

Fig. 55.1 Localized type I GV. (**a**) Endoscopic image of GV (IGV1). (**b**) Endosonographic appearance of GV. (**c** and **d**) MRI images showing large GV (yellow arrow) and a huge gastrorenal shunt (white arrow)

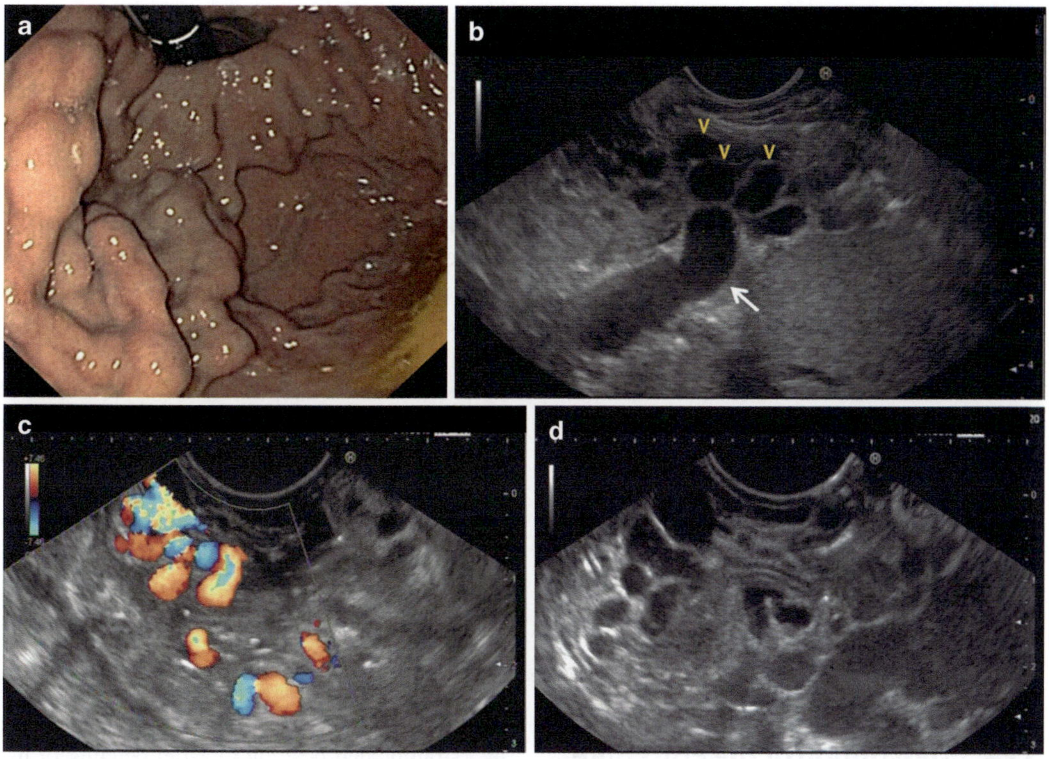

Fig. 55.2 Diffuse type II GV. (**a**) Endoscopic image. (**b**) Endosonographic appearance of diffuse GV showing the perforating feeding vein (white arrow) and the network of vessels within the gastric wall (yellow arrowheads). (**c** and **d**) Another examples of diffuse GV

Table 55.3 Gastric varices (Type I: IGV1, IGV2, and GOV2) amenable for EUS-guided treatment and therapeutic approaches

EUS-Guided approach	
Target	*Perforant* feeding vein puncture
	Gastric varices puncture
Obliteration methods	Injection of CYA
	Coil deployment
	Combined method: Coils + CYA

The combined method targeting gastric varices developed by Binmoeller et al. [14] is the most popular method with the largest worldwide experience [15], and EUS-guided therapy is increasingly performed worldwide as it is safe and accurate [9, 10, 16–18]. However, concerns on safety were raised after the results of two studies using CYA mixed with lipiodol and performing a chest CT-scan later. In one multicenter study [19] comparing EUS-guided injection of CYA plus lipiodol with EUS-guided deployment of coils, a statistically significant higher rate of adverse events in the CYA group (58% vs. 9%) was observed, with 9 out of 19 patients (47%) developing pulmonary glue embolism. One randomized study [20] comparing patients treated with endoscopic injection of CYA with patients treated with the combination technique of coil deployment and injection of CYA found pulmonary glue embolism in 50% and 25%, respectively. Although all the patients in both studies remained asymptomatic, this is still a potentially harmful adverse event.

We present some hemodynamics and anatomic findings of EUS-guided venography performed during several procedures of EUS-guided therapy of GV employing only coils.

55.2 Case History

Patients referred for EUS-guided therapy for active or recent episodes of bleeding GV, localized type I and IGV1 or GOV2.

55.3 Procedural Plan

Options of GV treatment include endoscopic, interventional vascular radiology and surgical procedures. In our referral center, due to its safety profile, accuracy, and availability, EUS-guided therapy (targeting the perforator and deploying coils exclusively) is the first-line therapy for active bleeding GV in the emergency setting or in case of secondary prophylaxis after a bleeding episode. In cases of large GV with red signs and patients with poor liver function, primary prophylaxis is also offered.

55.4 Description of the Procedure

The procedure is performed in an endoscopic suite under fluoroscopy with deep sedation controlled by an anesthesiologist and antibiotic prophylaxis. The feeding vessel is targeted, usually following the celiac trunk and rotating the probe in clock and counter-clockwise movements, at the level of the upper stomach or lower part of the esophagus (Fig. 55.3, Video 55.1). Povidone-iodine is instilled in the working channel of a therapeutic linear array echoendoscope. EUS-guided venography is performed after the puncture of the feeding vessel with a 19-gauge needle immediately before its entry into the gastric wall forming the GV. Then, we inject pure contrast or lipiodol to assess the blood flow direction (Video 55.1). We usually employed 0.035″ haired coils (Nester, Cook Medical, Limerick Ireland). We deploy the coils in the perforating feeding vessel just before it penetrates the muscle layer aiming that the thick gastric wall itself facilitates the obliteration of the blood flow. The diameter of the coils should be 20% more than the feeding vein and are deployed as much as needed to obtain a thick mesh that blocks the afferent flow. The length of the coils are usually 20 cm to create a thick mesh and employing lesser number of coils. The procedure is finished when a thick mesh of coils is observed and there is no more room to deploy more coils, even of smaller diameters. All of these endoscopic maneuvers have to be performed with the echoendoscope in a straightened position to avoid bending of the needle. Also, one should avoid up and down movements when the needle is inside the vessel in order to avoid its tearing of the vessel.

Then, another EUS-guided venography is performed to check blood is clotted in the vessel before ending the procedure and removing the needle. Occasionally, in some cases, even after a thick mesh was placed (even after deploying up to eight coils), blood flow still remained patent

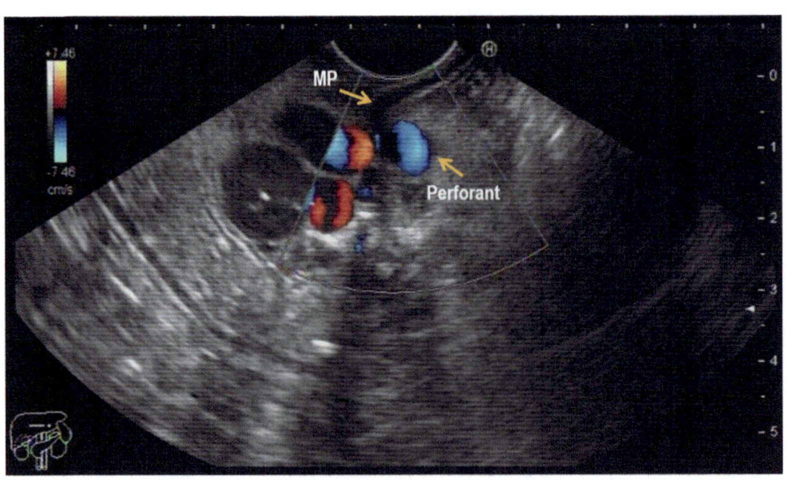

Fig. 55.3 Perforating feeding vein entering the muscularis propria (MP) of the gastric wall in type I localized GV (MP: muscularis propria)

(Figs. 55.4 and 55.5, Video 55.1). For this reason, we avoid the use of CYA in order to nullify any possibility of potential harmful glue embolism. EUS-guided therapy of GV also has the added advantage to accurately display the veins even in cases with massive hemorrhage without the need for endoscopic vision as blood and clots will not hamper the EUS images.

55.5 Post-Procedural Management

Management takes place in a multidisciplinary setting to also treat the underlying syndrome of portal hypertension [21]. One second EUS is scheduled one week later. If there are still patent GV, another EUS-guided therapy with coils is performed and the patient enters in a follow-up program.

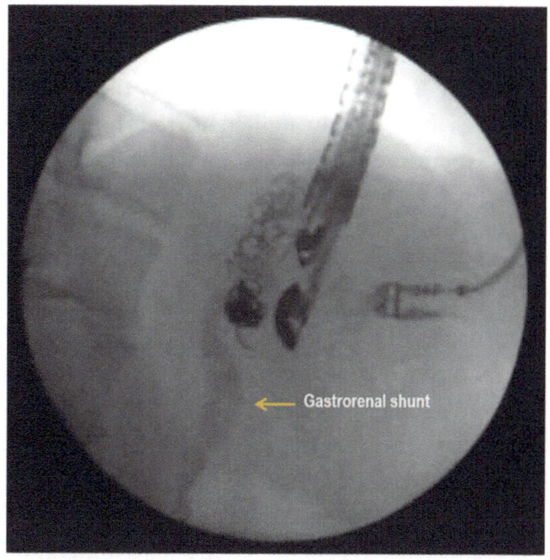

Fig. 55.4 EUS-guided venography displaying a gastrorenal shunt. Contrast flows through eight previously deployed coils. One week later, complete thrombosis and obliteration of GV was confirmed by endoscopy and endosonography with color Doppler

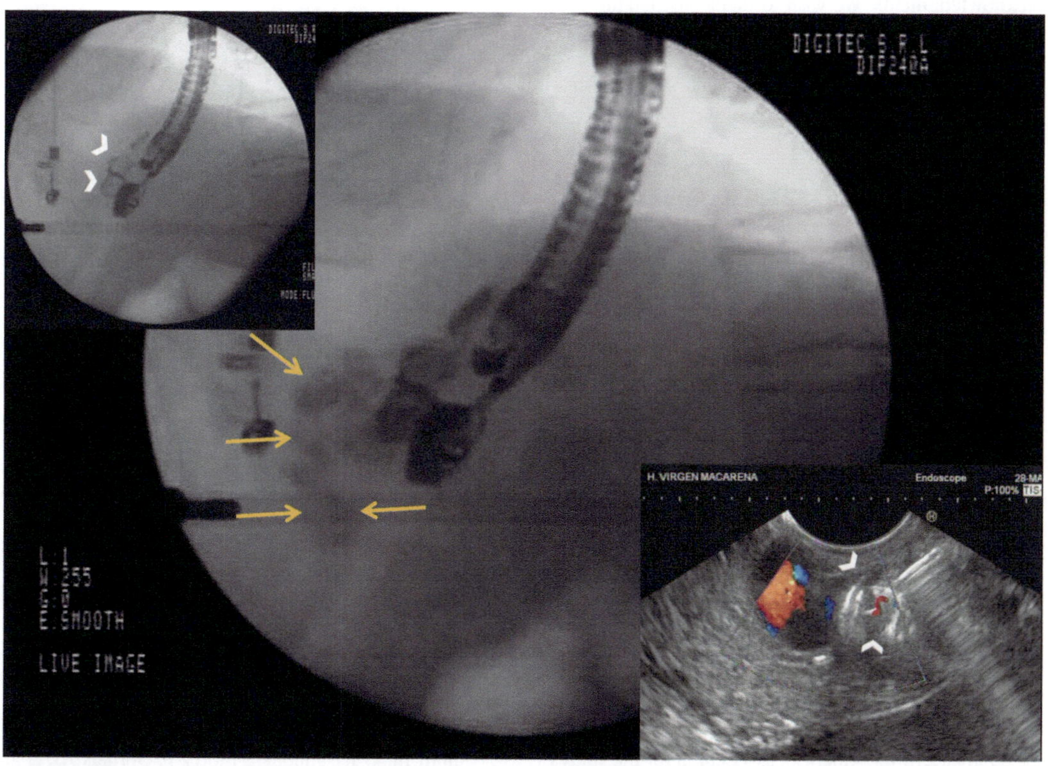

Fig. 55.5 Despite the deployment of eight coils (white arrowheads), there is still patent blood flow and the contrast flows towards the gastrorenal shunt (yellow arrows) as shown by EUS-guided venography. Complete thrombosis and obliteration of GV was confirmed by endoscopy and endosonography with Doppler during scheduled EUS performed one week later

55.6 Potential Pitfalls

The main drawback is the availability of the technique as it is mainly limited to referral centers with experienced endosonographers and auxiliary personnel and endoscopic rooms with fluoroscopy. However, these procedures are increasingly performed [9, 10, 17, 18, 22]. The afferent feeding vein is accurately identified, usually located around the celiac trunk area in the upper part of the fundus and confirmed by EUS-guided venography. We think these hemodynamic and anatomical findings raise some theoretical concerns on the use of CYA, even when combined with previously deployed coils. We should be aware of what could happen when CYA is injected in such a high blood flow volume system, even when a large number of coils are deployed. Well-designed controlled studies would clarify what is the safest EUS-guided approach.

Acknowledgments We wish to thank Ms. Ursula Feore for her kind revision of the English manuscript.

We are devoted to the loving memory of professor Juan Manuel Herrerias-Gutierrez and Dr. Francisco Marcos-Sanchez.

References

1. Fockens P, Meenan J, van Dullemen HM, Bolwerk CJ, Tytgat GN. Dieulafoy's disease: endosonographic detection and endosonography-guided treatment. Gastrointest Endosc. 1996;44(4):437–42.
2. Romero-Castro R, Rios-Martin JJ, Jimenez-Garcia VA, Pellicer-Bautista F, Hergueta-Delgado P. EUS-FNA of 2 right atrial masses. VideoGIE. 2019;4(7):323–4.
3. Soehendra N, Nam VC, Grimm H, Kempeneers I. Endoscopic obliteration of large esophagogastric varices with bucrylate. Endoscopy. 1986;18(1):25–6.
4. de Franchis R. Expanding consensus in portal hypertension: report of the Baveno VI consensus workshop: stratifying risk and individualizing care for portal hypertension. J Hepatol. 2015;63(3):743–52.
5. Garcia-Tsao G, Abraldes JG, Berzigotti A, Bosch J. Portal hypertensive bleeding in cirrhosis: risk stratification, diagnosis, and management: 2016 practice guidance by the American association for the study of liver diseases. Hepatology. 2017;65(1):310–35.
6. Romero-Castro R, Pellicer-Bautista FJ, Jimenez-Saenz M, Marcos-Sanchez F, Caunedo-Alvarez A, Ortiz-Moyano C, et al. EUS-guided injection of cyanoacrylate in perforating feeding veins in gastric varices: results in 5 cases. Gastrointest Endosc. 2007;66(2):402–7.
7. Romero-Castro R, Pellicer-Bautista F, Giovannini M, Marcos-Sanchez F, Caparros-Escudero C, Jimenez-Saenz M, et al. Endoscopic ultrasound (EUS)-guided coil embolization therapy in gastric varices. Endoscopy. 2010;42(Suppl 2):E35–6.
8. Levy MJ, Wong Kee Song LM, Kendrick ML, Misra S, Gostout CJ. EUS-guided coil embolization for refractory ectopic variceal bleeding (with videos). Gastrointest Endosc. 2008;67(3):572–4.
9. Hall PS, Teshima C, May GR, Mosko JD. Endoscopic ultrasound-guided vascular therapy: the present and the future. Clin Endosc. 2017;50(2):138–42.
10. Mohan BP, Chandan S, Khan SR, Kassab LL, Trakroo S, Ponnada S, et al. Efficacy and safety of endoscopic ultrasound-guided therapy versus direct endoscopic glue injection therapy for gastric varices: systematic review and meta-analysis. Endoscopy. 2020;52(4):259–67.
11. Sarin SK, Kumar A. Gastric varices: profile, classification, and management. Am J Gastroenterol. 1989;84(10):1244–9.
12. Arakawa M, Masuzaki T, Okuda K. Pathomorphology of esophageal and gastric varices. Semin Liver Dis. 2002;22(1):73–82.
13. Imamura H, Irisawa A, Shibukawa G, Takagi T, Hikichi T, Obara K, et al. Echo-endoscopic analysis of variceal hemodynamics in patient with isolated gastric varices. Endosc Ultrasound. 2014;3(4):238–44.
14. Binmoeller KF, Weilert F, Shah JN, Kim J. EUS-guided transesophageal treatment of gastric fundal varices with combined coiling and cyanoacrylate glue injection (with videos). Gastrointest Endosc. 2011;74(5):1019–25.
15. Bhat YM, Weilert F, Fredrick RT, Kane SD, Shah JN, Hamerski CM, et al. EUS-guided treatment of gastric fundal varices with combined injection of coils and cyanoacrylate glue: a large U.S. experience over 6 years (with video). Gastrointest Endosc. 2016;83(6):1164–72.
16. Levy I, Binmoeller KF. EUS-guided vascular interventions. Endosc Ultrasound. 2018;7(4):228–35.
17. Oleas R, Robles-Medranda C. Insights into the role of endoscopic ultrasound-guided vascular therapy. Ther Adv Gastrointest Endosc. 2019;12:2631774519878282.
18. McCarty TR, Bazarbashi AN, Hathorn KE, Thompson CC, Ryou M. Combination therapy versus monotherapy for EUS-guided management of gastric varices: a systematic review and meta-analysis. Endosc Ultrasound. 2020;9(1):6–15.
19. Romero-Castro R, Ellrichmann M, Ortiz-Moyano C, Subtil-Inigo JC, Junquera-Florez F, Gornals JB, et al. EUS-guided coil versus cyanoacrylate therapy for the treatment of gastric varices: a multicenter study (with videos). Gastrointest Endosc. 2013;78(5):711–21.

20. Lobo MRA, Chaves DM, DE Moura DTH, Ribeiro IB, Ikari E, DE Moura EGH. Safety and efficacy of EUS-guided coil plus cyanoacrylate versus conventional cyanoacrylate technique in the treatment of gastric varices: a randomized controlled trial. Arq Gastroenterol. 2019;56:99–105.
21. Laleman W. Endoscopic ultrasound-guided intervention for gastric varices: sticky stuff might not (yet) be enough. Endoscopy. 2020;52(4):244–6.
22. Siddiqui UD, Levy MJ. EUS-guided transluminal interventions. Gastroenterology. 2018;154(7):1911–24.

56 EUS-Guided Gastric Variceal Ablation with Coils

Rajesh Puri and Zubin Sharma

56.1 Background

EUS-guided variceal therapy has emerged in the last decade as it offers significant advantages over the conventional endoscopic therapy. Bleeding from gastric varices is usually severe and is associated with significant mortality and morbidity. It is also associated with significant rebleeding rates with conventional therapy [1, 2]. The current standard of care is endoscopic injection using cyanoacrylate, which is associated with higher homeostasis rate and lower rebleeding as compared to band ligation or sclerotherapy. But at the same time, it is also associated with adverse events like embolization, fever, rebleeding, and rarely death [3]. Scope damage, inadequate obliteration and multiple therapeutic sessions are added difficulties in conventional therapy.

EUS-guided Ablation therapy using coils is associated with fewer adverse events. It was initially described by Romero-Castro et al. in five cases [4] as independent therapy. It can be combined with cyanoacrylate therapy leading to higher obliteration rate and less adverse events. The first study for the same was done by Binmoeller et al. [5], who showed in 30 patients that the procedure is highly successful with 95.8% Obliteration rate. Subsequently in another large group of 152 patients by Bhat et al. [6], this combined approach was shown to have 93% success rate and only a 3% rebleeding rate. However, this was a retrospective study. In 2020, a randomized controlled trial was done by Carlos Robles-Medranda et al. [7], which compared two groups of 30 patients, each randomized to EUS-guided Coil Embolization and cyanoacrylate injection or coil embolization alone. The technical success rate was 100% in both the groups. With combined treatment, 83.3% of patients were free from reintervention versus 60% with coils alone. They concluded that combination therapy is better for lower rates of rebleeding and reintervention rate. This was a single center study, but still provides strong evidence towards combination therapy.

56.2 Case History

A 56-year-old male patient with known history of hepatitis B induced cirrhosis with hepatocellular carcinoma and portal vein thrombosis. His cirrhosis was Child's C decompensated cirrhosis with ascites with portal hypertension. The patient presented with hematemesis. Patient had previously bled from gastric varices for which endotherapy

Supplementary Information The online version contains supplementary material available at [https://doi.org/10.1007/978-981-16-9340-3_56].

R. Puri (✉) · Z. Sharma
Institute of Digestive and Hepatobiliary Sciences, Medanta Hospital, Gurugram, India

A. Y.B. Teoh et al. (eds.), *Atlas of Interventional EUS*, https://doi.org/10.1007/978-981-16-9340-3_56

using cyanoacrylate glue was performed twice. TIPS was not offered due to the presence of portal vein thrombosis. Patient was initially managed in the emergency with fluid resuscitation, blood replacement and antibiotics. After stabilization, the patient was taken up for Upper endoscopy, which showed large GOV2 gastric varices with size more than 2 cm and signs of recent bleed. In view of large size, EUS-guided coil and glue injection were offered to the patient.

56.3 Procedural Plan

Initially the varices are to be evaluated with standard endoscopy. After evaluation, EUS examination is done. The stomach is usually filled approximately 125–150 ml of saline, and the varices are assessed on their size, flow rates on color doppler and location of perforating vessels supply the varices. Then, the optimal method of EUS-guided coil ablation can be decided—the trans-esophageal-trans crural approach or the trans-gastric approach. In trans-esophageal approach, the scope is relatively stable and facilitates the puncture. It is beneficial only for varices near to cardia. For all other varices, trans-gastric approach is needed.

The choice of needle is made depending on the coil we are using. Coils are synthetic strands attached to metal coils. They lead to coagulation in the varix and also provide a scaffold for the glue to act locally. As coil diameters range from 2 mm to 20 mm, a 19G needle is needed if we intend to use >10 mm coils. The size of coil used is approximately 1.2 times bigger than the diameter of varix. N-actyl cyanoacrylate or N-octyl cyanoacrylate can be used as glue through the same needle used for puncture. N-actyl cyanoacrylate may require prior lipoidal injection along with the glue to delay polymerization.

56.4 Description of the Procedure

After ascertaining the appropriate approach, the puncture is made (Video 56.1). The needle used is dependent on size of varix. In our case, as the size of varix is 3.5 cm with septa, we used a 19G needle. The needle is primed with 5% dextrose. After puncturing the varix, aspiration can be done to confirm the presence of blood which confirms the right position. The needle is reflushed with 5% dextrose to prevent clotting. We use the embolization coils which are between 5–18 mm in diameter and 7–14 cm in length (Cook Medical, Bloomington, USA). Following this, the needle style is used to push the coils into the varix. Using the same needle, cyanoacrylate glue diluted with lipoidal in a 1:1 ratio is injected into the lumen, which is to be done slowly. After the procedure, hemostasis is checked and flow of the blood in varix is checked using doppler. There should be a lack of active bleeding and absent flow during doppler examination. The needle is withdrawn into the sheath. Following this, the entire scope is taken out to prevent any scope damage.

56.5 Post-Procedural Management

Diets are usually resumed 6 h after the procedure as it is done under anesthesia. Clear liquid diet is initially started and increased as tolerated. Hemoglobin is monitored. One more dose of antibiotics (third-generation cephalosporin) is usually given. If the patient remains stable, they can be usually discharged by the second day. Repeat endoscopy after 4 weeks is usually arranged to assess for the presence of residue varices.

56.6 Potential Pitfalls

The potential pitfalls for EUS-guided coil deployment are few. The first pressure point would be localization of the feeder vessels for which proper anatomic evaluation should be done. Secondly, the puncture has to be appropriate. Glue injection has its associated issues of embolization and local extrusion. Rarely, bleeding can happen from the puncture site. It is usually mild and controlled. Scope damage due to glue is another issue (Figs. 56.1, 56.2, 56.3, 56.4, 56.5, 56.6, 56.7 and 56.8).

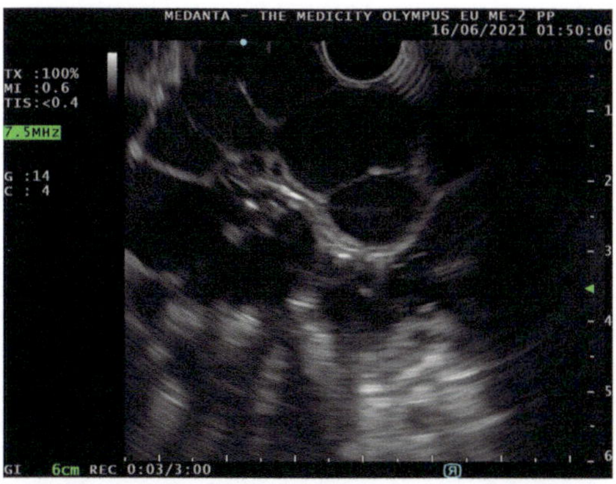

Fig. 56.1 EUS image showing gastric varices

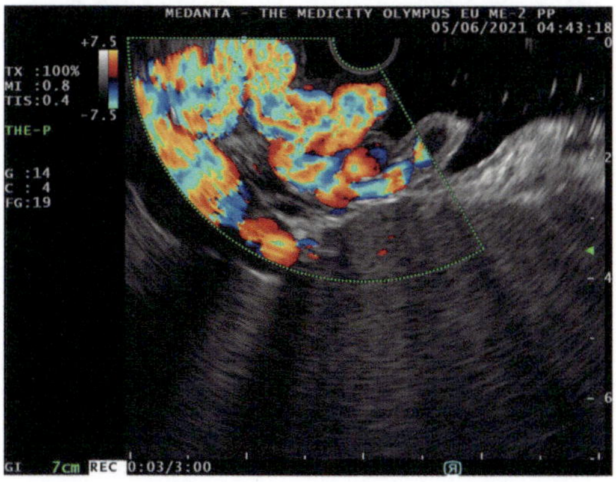

Fig. 56.2 EUS doppler image showing similar varices

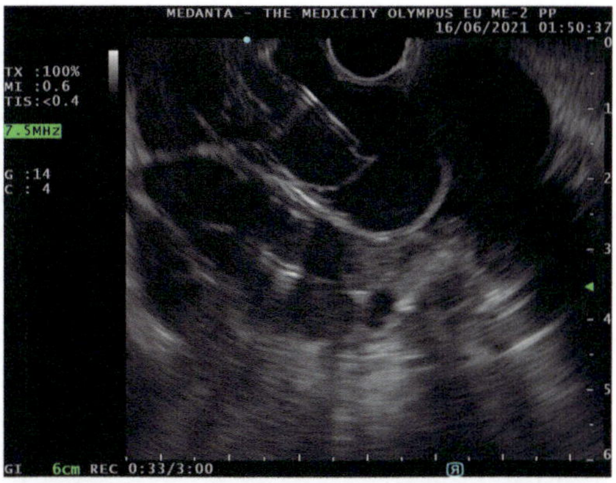

Fig. 56.3 EUS image showing needle puncture of varix

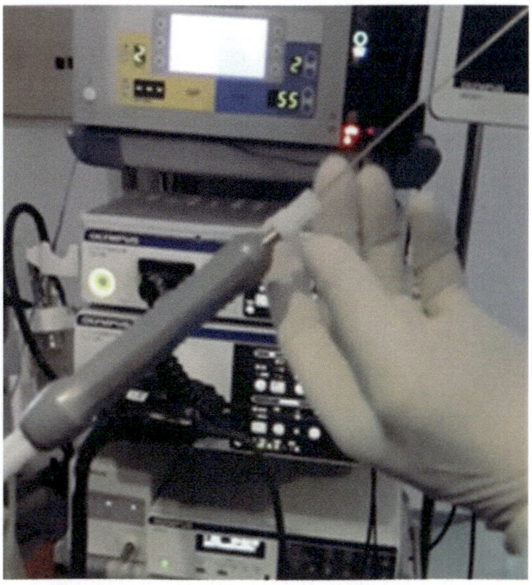

Fig. 56.4 Insertion of coils in the needle

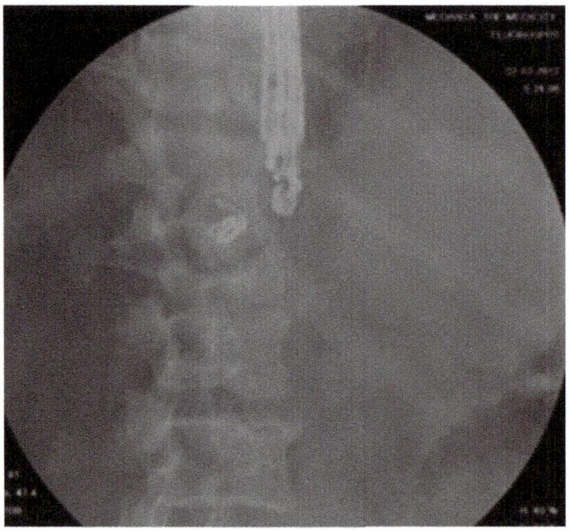

Fig. 56.5 Fluoroscopy image showing coils being deployed

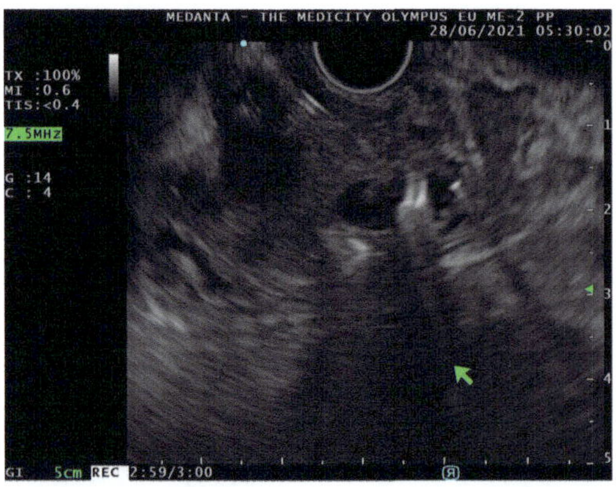

Fig. 56.6 EUS image showing coil being deployed

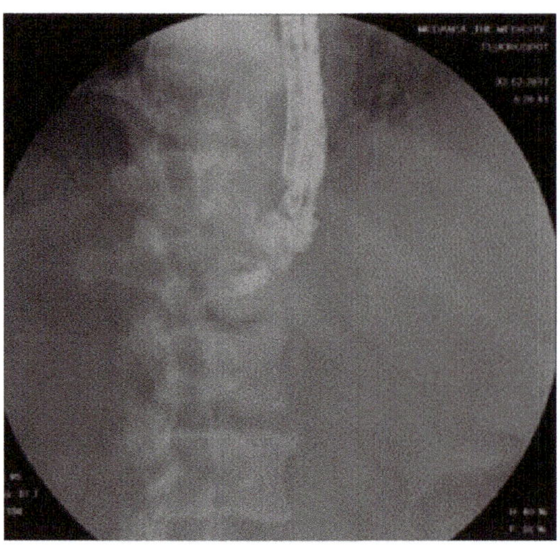

Fig. 56.7 Fluoroscopy image showing glue being injected

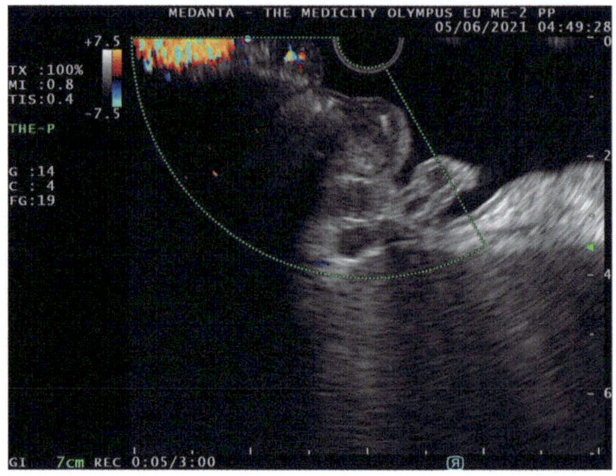

Fig. 56.8 Obliteration of previously seen varix on EUS

References

1. Dagradi AE. The natural history of esophageal varices in patients with alcoholic liver cirrhosis. An endoscopic and clinical study. Am J Gastroenterol. 1972;57:520–40.
2. Sarin SK, Lahoti D, Saxena SP, et al. Prevalence, classification and natural history of gastric varices: a long-term follow-up study in 568 portal hypertension patients. Hepatology. 1992;16:1343–9.
3. Sarin SK, Kumar A. Gastric varices: profile, classification, and management. Am J Gastroenterol. 1989;84:1244–9.
4. Romero-Castro R, Pellicer-Bautista FJ, Jimenez-Saenz M, et al. EUS-guided injection of cyanoacrylate in perforating feeding veins in gastric varices: results in 5 cases. Gastrointest Endosc. 2007;66:402–7.
5. Binmoeller KF, Weilert F, Shah JN, et al. EUS-guided transesophageal treatment of gastric fundal varices with combined coiling and cyanoacrylate glue injection. Gastrointest Endosc. 2011;74:1019–25.
6. Bhat YM, Weilert F, Fredrick RT, Kane SD, Shah JN, Hamerski CM, Binmoeller KF. EUS-guided treatment of gastric fundal varices with combined injection of coils and cyanoacrylate glue: a large U.S. experience over 6 years (with video). Gastrointest Endosc. 2016;83:1164–72.
7. Carlos, et al. Endoscopic ultrasonography-guided deployment of embolization coils and cyanoacrylate injection in gastric varices versus coiling alone: a randomized trial. Endoscopy. 2020;52(4):v15.

Part XV

EUS-Guided Arterial Embolization

57 EUS-Guided Arterial Embolization

Marc Barthet

57.1 Background

Therapeutic endoscopic ultrasounds have growing indications as EUS-guided biliary or pancreatic drainage, drainage of pancreatic collections, and more recently EUS-guided gastrojejunal anastomosis. EUS-guided management of refractory or severe gastrointestinal bleedings represents a new alternative to endoluminal or radiological approaches [1–3]. Endoluminal conventional endoscopic approach failed to stop gastrointestinal bleeding immediately or with early recurrences in about 10–15% of cases [4]. To date, a limited number of human studies with small patient cohorts [1–3] have been reported in the literature. Thirteen series including at least 242 patients have been published [3]. Nevertheless, the effectiveness and possible complications of the EUS-guided vascular approach in the treatment of refractory gastrointestinal bleeding have been poorly assessed in the literature [5–15].

Most of the cases with recurrent bleeding of gastric or perianastomotic varices have been treated with injection of polidocanol or cyanoacrylate, with a satisfactory final success rate [8, 11, 13, 15]. More recently, EUS-guided vascular embolization with microcoils has been promoted to decrease the risk of pulmonary embolism [12, 15]. Bleeding related to ulceration of gastrointestinal stromal ulceration (GIST) has also been managed under EUS guidance [5, 8, 14]. EUS-guided Cyanoacrylate injections have been performed in at least 3 cases and successful in all the cases [8, 13, 14].

The potential limitations of this new application of therapeutic EUS are numerous [1–3, 5–15] and include the limited visual field of the scope, the risk of damaging the operating channel, and the risk of induced infections and pulmonary embolism.

57.2 Case History

We report there two cases of arterial embolization using lipiodol and cyanoacrylate. Both patients with refractory bleeding were treated under EUS guidance.

The first patient was an 83-year-old patient presenting with recurrent hematemesis and melena. Endoscopy showed a huge gastric cancer located to the lesser curve and CT scan multiple liver metastases. The lesion was a large deeply excavated ulcer measuring at least 3 cm. He underwent two attempts of conventional hemostatic endoscopic procedures with either

Supplementary Information The online version contains supplementary material available at [https://doi.org/10.1007/978-981-16-9340-3_57].

M. Barthet (✉)
Service de Gastro-entérologie, Aix Marseille Université, Hôpital Nord, Marseille, France
e-mail: marc.barthet@ap-hm.fr

A. Y.B. Teoh et al. (eds.), *Atlas of Interventional EUS*, https://doi.org/10.1007/978-981-16-9340-3_57

coagulation or clips. As he was unfit for surgery, it was decided to perform EUS-guided vascular treatment.

The second patient was a 48-year-old patient with early alcoholic chronic pancreatitis without calcifications. It was the second attack of acute pancreatitis which was necrotizing acute pancreatitis. The patient was hospitalized in the intensive care unit and on day 4, massive bleeding occurred. At endoscopy, no mucosal lesion could be demonstrated but CT scan showed a pseudoaneurysm located to the head of the pancreas. After reaching hemodynamic stability, EUS-guided vascular treatment was indicated for him.

57.3 Procedural Plan

All procedures were performed on hemodynamically stable patients who received systemic antibiotic prophylaxis (2 g of amoxicillin and clavulanate) 30 minutes previously. PPI infusion was administrated for one week. Patients were under general anesthesia within the operating room with X-ray control. Following conventional endoscopy, a linear endoscope with a large working channel (3.8 mm; Pentax UTK, Japan) with Doppler-enhanced EUS was used. The procedure involved the puncture of the target vessel with a 19-gauge needle (EchoTip; Cook, Winston Salem, USA), followed by the injection of a combination of cyanoacrylate and Lipiodol (2 mL) under direct visualization. The agent used was a combination of cyanoacrylate glue and Lipiodol (2 mL) in both patients since microcoils embolization was not available in our hospital. Doppler monitoring was performed at the end of the procedure to ensure the disappearance of the Doppler signal.

57.4 Description of the Procedure

In the first patient, after endoscopic assessment of the tumor ulceration directly with the EUS scope, the gastric lumen was completely sucked until air disappeared (Video 57.1). Then US assessment was cautiously performed until the feeding artery of the tumor could be shown. Then the vessel was targeted with a 19-G needle with doppler control. The combination of lipiodol (1 ml) and cyanoacrylate (1 ml) was injected directly into the vessel, followed by the injection of 2 ml of pure lipiodol to rinse the content of the 19-G needle. Complete disappearance of the Doppler signal was checked at the end of the procedure.

The second patient was carefully checked with EUS approach until the pseudoaneurysm could be located in the head of the pancreas (Video 57.2). The pancreatic artery within the pseudoaneurysm was targeted with US and doppler and the 19-G needle was advanced cautiously in the artery lumen. The mixture of lipiodol and cyanoacrylate glue was injected followed by 2 ml of pure lipiodol. X-ray control showed a partial reflux in the gastroduodenal artery than hepatic artery without any clinical or biological consequences.

57.5 Post-Procedural Management

Patients were allowed to eat again 3 days after the procedure. Clinical and laboratory evaluations were performed daily for 1 week, with computed tomography (CT) scans performed within the first-week post-procedure. CT scan in the second patient showed complete occlusion of the pseudoaneurysm, highlighted by the lipiodol injection.

No recurrence of bleeding occurred during the follow-up of these patients. No infection or liver damages occurred based on clinical and biological examinations.

57.6 Potential Pitfalls

Few complications occurred in most of the series, in which the patients received antibiotic prophylaxis [1–3, 5–15]. The technical procedure requires to target the vessel color doppler ultrasound then puncture it with a 19-G needle. Injection of the embolization agent is possible in all the cases throughout the 19-G needle without damaging the scope by stopping the suction on the connecting tube. The goal of the procedure is to obtain a complete disappearance of the Doppler signal at the level of the targeted vessel. This is required to decrease the risk of recurrence as we previously reported in our series including eight patients and also demonstrated in series evaluating endoscopic treatment of bleeding ulcers [1, 16] (Figs. 57.1 and 57.2).

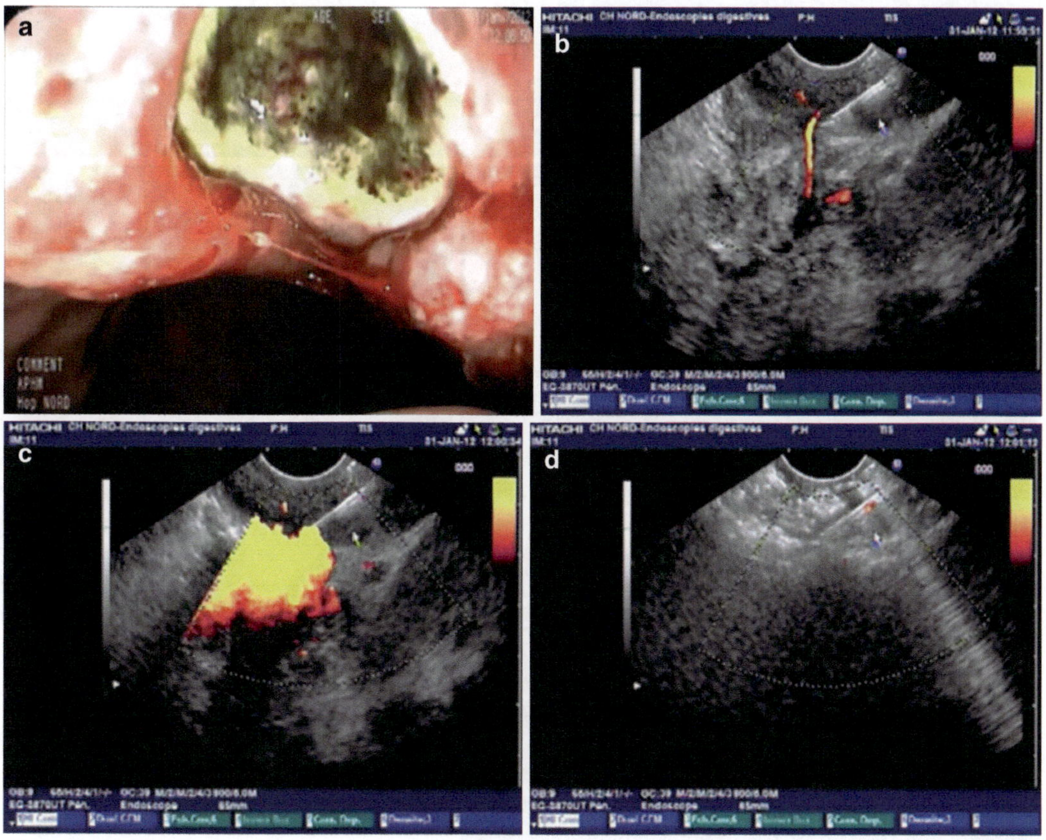

Fig. 57.1 Patient with refractory bleeding due to gastric cancer. (**a**) Bleeding gastric cancer to the lesser curve. (**b**) Feeding artery with 19 G needle in close contact. (**c**) Injection of a combination of lipiodol and cyanoacrylate glue. (**d**) Disappearance of the Doppler signal

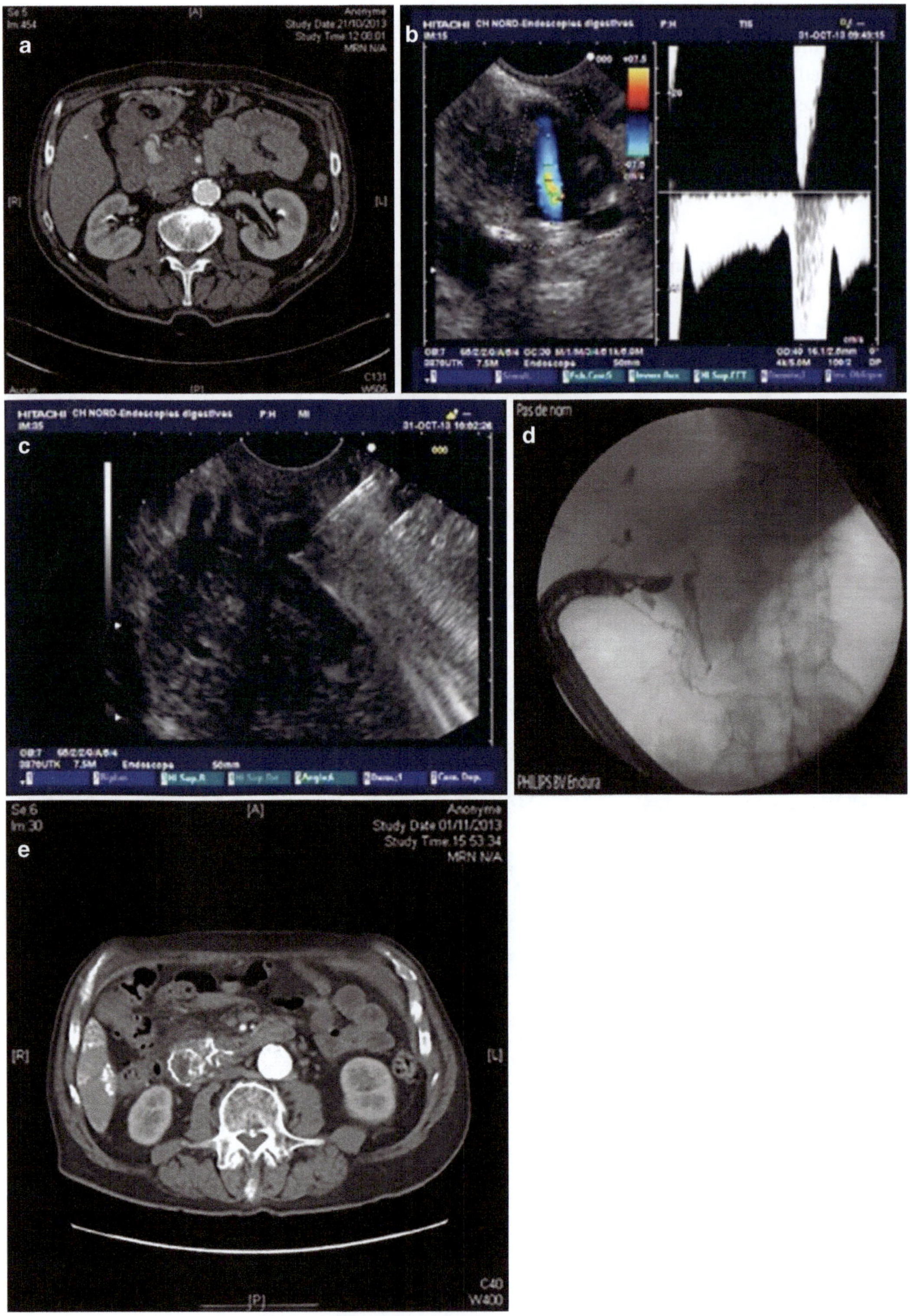

Fig. 57.2 Patient with bleeding pseudoaneurysm located to the pancreatic head. (**a**) CT scan view of the pseudoaneurysm in the pancreatic head. (**b**) EUS view with Doppler. (**c**) Insertion of the 19-G needle inside the pseudoaneurysm. (**d**) Injection of the combination of Lipiodol and cyanoacrylate glue under X-ray control. (**e**) Postoperative CT scan showing efficient embolization of the pseudoaneurysm

References

1. Gonzalez JM, Giacino C, Pioche M, et al. EUS-guided vascular therapies: is it safe and effective? Endoscopy. 2012;44:539–42.
2. Siddiqui UM, Levy MJ. EUS-guided transluminal interventions. Gastroenterology. 2018;154:1911–24.
3. Dain D, Thosani N, Shingal S, et al. EUS-assisted gastrointestinal hemostasis: an evolving technique. Therap Adv Gastroenterol. 2016;9:635–47.
4. Laine L. Endoscopic therapy for bleeding ulcers: room for improvement. Gastrointest Endosc. 2003;57:557–60.
5. Law R, Fujii L, Wong Kee Song LM, et al. Efficacy of EUS-guided hemostatic interventions for resistant non-variceal bleedings. Clin Gastroenterol Hepatol. 2014;13:808–12.
6. Magno P, Ko CW, Buscaglia JM, et al. EUS-guided angiography: a novel approach to diagnostic and therapeutic interventions in the vascular system. Gastrointest Endosc. 2007;66:587–91.
7. Giday SA, Clarke JO, Buscaglia JM, et al. EUS-guided portal vein catheterization: a promising novel approach for portal angiography and portal vein pressure measurements. Gastrointest Endosc. 2008;67:338–42.
8. Levy MJ, Chak A. EUS 2008 working group document: evaluation of EUS-guided vascular therapy. Gastrointest Endosc. 2009;69:37–42.
9. Buscaglia JM, Dray X, Shin EJ, et al. A new alternative for a transjugular intrahepatic portosystemic shunt: EUS-guided creation of an intrahepatic portosystemic shunt. Gastrointest Endosc. 2009;69:941–7.
10. Fockens P, Meenan J, Van Dullemen HM, et al. Dieulafoy's disease: endosonographic detection and endosonography-guided treatment. Gastrointest Endosc. 1996;44:437–42.
11. Romero-Castro R, Pellicer-Bautista FJ, Jimenez-Saenz M, et al. EUS-guided injection of cyanoacrylate in perforating feeding veins in gastric varices: results in 5 cases. Gastrointest Endosc. 2007;66:402–7.
12. Levy MJ, Wong Kee Song LM, Kendrick ML, et al. EUS-guided coil embolization for refractory ectopic variceal bleeding. Gastrointest Endosc. 2008;67:572–4.
13. Gonzales JM, Ezzedine S, Vitton V, et al. Endoscopic ultrasound treatment of vascular complications in acute pancreatitis. Endoscopy. 2009;41:721–4.
14. Levy MJ, Wong Kee Song LM, Farnell MB, et al. Endoscopic ultrasound (EUS)-guided angiotherapy of refractory gastrointestinal bleeding. Am J Gastroenterol. 2008;103:352–9.
15. Baht Y, Weilert F, Freidrick R, et al. EUS-guided treatment of gastric fundal varices with combined injection of coils and cyanoacrylate glue: a large U.S. experience over 6 years (with Video). Gastrointest Endosc. 2016;83:1164–72.
16. Wong RC. Endoscopic Doppler US probe for acute peptic ulcer hemorrhage. Gastrointest Endosc. 2004;60:804–12.

Part XVI

Management of Adverse Events After EUS-Guided Interventions

How to Salvage a Mis-Deployed EUS-Guided Hepaticogastrostomy Stent

58

Hon Chi Yip and Anthony Y.B. Teoh

58.1 Background

Endoscopic retrograde cholangio-pancreatography (ERCP) and self-expandable metallic stent (SEMS) insertion have been the preferred mode of biliary drainage in patients suffering from malignant distal biliary obstruction [1, 2]. However, transpapillary access can be difficult in patients with gastric outlet obstruction or surgically altered anatomy. Traditionally, these patients would be managed by percutaneous biliary drainage that is associated with drain-associated morbidities. To avoid this, EUS-guided biliary drainage (EUS-BD) is increasingly performed as an alternative to percutaneous drainage in patients with malignant biliary obstruction that are not amenable to ERCP or had failed ERCP. A meta-analysis of EUS-BD showed significantly better clinical success, lower rate of post-procedure adverse events, and fewer re-interventions as compared with percutaneous biliary drainage in patients with distal biliary obstruction and when ERCP failed [3]. In addition, EUS-BD was found to have comparable technical and clinical success rates as compared to ERCP for malignant biliary obstruction [4, 5]. EUS-BD avoids the need for placing the metallic stent through the tumor, reducing the risk of tumor ingrowth. A lower rate of post-procedure pancreatitis, re-interventions, and a higher rate of stent patency were also found in a prospective randomized study of EUS-BD versus ERCP guided biliary drainage for malignant biliary obstruction [4].

As with any endoscopic procedure, adverse events (AE) can occur during EUS-BD and rates of up to 23% have been reported for EUS-guided hepaticogastrostomy (HGS) [6]. Mis-deployment or migration of the stent is one of the most feared AE as it may be difficult to salvage endoscopically and be fatal to the patient. Prevention is the key to management and several points should be noted. Firstly, SEMS with longer lengths (10–12 cm) are preferred and the length of the intragastric portion should be more than 4 cm [7]. Some metal stents also possess anti-migratory flaps and these may further prevent migration [8]. When deploying the proximal part of the stent, an intrascope channel release method is preferred [9]. The technique involves releasing the stent within the endoscope channel. Followed-up progressive withdrawal of the endoscope and simultaneously pushing the stent delivery system. The technique can reduce the length of the stent between the liver parenchyma and the stomach and also reduce the risk of migration. Finally, if

Supplementary Information The online version contains supplementary material available at [https://doi.org/10.1007/978-981-16-9340-3_58].

H. C. Yip · A. Y.B. Teoh (✉)
Department of Surgery, The Prince of Wales Hospital, The Chinese University of Hong Kong, Shatin, Hong Kong SAR, China
e-mail: hcyip@surgery.cuhk.edu.hk; anthonyteoh@surgery.cuhk.edu.hk

A. Y.B. Teoh et al. (eds.), *Atlas of Interventional EUS*, https://doi.org/10.1007/978-981-16-9340-3_58

the stent is deployed in the peritoneal cavity, it is extremely important to maintain guidewire access to the bile duct so as to facilitate insertion of an additional SEMS to bridge the mis-deployed SEMS to the stomach. However, if guidewire access is lost then, endoscopic salvage may not be possible. In the current case, we described our technique of salvaging a mis-deployed HGS stent with the lost of guidewire access.

58.2 Case History

A 70 years old gentleman had known history of metastatic cancer of the gastric antrum. He received endoscopic stenting for gastric outlet obstruction few months before this admission. He presented with malignant biliary obstruction and trans-abdominal ultrasound showed dilated common bile duct to 1.3 cm and dilated bilateral intrahepatic ducts to 4 mm. After discussion on the mode of biliary drainage, EUS-guided biliary drainage was decided.

58.3 Procedural Plan

In the current case, EUS-HGS was the chosen procedure as a gastroduodenal stent made EUS-CDS impossible. When the HGS stent was being deployed, the endoscopist attempted to obtain endoscopic view of the stent by pushing the endoscope forward. During this maneuver, the stent and the delivery system was pushed out of the stomach at the same time. After mis-deployment was recognized, the guidewire was left in-situ in an attempt to insert an addition SEMS to bridge the mis-deployed stent. However, the guidewire was also dislodged during manipulation. Then, there were two problems to deal with—a gastric opening and a mis-deployed HGS. The gastric opening was first closed endoscopically followed by an attempt to visualize the opening of the mis-deployed stent by EUS. A stable position and view were obtained by EUS and the opening of stent could be punctured with EUS followed by insertion of an additional SEMS.

58.4 Description of the Procedure

EUS-HGS was performed with a linear echoendoscope (Video 58.1). The known gastric cancer was located in the distal stomach, causing obstruction where the endoscope could not pass through. On EUS view, segment III bile ducts were dilated to 5 mm in size. A branch of the duct was punctured with 19-gauge needle (Expect™, Boston Scientific Corp, USA). After confirming the position by contrast cholangiogram, a 0.025″ guidewire was inserted into the common bile duct through the needle. The tract was dilated with 6Fr cystotome and an 8 mm × 10 cm partially covered stent (GIOBOR™, Taewoong Medical Corporations, Korea) was introduced. As the stent was being deployed under fluoroscopic guidance, the stent was mis-deployed outside of the stomach during adjustment of its position (Fig. 58.1). An attempt to place a fully covered stent to bridge the gastric side through the original guidewire was not successful due to looping and angulation. The guidewire migrated outside of the stent as well during manipulation (Fig. 58.2). The stent was no longer visible inside the lumen of the stomach and attempt to pass guidewire into the stent and the bile duct was not successful.

To salvage the situation, an end-view gastroscope mounted with an over-the-scope clip (OTSC, Ovesco Endoscopy GmbH, Tübingen, Germany) was inserted into the stomach, and the gastric puncture site was closed completely by the clip (Fig. 58.3). A linear echoendoscope was re-introduced afterwards, with the stent visualized outside of the stomach on EUS and fluoroscopic view. The proximal end of the stent was punctured with a 19G needle, and an angled tipped guidewire was passed into the common bile duct (Figs. 58.4 and 58.5). The tract was dilated again with 6Fr cystotome and an additional fully covered biliary SEMS (10 mm × 80 mm, Wallflex™ biliary fully covered stent, Boston Scientific Corp, USA) was inserted to bridge the entire tract of the partially covered stent, with the proximal 3 cm of the stent inside the stomach. Contrast injection through

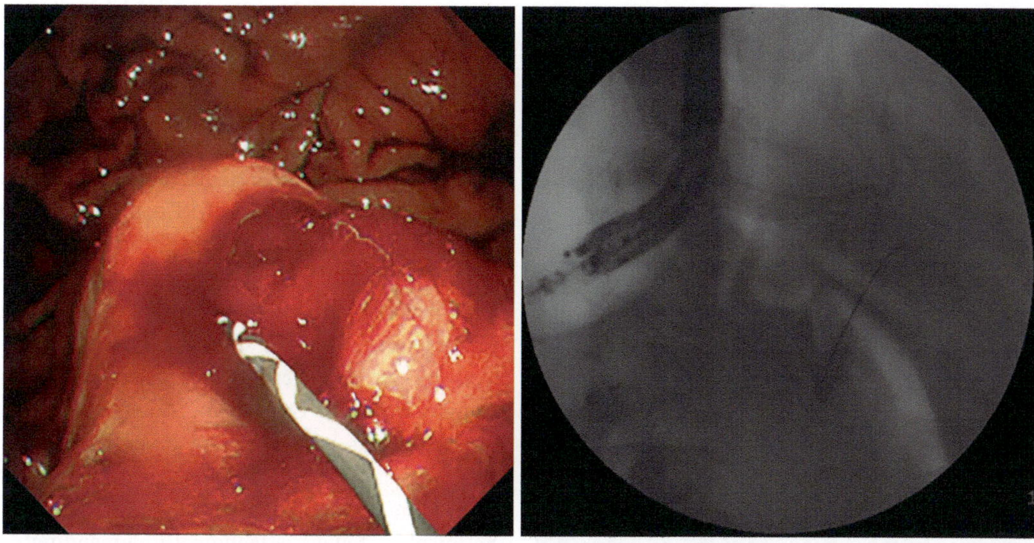

Fig. 58.1 Mis-deployed HGS completely outside of gastric lumen

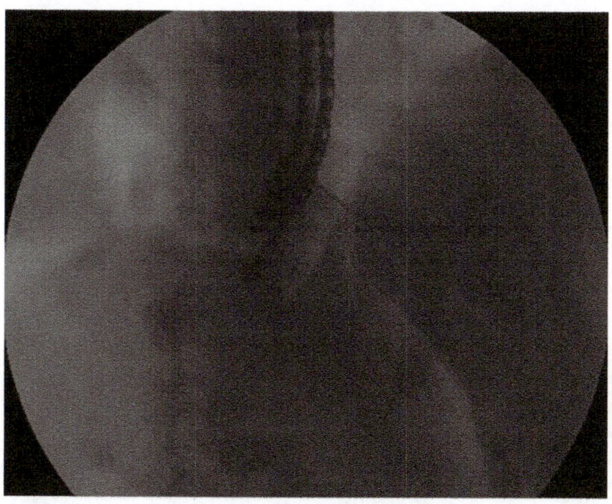

Fig. 58.2 EUS puncture of the migrated HGS stent, with guidewire repositioned inside common bile duct

the newly inserted stents showed no leakage into the peritoneal cavity (Fig. 58.6).

58.5 Post-Procedural Management

The patient was put on one-week course of broad-spectrum antibiotics. He had an episode of fever that subsided spontaneously. A follow-up computed tomography showed no evidence of bile leakage or intra-abdominal collection. His liver functions gradually improved and the patient was subsequently discharged home.

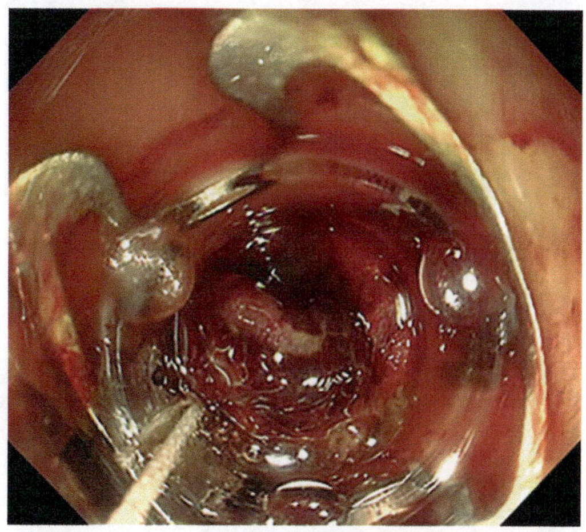

Fig. 58.3 The gastric opening closed with OTSC

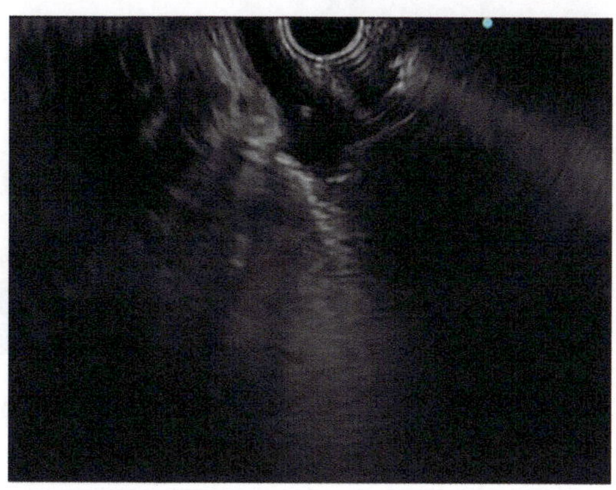

Fig. 58.4 The opening of the mis-deployed stent punctured under EUS guidance

58.6 Potential Pitfalls

Migration of stent during EUS-HGS is one of the potential adverse events; the stent could migrate inward, as in the current case, or outward from the liver into the stomach. Recently, intrascope channel deployment of the SEMS is advised by many experts to reduce the risk of inward stent migration [10, 11] The stent position should also be checked frequently both in the fluoroscopic and endoscopic view throughout the procedure. If the guidewire is still within the stent and the biliary system when stent migration occurs, an additional fully covered SEMS could be placed to bridge the two lumens. In the unfortunate event that the guidewire no longer in-situ, the situation could become lethal with risk of both gastric and biliary leakage, and the situation should be managed by an experienced interventional endosonographer [12]. Endoscopic salvage may still be possible, as in the current case. The gastric entry site can usually be closed completely by endoscopic means, but EUS-guided puncture of the misplaced stent is technically demanding. If EUS-guided puncture is not possible, a transgastric NOTES approach to retrieve the stent has also been described, but this requires expert endoscopic skills [13]. If endoscopic salvage is unsuccessful, then percutaneous biliary drainage could be performed to divert bile flow, but surgical salvage may be required if the sepsis could not be controlled [14].

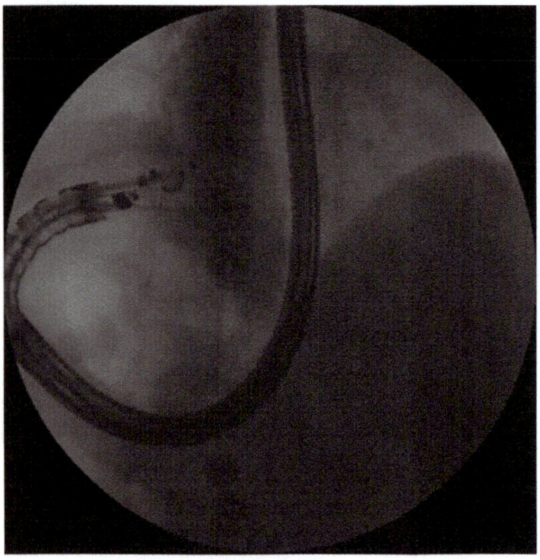

Fig. 58.5 Guidewire passed through the mis-deployed stent in to the bile duct

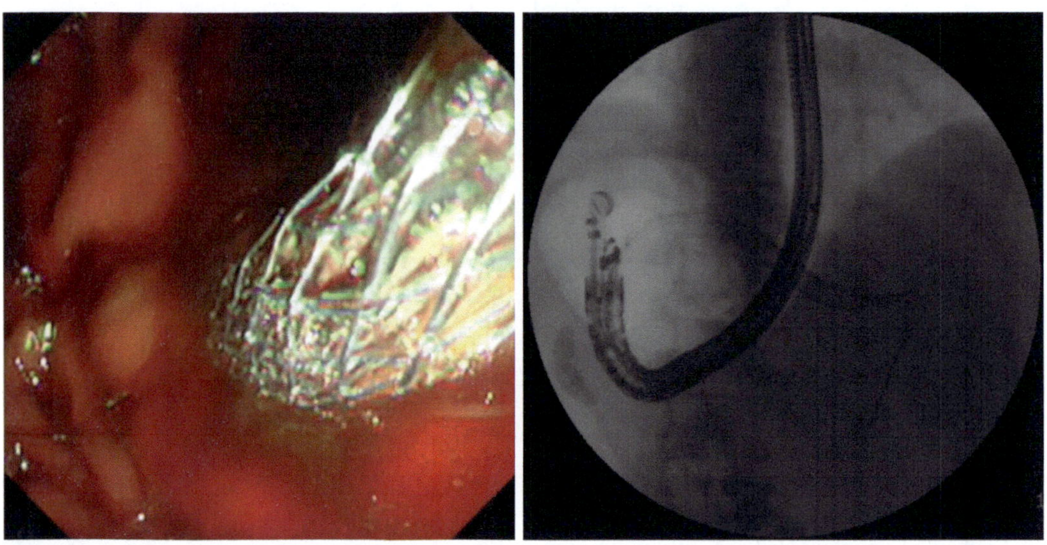

Fig. 58.6 A fully covered SEMS bridging the mis-deployed stent to the stomach was inserted

References

1. Das A, Sivak MV. Endoscopic palliation for inoperable pancreatic cancer. Cancer Control. 2000;7(5):452–7.
2. Castaño R, Lopes TL, Alvarez O, Calvo V, Luz LP, Artifon ELA. Nitinol biliary stent versus surgery for palliation of distal malignant biliary obstruction. Surg Endosc. 2010;24(9):2092–8.
3. Sharaiha RZ, Khan MA, Kamal F, Tyberg A, Tombazzi CR, Ali B, et al. Efficacy and safety of EUS-guided biliary drainage in comparison with percutaneous biliary drainage when ERCP fails: a systematic review and meta-analysis. Gastrointest Endosc. 2017;85(5):904–14.
4. Paik WH, Lee TH, Park DH, Choi JH, Kim SO, Jang S, et al. EUS-guided biliary drainage versus ERCP for the primary palliation of malignant biliary obstruction: a multicenter randomized clinical trial. Am J Gastroenterol. 2018;113(7):987–97.
5. Jin Z, Wei Y, Lin H, Yang J, Jin H, Shen S, et al. Endoscopic ultrasound-guided versus endoscopic retrograde cholangiopancreatography-guided biliary drainage for primary treatment of distal malignant biliary obstruction: a systematic review and meta-analysis. Dig Endosc. 2020;32(1):16–26.
6. Ogura T, Higuchi K. Technical tips for endoscopic ultrasound-guided hepaticogastrostomy. World J Gastroenterol. 2016;22(15):3945–51.
7. Ogura T, Yamamoto K, Sano T, Onda S, Imoto A, Masuda D, et al. Stent length is impact factor associated with stent patency in endoscopic ultrasound-guided hepaticogastrostomy. J Gastroenterol Hepatol. 2015;30(12):1748–52.
8. Song TJ, Lee SS, Park DH, Seo DW, Lee SK, Kim MH. Preliminary report on a new hybrid metal stent for EUS-guided biliary drainage (with videos). Gastrointest Endosc. 2014;80(4):707–11.
9. Miyano A, Ogura T, Yamamoto K, Okuda A, Nishioka N, Higuchi K. Clinical impact of the intra-scope channel stent release technique in preventing stent migration during EUS-guided hepaticogastrostomy. J Gastrointest Surg. 2018;22(7):1312–8.
10. Uchida D, Kawamoto H, Kato H, Goto D, Tomoda T, Matsumoto K, et al. The intra-conduit release method is useful for avoiding migration of metallic stents during EUS-guided hepaticogastrostomy (with video). J Med Ultrason (2001). 2018;45(3):399–403.
11. Mandai K, Uno K, Yasuda K. Relationship between the intraperitoneal stent length in endoscopic ultrasound-guided hepaticogastrostomy and surgically altered upper gastrointestinal anatomy in patients with malignant biliary obstruction. Gastroenterology Res. 2018;11:305–8.
12. Martins FP, Rossini LG, Ferrari AP. Migration of a covered metallic stent following endoscopic ultrasound-guided hepaticogastrostomy: fatal complication. Endoscopy. 2010;42(Suppl 2):E126–7.
13. Pham KD, Hoem D, Horn A, Dimcevski GG. Salvage of a dislodged hepaticogastrostomy stent in the peritoneum with NOTES. Endoscopy. 2017;49(9):919–20.
14. Itoi T, Isayama H, Sofuni A, Itokawa F, Kurihara T, Tsuchiya T, et al. Stent selection and tips on placement technique of EUS-guided biliary drainage: transduodenal and transgastric stenting. J Hepatobiliary Pancreat Sci. 2011;18(5):664–72.

59 Endoscopic Salvage of a Mis-Deployed Choledochoduodenostomy Stent

Anish A. Patel, Nicholas G. Brown, and Amrita Sethi

59.1 Background

Endoscopic biliary drainage is a well-established technique for providing biliary decompression in patients with obstructive jaundice. Endoscopic transpapillary biliary stenting is the most common procedure for biliary drainage in patients with obstructive jaundice. However, failure to achieve bile duct access still occurs in some patients due to failed biliary cannulation, inaccessible papilla because of severe duodenal stenosis caused by tumor invasion, other anatomical issues. In these cases, percutaneous transhepatic biliary drainage (PTBD) or surgical intervention is required. However, both methods have been associated with significant morbidity and mortality rates. Endoscopic ultrasound (EUS)-guided biliary drainage (EUS-BD) has emerged as an alternative in cases of endoscopic retrograde cholangiopancreatography (ERCP) failure. EUS-BD includes a rendezvous technique and a direct access technique. The direct access technique includes two major methodologies: EUS-guided choledochoduodenostomy (EUS-CDS) and EUS-guided hepatogastrostomy [1].

Supplementary Information The online version contains supplementary material available at [https://doi.org/10.1007/978-981-16-9340-3_59].

A. A. Patel
VMG—Center For Digestive Health, Valley Health System, Ridgewood, NJ, USA

N. G. Brown · A. Sethi (✉)
Division of Digestive and Liver Diseases, Columbia University Irving Medical Center, New York, NY, USA
e-mail: nb2931@cumc.columbia.edu; as3614@cumc.columbia.edu

59.2 Case History

An 85-year-old woman with multiple comorbidities admitted to the intensive care unit with septic shock. Physical examination showed right upper quadrant pain. Blood culture showed multi-drug-resistant *Escherichia coli*. Computed tomography showed a persistently dilated common bile duct status post cholecystectomy, with a focal cutoff at the level of a lesion within the distal common bile duct (Fig. 59.1). The features are compatible with septic shock secondary to choledocholithiasis (Fig. 59.2). EUS-CDS was offered to the patient due to failed ERCP.

59.3 Procedural Plan

EUS-BD includes a rendezvous technique and a direct access technique. A rendezvous technique may be considered whereby a wire is placed into an intrahepatic or extrahepatic bile duct, passed through the papilla, and retrieved by a duodenoscope for transpapillary interventions. The direct

A. Y.B. Teoh et al. (eds.), *Atlas of Interventional EUS*, https://doi.org/10.1007/978-981-16-9340-3_59

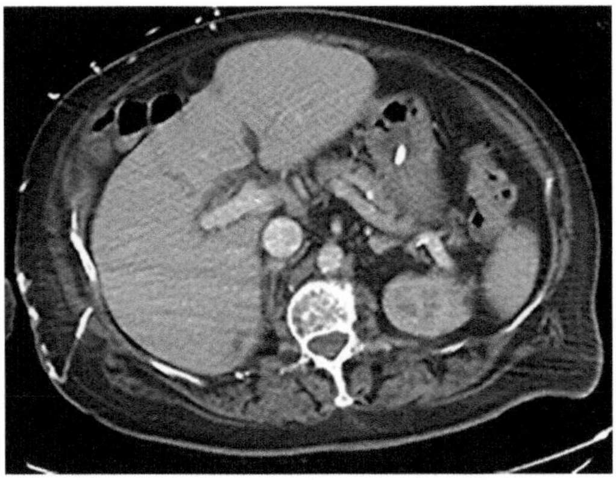

Fig. 59.1 Computed tomography demonstrating choledocholithiasis

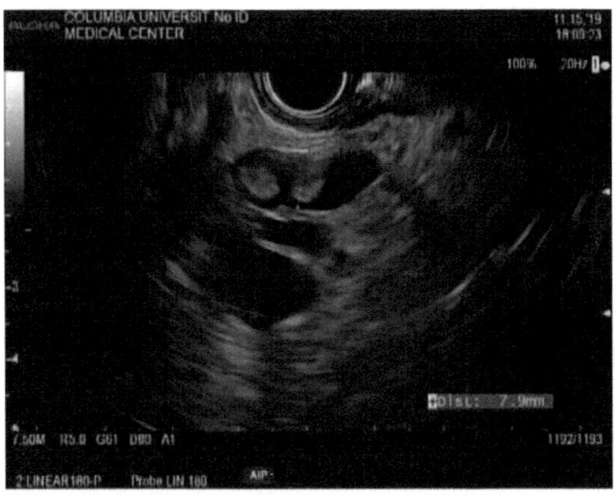

Fig. 59.2 Choledocholithiasis as noted on EUS

access technique includes two major methodologies: EUS-guided choledochoduodenostomy (EUS-CDS) and EUS-guided hepatogastrostomy. Both are performed without accessing the papilla. Recent studies have shown that both approaches are effective and safe for the treatment of distal biliary obstruction after failed ERCP [2, 3]. A recent meta-analysis demonstrated equal efficacy and safety, with very high technical and clinical success rates [4]. Some studies have shown that metallic stents should be placed whenever feasible, and non-coaxial electrocautery should be avoided when possible as plastic stenting and non-coaxial electrocautery were independently associated with adverse events [5].

59.4 Description of the Procedure

EUS-CDS was performed initially with a cautery-enhanced fully covered self-expandable metal stent (SEMS) via the transduodenal approach using a linear echoendoscope. Endoscopic observation was initially performed to confirm the absence of any lesions in the duodenal bulb. The extrahepatic bile duct was visualized along the long axis from the duodenal bulb. The location of the echoendoscope was adjusted so that the puncture needle faced toward the hepatic hilum. Color and power Doppler mode was used to confirm lack of blood vessels between the transducer and the extrahepatic bile duct. The duodenal wall and the common bile duct were punctured under endosonographic guidance with the 19-guage needle (Fig. 59.3). Bile was aspirated. Contrast was injected to perform a cholangiogram. Initially, a 0.025 inch straight standard wire was inserted into the extrahepatic bile duct under fluoroscopic guidance to attempt a rendezvous approach; however, the wire could not be passed into the duodenum across the papilla in an antegrade fashion. Therefore, it was decided to perform a direct access approach with a choledochoduodenostomy. Freehand access was attempted using a 10 mm × 10 mm electrocautery-enhanced lumen apposing metal stent (ECE-LAMS, Axios, Boston Scientific, Marlborough,

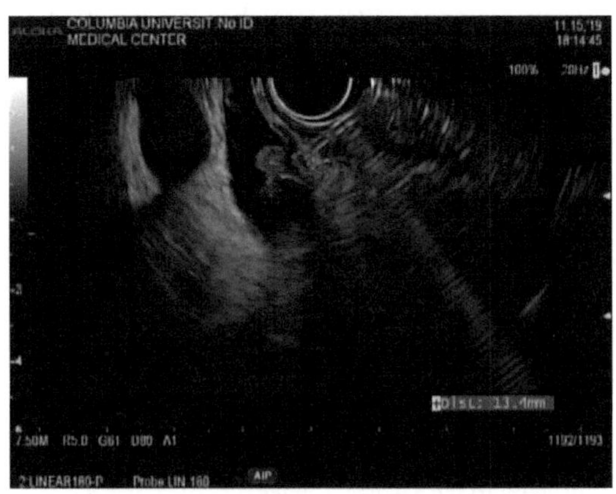

Fig. 59.3 Dilated common bile duct punctured with a 19-gauge needle

MA). The catheter was introduced through the working channel and advanced to the duodenal mucosa under EUS guidance. Current was applied to the cautery tip, and the catheter was advanced into the bile duct. The first flange of the LAMS was then deployed within the lumen of the bile duct, and the catheter was withdrawn slightly to appose the wall of the bile duct and the duodenum. There was some concern that the flange itself may have been exiting the bile duct wall; however, deployment was continued with the release of the second flange within the duodenal lumen, confirmed on endoscopic view. Given the concern for potential misdeployment, a wire was passed through the introducer into the bile duct prior to removal of the LAMS system. A balloon catheter was inserted and contrast injected, which demonstrated a cholangiogram with bile entirely with the biliary tree, however, with only the tip of the LAMS remaining within the duct lumen while the flange itself was between the wall of the duodenum and the bile duct. The wire access was lost at that time. In anticipation of complete stent migration out of the duct and resulting perforation, a salvage technique was planned. The linear echoendoscope was exchanged for a duodenoscope, which allowed for visualization of the SEMS (Fig. 59.4). A small hole was visualized through the LAMS and felt to be the defect in the bile duct wall. A wire was passed through the LAMS and advanced into the intrahepatic duct. A 10 mm × 60 mm FCSEMS was placed over the wire, through the SEMS under fluoroscopic guidance. A final balloon occlusion cholangiogram was performed within the stents to ensure appropriate filling of the biliary tree. There was adequate filling of the entire biliary tree and no extravasation of contrast on the final cholangiogram.

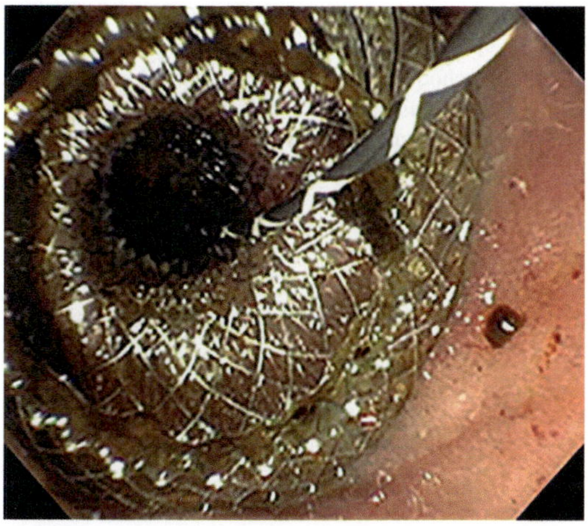

Fig. 59.4 Proximal flange of LAMS deployed in the duodenal bulb

59.5 Post-procedure Management

Patients should be closely monitored for adverse events related to the procedure. Follow-up imaging is reasonable if patients do not improve clinically and continue to demonstrate signs of infection. If the patient develops signs of peritonitis or abscess formation, interventional radiological or surgical intervention may be indicated.

59.6 Potential Pitfalls

The potential adverse events related to EUS-CDS include infection (peritonitis, cholangitis), pneumoperitoneum, bile leak, biloma, bleeding, abdominal pain, perforation, stent migration, and stent misdeployment [6]. In the case of stent misdeployment, management depends on which flange has been misdeployed and whether a guidewire is present. Early recognition and placement of a wire into the intended target lumen is critical to further salvage techniques, although NOTES-type procedures can also be deployed. A bridging covered metal stent of either similar or larger diameter can be placed to bridge the two lumens (Fig. 59.5).

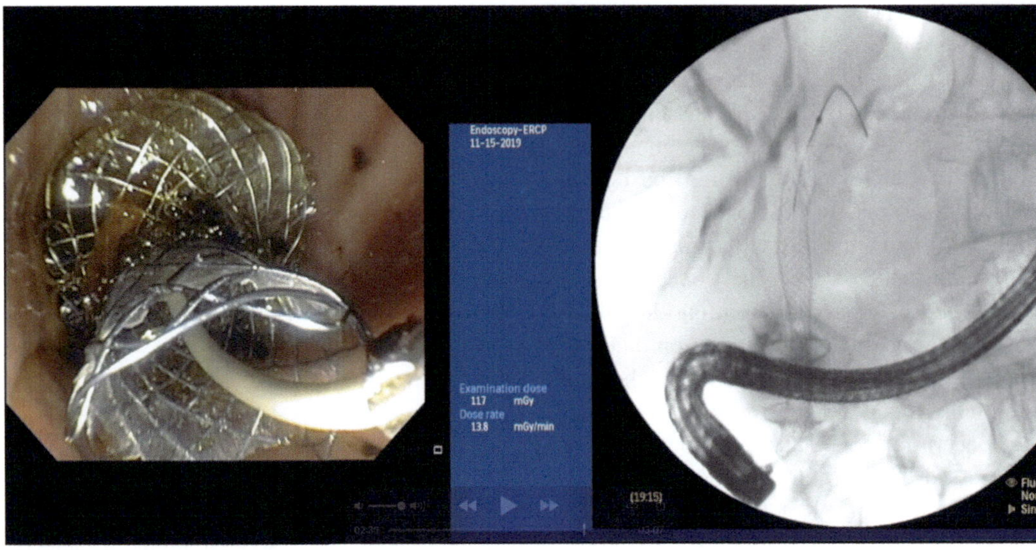

Fig. 59.5 FCSEMS deployed through lumen of LAMS

References

1. Itoi T, Itokawa F, Sofuni A, Kurihara T, Tsuchiya T, Ishii K, Tsuji S, Ikeuchi N, Moriyasu F. Endoscopic ultrasound-guided choledochoduodenostomy in patients with failed endoscopic retrograde cholangiopancreatography. World J Gastroenterol. 2008;14(39):6078–82.
2. Minaga K, Ogura T, Shiomi H, Imai H, Hoki N, Takenaka M, Nishikiori H, Yamashita Y, Hisa T, Kato H, Kamada H, Okuda A, Sagami R, Hashimoto H, Higuchi K, Chiba Y, Kudo M, Kitano M. Comparison of the efficacy and safety of endoscopic ultrasound-guided choledochoduodenostomy and hepaticogastrostomy for malignant distal biliary obstruction: Multicenter, randomized, clinical trial. Dig Endosco: Official Journal of the Japan Gastroenterological Endoscopy Society. 2019;31(5):575–82.
3. Khan MA, Akbar A, Baron TH, Khan S, Kocak M, Alastal Y, Hammad T, Lee WM, Sofi A, Artifon ELA, Nawras A, Ismail MK. Endoscopic ultrasound-guided biliary drainage: a systematic review and meta-analysis. Dig Dis Sci. 2016;61(3):684–703.
4. Uemura RS, Khan MA, Otoch JP, Kahaleh M, Montero EF, Artifon ELA. EUS-guided Choledochoduodenostomy Versus Hepaticogastrostomy: A Systematic Review and Meta-analysis. J Clin Gastroenterol. 2018;52(2):123–30.
5. Khashab MA, Messallam AA, Penas I, Nakai Y, Modayil RJ, De la Serna C, Hara K, El Zein M, Stavropoulos SN, Perez-Miranda M, Kumbhari V, Ngamruengphong S, Dhir VK, Park DH. International multicenter comparative trial of transluminal EUS-guided biliary drainage via hepatogastrostomy vs. choledochoduodenostomy approaches. Endoscopy Int Open. 2016;4(2):E175–81.
6. Ogura T, Higuchi K. Technical tips of endoscopic ultrasound-guided choledochoduodenostomy. World J Gastroenterol. 2015;21(3):820–8.

Endoscopic Salvage of a Dislodged Gastro-Gastrostomy Stent

60

Qais Dawod and Reem Z. Sharaiha

60.1 Background

Patients with altered anatomy including those who underwent Roux-en-Y gastric bypass pose distinct challenges to performing endoscopic retrograde cholangiopancreatography (ERCP). Multiple different techniques, including enteroscopy-assisted ERCP, laparoscopy-assisted ERCP, and EUS-directed transgastric ERCP (EDGE), have been described [1].

EDGE is an emerging endoscopic procedure which allows ERCP in patients who underwent Roux-en-Y gastric bypass. In an EDGE procedure, a lumen-apposing metal stent (LAMS) is used to create a temporary connection between the excluded stomach and the gastric pouch, allowing a direct pathway for the performance of ERCP [2].

Supplementary Information The online version contains supplementary material available at [https://doi.org/10.1007/978-981-16-9340-3_60].

Q. Dawod · R. Z. Sharaiha (✉)
Division of Gastroenterology and Hepatology, New York Presbyterian Hospital/Weill Cornell Medical Centre, New York, NY, USA
e-mail: qad2001@med.cornell.edu; rzs9001@med.cornell.edu

60.2 Case History

A 56-year-old women with a history of Roux-en-Y gastric bypass surgery in 2001 for obesity presented with abdominal pain and fevers. MRI/MRCP showed a newly dilated biliary and pancreatic duct (Fig. 60.1). The patient's course was notable for Klebsiella bacteremia concerning for cholangitis. Decision was made to proceed with an EDGE, in which a LAMS is used to create a gastrogastrostomy to facilitate ERCP with a duodenoscope.

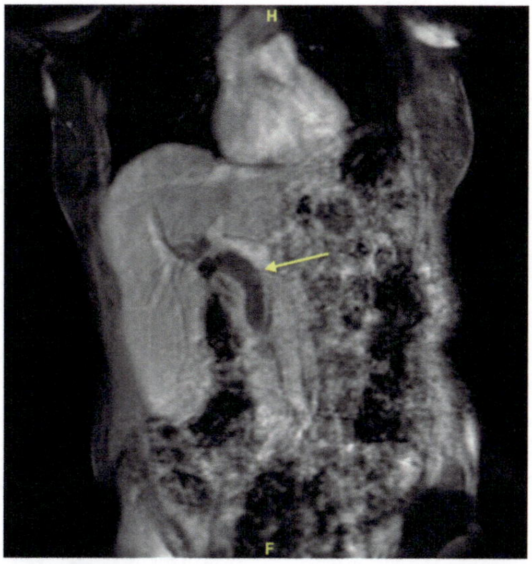

Fig. 60.1 MRI/MRCP showed a newly dilated biliary and pancreatic duct

A. Y.B. Teoh et al. (eds.), *Atlas of Interventional EUS*, https://doi.org/10.1007/978-981-16-9340-3_60

60.3 Procedural Plan

The EDGE technique is divided into two stages performed either in one session in cases of emergent ERCP or in separate endoscopic sessions, with studies showing a mean procedure times of 81 and 98 mins [3]. The first stage of the procedure involves placement of a LAMS into the excluded stomach by using EUS guidance. During the second stage, which can occur anywhere from 2 to 4 weeks post stage 1, a duodenoscope is advanced through the LAMS to the major papilla to perform the ERCP.

60.4 Description of the Procedure

The patient underwent upper endoscopy, using a linear echo endoscope for ultrasonographic guidance, and the excluded stomach was identified. A 19-gauge EUS-FNA needle was used to puncture the remnant stomach from the jejunal wall, and contrast was injected which confirmed filling of the remnant stomach under fluoroscopic and sonographic visualization.

After distension, a 15 mm cautery-enhanced LAMS was deployed under endosonographic and fluoroscopic guidance with the distal flange into the excluded stomach and the proximal flange into the jejunal loop of bowel. The stent was then dilated with a CRE balloon sequentially to 15 mm under endoscopic guidance (Fig. 60.2). A wire was left in place, and subsequently, a duodenoscope was inserted (alongside the wire) through the metal stent to perform an ERCP; the ampulla was identified in normal position. Cannulation of the bile duct was performed using sphincterotome with a preloaded 0.035″ hydrajag guidewire. Contrast was injected to confirm location within the duct. The sphincterotome was then used to create a biliary sphincterotomy. An occlusion cholangiogram was then performed demonstrating a distal CBD stricture with an upstream dilated common bile duct measuring ~2 cm with dilated intrahepatic ducts (Fig. 60.3). No filling defect was identified. The distal stricture was then brushed with a cytology brush given sluggish drainage and concern for cholangitis; a 10 cm × 4 cm FCSEMS was deployed into the CBD. Bile was seen draining upon stent deployment, and position was confirmed on fluoroscopy.

Upon withdrawing the duodenoscope, it became clear that the proximal flange of the LAMS had migrated into the peritoneum (Fig. 60.4). A wire was left in the remnant stomach, and along the wire, a through-the-scope 20 mm × 60 mm fully covered esophageal stent was deployed with the distal flange within the LAMS and the proximal flange in the jejunal loop of bowel (from patient's gastrojejunostomy; Fig. 60.5). Contrast was then injected and demonstrated no evidence of a leak. The esophageal stent was the sutured in place to the jejunal loop

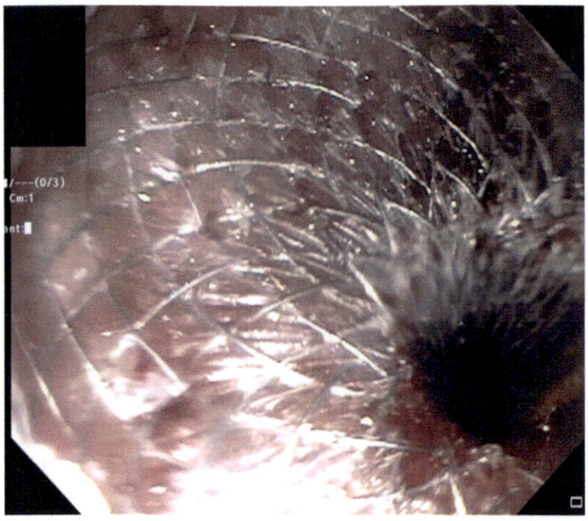

Fig. 60.2 15 mm Lumen-apposing metal stent after dilation

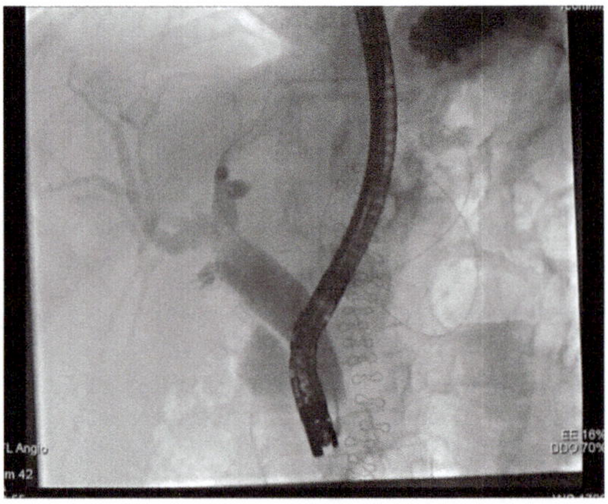

Fig. 60.3 Occlusion cholangiogram demonstrating a distal CBD stricture with an upstream dilated common bile duct measuring ~2 cm with dilated intrahepatic ducts

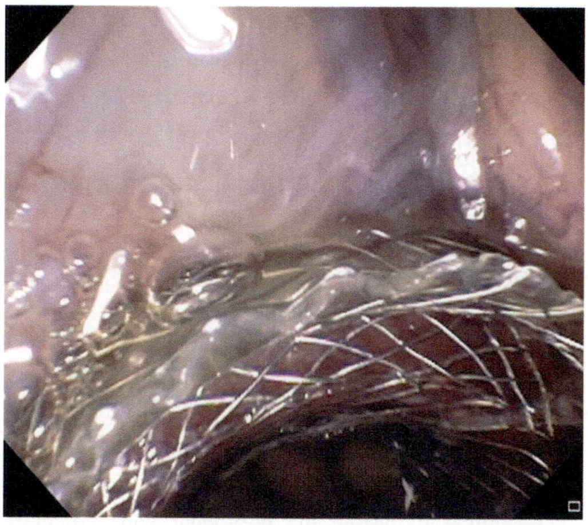

Fig. 60.4 The proximal flange of the LAMS had migrated into the peritoneum

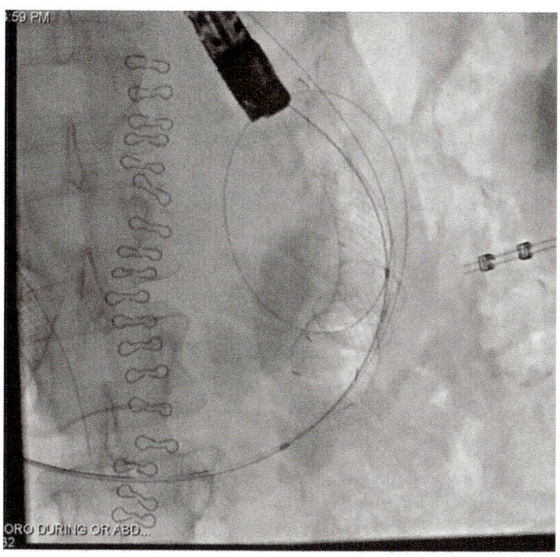

Fig. 60.5 Fully covered esophageal stent was deployed with the distal flange within the LAMS and the proximal flange in the jejunal loop of bowel (from patient's gastrojejunostomy)

of bowel with two sutures using an endoscopic suturing device (Fig. 60.6).

60.5 Post-procedural Management

The patient was kept in the hospital for the next 24 hours for further observation. She remained stable. She was started on clears the next day and

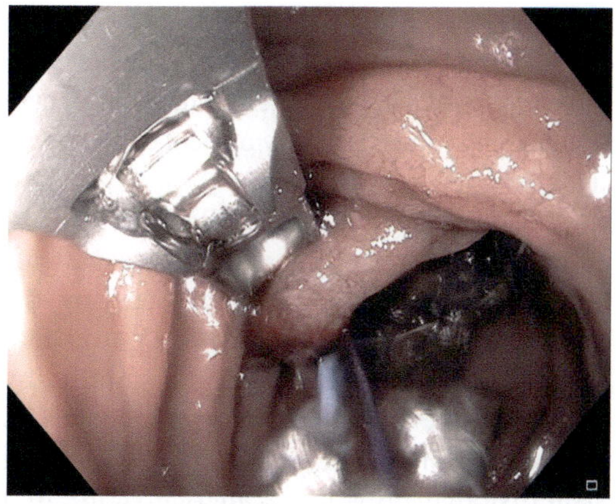

Fig. 60.6 The esophageal stent was the sutured in place to the jejunal loop of bowel

was discharged on a 10-day course of antibiotics. She advanced her diet slowly and remained asymptomatic. She had a follow-up ERCP with stent removal, and at that time both her esophageal stent and lumen-apposing stent were removed. Her gastro-gastric fistula was closed with sutures.

60.6 Potential Pitfalls

There are notable concerns associated with the utilization of EDGE, including the risk of stent-related adverse events and the risk of weight regain after creating the fistula, in effect reversing the benefit of the surgical bypass. Stent-related adverse events include mis-deployment of the stent or dislodgment, which might lead to peritonitis. Most cases of LAMS dislodgment have been endoscopically managed, with LAMS repositioning or placement of a second LAMS, although surgery has been needed in a few cases [4].

In this particular case performing the ERCP alongside a wire helped maintain access into the excluded limb despite the stent dislodgment and facilitated the salvage of the procedure in order to maintain access. Using the through-the-scope esophageal stent also aided in immediate resolution of the dislodged stent thereby decreasing peritoneal exposure and increasing the risk of contamination.

Consideration for ERCP after maturation of the gastro-gastric fistula should be made if the indication is of a less emergent nature and if there is concern for the possibility of stent dislodgment during the index procedure [1, 4].

A safe, single-stage EDGE can be performed in Roux-en-Y gastric bypass patients without LAMS dislodgment by securing the stent to the gastric pouch with an over-the-scope clip (OTSC) or endoscopic suturing by fixation of the stent to the gastric mucosa [5]. We expect a significant reduction in the risk of stent dislodgment with the alternative use of a pediatric duodenoscope through a 15-mm LAMS or the use of a 20-mm LAMS which would allow for the easier passage of the duodenoscope [1, 6].

In summary, the EDGE procedure may offer a cost-effective, minimally invasive option with few adverse events for a common problem in a growing patient demographic. Dealing with potential pitfalls and their immediate recognition during this procedure is of utmost importance in decreasing downstream morbidity.

References

1. Kedia P, Tyberg A, Kumta NA, Gaidhane M, Karia K, Sharaiha RZ, et al. EUS-directed transgastric ERCP for Roux-en-Y gastric bypass anatomy: a minimally invasive approach. Gastrointest Endosc. 2015 Sep 1;82(3):560–5.
2. Mendoza LA. EUS-directed transgastric ERCP. VideoGIE Off Video J Am Soc Gastrointest Endosc. 2018 May 29;3(6):175–6.
3. Kedia P, Kumta NA, Sharaiha R, Kahaleh M. Bypassing the bypass: EUS-directed transgastric ERCP for Roux-en-Y anatomy. Gastrointest Endosc. 2015 Jan 1;81(1):223–4.
4. Duloy A, Hammad H, Shah RJ. An adverse event of EUS-directed transgastric ERCP: stent-in-stent technique to bridge the peritoneal gap. VideoGIE Off Video J Am Soc Gastrointest Endosc. 2019 Sep 6;4(11):508–11.
5. Ichkhanian Y, Runge T, Jovani M, Vosoughi K, Brewer Gutierrez OI, Khashab MA. Management of adverse events of EUS-directed transgastric ERCP procedure. VideoGIE Off Video J Am Soc Gastrointest Endosc. 2020 Mar 20;5(6):260–3.
6. Irani S, Yang J, Khashab MA. Mitigating lumen-apposing metal stent dislodgment and allowing safe, single-stage EUS-directed transgastric ERCP. VideoGIE Off Video J Am Soc Gastrointest Endosc. 2018 Aug 3;3(10):322–4.

Management of Hemorrhage During EUS-Guided Pancreatic Fluid Collection Drainage: Thinking on Your Feet

61

Sundeep Lakhtakia and Shujaath Asif

61.1 Background

EUS-guided drainage of pancreatic fluid collection is the standard of care with high success rate, but it is not devoid of complications. Reported adverse events vary from 5–30% [1–3], with mortality ranging from 1 to 11% [4–6]. Hemorrhage, a common adverse event, associated with EUS-guided drainage of PFC can present either as intra-procedural or post-procedural bleeding. *Intra-procedural bleeding* events are usually caused by rupture of pseudoaneurysm, or collateral vessels, inadvertent puncture of major vessels, or intra-cavitary vessel bleed. *Post-procedural bleeding* events are associated with stent erosion of major vessels adjoining the collapsed PFC and in coagulation disorders [7]. The main methods for confirming hemorrhage are Endoscopy and CT angiogram [6, 8]. Based on clinical situation, the four major hemostatic management approaches include: conventional treatment [9], endoscopic treatment [10, 11], interventional radiology-guided embolization [12, 13], and surgery [14]. Among the endoscopic methods considered to control bleeding during or after EUS drainage include medicine injection (dilute epinephrine, hemostatic powder), endoscopic clip application, electrocautery, balloon tamponade, and the placement of large-diameter FCSEMS [15].

61.2 Case History

A 36-year-old male patient with ethanol related liver cirrhosis and recent episode of acute pancreatitis, presented with abdominal distension and pain along with vomiting. Investigations revealed mild increase in alkaline phosphatase, raised serum amylase and low serum albumin. MRI/MRCP abdomen showed thrombosed portal and splenic vein with multiple periportal collaterals and moderate ascites, along with dilated MPD. There were multiple peri-pancreatic collections—one large (163 × 92 × 91 mm) in lesser sac and a smaller collection (46 × 46 × 34 mm) in pancreatic head (Fig. 61.1). Ascitic fluid analysis showed high serum albumin-ascites gradient (SAAG) and high fluid amylase (966 U/L).

EUS-guided drainage of PFC was contemplated after therapeutic ascitic fluid paracentesis and few days of albumin infusion and diuretics.

Supplementary Information The online version contains supplementary material available at [https://doi.org/10.1007/978-981-16-9340-3_61].

S. Lakhtakia (✉) · S. Asif
Asian Institute of Gastroenterology, AIG Hospitals, Hyderabad, India

A. Y.B. Teoh et al. (eds.), *Atlas of Interventional EUS*, https://doi.org/10.1007/978-981-16-9340-3_61

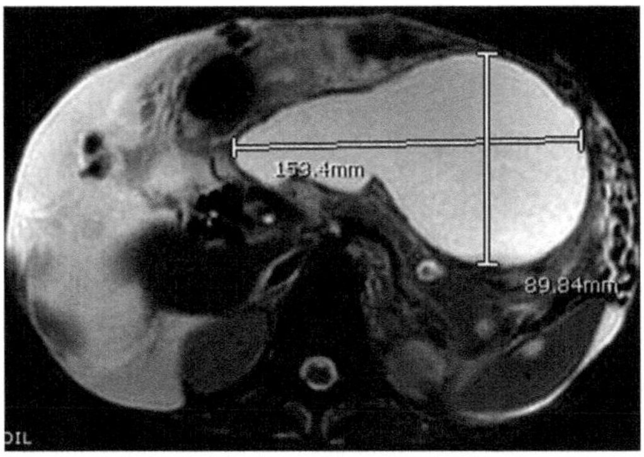

Fig. 61.1 MRI image showing large pancreatic fluid collection (153 × 89 mm) in the lesser sac, ascites

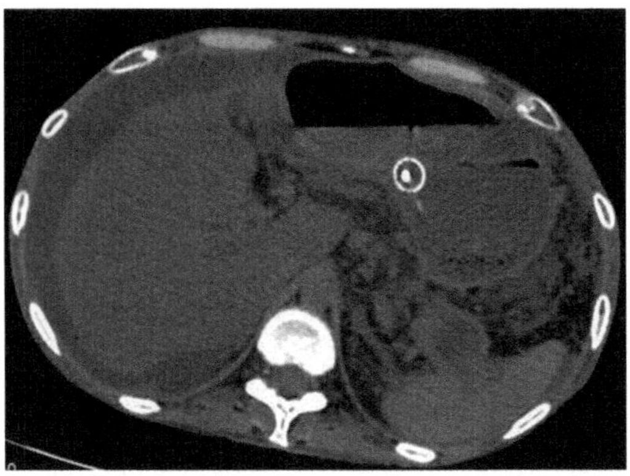

Fig. 61.2 CT image (at 24 hours): substantial decrease in size of collection, BFMS in situ, minimal ascites, no bleed

61.3 Procedure

The assessment of PFC using linear echoendoscope suggested likely communication between the two peri-pancreatic collections (Fig. 61.2). There were multiple periportal and peri-gastric collateral vessels. The larger collection in lesser sac was considered for EUS-guided drainage with plastic stents due to absent debris within the PFC (suggestive of pseudocyst).

A relatively avascular area avoiding the peri-gastric collaterals was selected for puncture with EUS for the large pseudocyst in lesser sac from the stomach (trans-gastric route). Pseudocyst was punctured using 19G needle and clear fluid was aspirated. While passing a 0.025" angled tip guidewire inside the PFC, internal bleeding was observed seen on EUS image as spurt into the cavity from the puncture site that was confirmed on Doppler.

61.4 Thinking on Your Feet

Immediate change of plan in further drainage was made from plastic stent to BFMS (Nagi stent). Instead of standard practice of using over-the-wire cystotome to create cysto-gastric fistula, a tapered bougie was used to avoid any thermal injury to the bleeding vessel. The tract was further dilated with 4 mm Titan balloon (Cook medical) and was kept inflated for one minute that provided immediate hemostasis by tamponade. This was followed by a self-expanding cysto-gastric metallic stent (16 mm Nagi) deployment that maintained the tamponade and stopped the brisk bleed. A 7 French 4 cm double pigtail plastic stent was placed within the BFMS (Video 61.1).

61.5 Post-Procedure Management

Patient was closely monitored for next 24 hours. There was no further bleeding or fall in hemoglobin. Computer tomography done after 24 hours showed reduction in size of collection and there was no bleed within the PFC (Fig. 61.3). Similar case has been earlier reported by our group [16].

61.6 Conclusion

Complications associated with endoscopic drainage of PFC include—bleeding, perforation, secondary infection and stent migration. EUS help to reduce the risk of bleeding by visualizing and avoiding any interposing vessels. However, even with EUS guidance, bleeding remains an important adverse event. This can be possibly explained by the fact that small vessels in PFC wall may have no flow on Doppler due to a relatively high pressure of fluid inside. Such compressed vessels

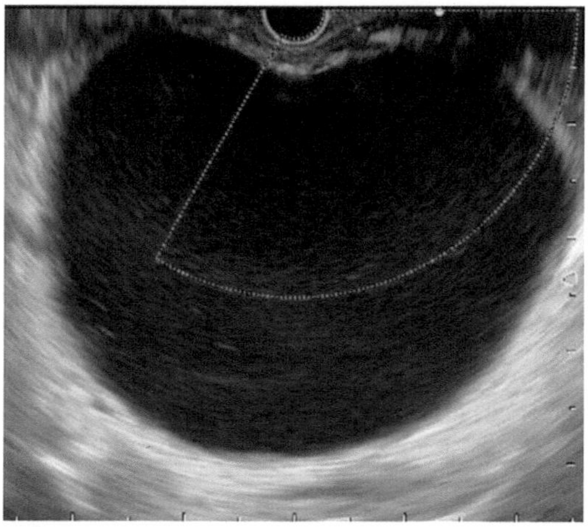

Fig. 61.3 EUS image—large pseudocyst in lesser sac with no obvious interposing vessel

can suddenly bleed when the critical pressure is released on drainage, as may have happened in the index case.

61.7 Intra-procedural Bleed

Mild bleed—are usually self-limited and reduce in intensity on continuous observation at drainage procedure.

Moderate to severe bleed—endoscopic therapy such as clip application, cautery, or balloon tamponade may be considered. Embolization of bleeding vessel by IR is the next step. Lastly, surgery is considered if all options fail. In the index case, a modification of plan (from plastic to metal stent) helped in achieving sustained hemostasis.

61.8 Post-Procedural Bleed

Bleeding is caused by erosion of major vessels from the internal end of LAMS as the cyst gradually collapses. This is typically observed at 3–4 weeks after index drainage. Hence, LAMS and all metals stent should be removed by this period. In such case, CT angiography is used to locate the culprit vessel or newly formed aneurysm, followed by angio-embolization.

References

1. Walter D, Will U, Sanchez-Yague A, Brenke D, Hampe J, Wollny H, López-Jamar JM, Jechart G, Vilmann P, Gornals JB, Ullrich S, Fähndrich M, de Tejada AH, Junquera F, Gonzalez-Huix F, Siersema PD, Vleggaar FP. A novel lumen-apposing metal stent for endoscopic ultrasound-guided drainage of pancreatic fluid collections: a prospective cohort study. Endoscopy. 2015;47:63–7.
2. Siddiqui AA, Kowalski TE, Loren DE, Khalid A, Soomro A, Mazhar SM, Isby L, Kahaleh M, Karia K, Yoo J, Ofosu A, Ng B, Sharaiha RZ. Fully covered self-expanding metal stents versus lumen-apposing fully covered self-expanding metal stent versus plastic stents for endoscopic drainage of pancreatic walled-off necrosis: clinical outcomes and success. Gastrointest Endosc. 2017;85:758–65.
3. Sharaiha RZ, DeFilippis EM, Kedia P, Gaidhane M, Boumitri C, Lim HW, Han E, Singh H, Ghumman SS, Kowalski T, Loren D, Kahaleh M, Siddiqui A. Metal versus plastic for pancreatic pseudocyst drainage: clinical outcomes and success. Gastrointest Endosc. 2015;82:822–7.
4. Rinninella E, Kunda R, Dollhopf M, Sanchez-Yague A, Will U, Tarantino I, Gornals Soler J, Ullrich S, Meining A, Esteban JM, Enz T, Vanbiervliet G, Vleggaar F, Attili F, Larghi A. EUS-guided drainage of pancreatic fluid collections using a novel lumen apposing metal stent on an electrocautery-enhanced delivery system: a large retrospective study (with video). Gastrointest Endosc. 2015;82:1039–46.
5. Mukai S, Itoi T, Baron TH, Sofuni A, Itokawa F, Kurihara T, Tsuchiya T, Ishii K, Tsuji S, Ikeuchi N, Tanaka R, Umeda J, Tonozuka R, Honjo M, Gotoda T, Moriyasu F, Yasuda I. Endoscopic ultrasound-guided placement of plastic vs. biflanged metal stents for therapy of walled-off necrosis: a retrospective single-center series. Endoscopy. 2015;47:47–55.
6. Cavallini A, Butturini G, Malleo G, Bertuzzo F, Angelini G, Abu Hilal M, Pederzoli P, Bassi C. Endoscopic transmural drainage of pseudocysts associated with pancreatic resections or pancreatitis: a comparative study. Surg Endosc. 2011;25:1518–25.
7. Varadarajulu S, Christein JD, Wilcox CM. Frequency of complications during EUS-guided drainage of pancreatic fluid collections in 148 consecutive patients. J Gastroenterol Hepatol. 2011;26:1504–8.
8. Bapaye A, Dubale NA, Sheth KA, Bapaye J, Ramesh J, Gadhikar H, Mahajani S, Date S, Pujari R, Gaadhe R. Endoscopic ultrasonography-guided transmural drainage of walled-off pancreatic necrosis: Comparison between a specially designed fully covered bi-flanged metal stent and multiple plastic stents. Dig Endosc. 2017;29:104–10.
9. Ang TL, Kongkam P, Kwek AB, Orkoonsawat P, Rerknimitr R, Fock KM. A two-center comparative

study of plastic and lumen-apposing large diameter self-expandable metallic stents in endoscopic ultrasound-guided drainage of pancreatic fluid collections. Endosc Ultrasound. 2016;5:320–7.

10. Vazquez-Sequeiros E, Baron TH, Pérez-Miranda M, SánchezYagüe A, Gornals J, Gonzalez-Huix F, de la Serna C, Gonzalez Martin JA, Gimeno-Garcia AZ, Marra-Lopez C, Castellot A, Alberca F, Fernandez-Urien I, Aparicio JR, Legaz ML, Sendino O, Loras C, Subtil JC, Nerin J, Perez-Carreras M, Diaz-Tasende J, Perez G, Repiso A, Vilella A, Dolz C, Alvarez A, Rodriguez S, Esteban JM, Juzgado D, Albillos A, Spanish Group for FCSEMS in Pancreas Collections. Evaluation of the short- and long-term effectiveness and safety of fully covered self-expandable metal stents for drainage of pancreatic fluid collections: results of a Spanish nationwide registry. Gastrointest Endosc. 2016;84:450–7.
11. Cohen M, Kedia P, Sharaiha R, Kahaleh M. Tamponade of a bleeding pseudocyst with a fully covered metal stent. Gastrointest Endosc. 2015;81:229–30.
12. Bang JY, Hasan M, Navaneethan U, Hawes R, Varadarajulu S. Lumen-apposing metal stents (LAMS) for pancreatic fluid collection (PFC) drainage: may not be business as usual. Gut. 2017;66:2054–6.
13. Yamamoto N, Isayama H, Kawakami H, Sasahira N, Hamada T, Ito Y, Takahara N, Uchino R, Miyabayashi K, Mizuno S, Kogure H, Sasaki T, Nakai Y, Kuwatani M, Hirano K, Tada M, Koike K. Preliminary report on a new, fully covered, metal stent designed for the treatment of pancreatic fluid collections. Gastrointest Endosc. 2013;77:809–14.
14. Lakhtakia S, Basha J, Talukdar R, Gupta R, Nabi Z, Ramchandani M, Kumar BVN, Pal P, Kalpala R, Reddy PM, Pradeep R, Singh JR, Rao GV, Reddy DN. Endoscopic "step-up approach" using a dedicated biflanged metal stent reduces the need for direct necrosectomy in walled-off necrosis (with videos). Gastrointest Endosc. 2017;85:1243–52.
15. Lakhtakia S. Complications of diagnostic and therapeutic Endoscopic Ultrasound. Best Pract Res Clin Gastroenterol. 2016;30:807–23.
16. Chavan R, Basha J, Lakhtakia S, Nabi Z, Reddy DN. Large-caliber metal stent controls significant entry site bleeding during EUS-guided drainage of walled-off necrosis. VideoGIE. 2019 Jan;4(1):27.

GPSR Compliance

The European Union's (EU) General Product Safety Regulation (GPSR) is a set of rules that requires consumer products to be safe and our obligations to ensure this.

If you have any concerns about our products, you can contact us on ProductSafety@springernature.com

In case Publisher is established outside the EU, the EU authorized representative is:

Springer Nature Customer Service Center GmbH
Europaplatz 3
69115 Heidelberg, Germany

Batch number: 08860018

Printed by Printforce, the Netherlands